THE HEALTH AND SAFETY OF WORKERS

THE HEALTH AND SAFETY OF WORKERS

Case Studies in the Politics of Professional Responsibility

EDITED BY

Ronald Bayer

The Hastings Center

New York Oxford
Oxford University Press
1988

Oxford University Press

Oxford   New York   Toronto
Delhi   Bombay   Calcutta   Madras   Karachi
Petaling Jaya   Singapore   Hong Kong   Tokyo
Nairobi   Dar es Salaam   Cape Town
Melbourne   Auckland

and associated companies in
Beirut   Berlin   Ibadan   Nicosia

Library of Congress Cataloging-in-Publication Data
The Health and Safety of Workers: Case Studies in the Politics
of Professional Responsibility / edited by Ronald Bayer.
p.   cm.   includes bibliographies and index.
ISBN 0-19-505365-6
1. Industrial hygiene—Social aspects.   2. Industrial hygiene—Case studies
3. Lead mines and mining—Health aspects.   4. Coal mines and mining—
Health aspects.   5. Asbestos mines and mining—Health aspects.   I. Bayer, Ronald.
[DNLM: 1. Accident Prevention.   2. Occupational Diseases—prevention & control.
3. Professional practice—trends.   4. Social responsibility.   WA 440 01485]
RC967.027 1988   363.1'1—dc19   87-28111   CIP

Portions of two chapters were previously published in slightly different form.
Chapter 1, by William Graebner, originally appeared in David Rosner and Gerald
Markowitz, eds., *Dying for Work: Workers' Safety and Health in Twentieth-Century
America:* "Hegemony Through Science: Information Engineering and Lead
Toxicology, 1925–1965" (Bloomington: Indiana University Press, 1987), pp. 140–159
and in *New York History:* "Ethyl in Manhattan: A Note on the Science and Politics
of Leaded Gasoline," 67 (October 1986), pp. 437–443. Chapter 4, by Ronald Bayer,
appeared in the National Academy of Engineering's *Hazards: Technology and
Fairness* (Washington, D.C.: National Academy Press, 1986).

9 8 7 6 5 4 3 2 1

Printed in the United States of America
on acid-free paper

Acknowledgments

The project from which the papers collected in this volume have come was made possible by a grant from the Program in Ethics and Values in Science and Technology of the National Science Foundation to The Hastings Center. The critical but supportive guidance provided by Rachelle Hollander was very helpful in fashioning the final design of our work. Support from the J.C. Penney Foundation made possible much of the effort expended in preparing this volume for publication. Both the design of this project and its execution were responsibilities I shared with my colleagues Willard Gaylin and Thomas Murray. The diligent research of Eric Feldman, aided by The Hastings Center's librarian Marna Howarth, proved to be of invaluable assistance. Finally, I as well as each of the authors represented in this volume benefited from the critical response to and reading of first and sometimes second drafts of the papers by project participants. Other than those whose work is included in this volume, the members of the Occupational Health Research Project who collaborated in this work were Brian Barry, Jacqueline Corn, Morton Corn, Harold Edgar, Vilma Hunt, Deborah Johnson, and Gilbert Omenn. Because of the energy with which he read and analyzed the work of his colleagues, a very special acknowledgment is due Edwin T. Layton, Jr.

Briarcliff Manor, New York   R.B.
September 1987

Contents

Contributors

RONALD BAYER, The Hastings Center, 255 Elm Road, Briarcliff Manor, New York 10510

ARTHUR L. DONOVAN, Department of Humanities, U.S. Merchant Marine Academy, Kingspoint, New York 11024

WILLIAM GRAEBNER, State University of New York at Fredonia, Department of History, Fredonia, New York 14063

THOMAS H. MURRAY, Center for Biomedical Ethics, Case Western Reserve University School of Medicine, Cleveland, Ohio 44106

DAVID OZONOFF, Environmental Health Section, School of Public Health, Boston University, Boston, Massachusetts 02118

CURTIS SELTZER, Virginia Center for Coal and Energy Research, Virginia Polytechnic Institute and State University, Blacksburg, Virginia 24061

THE HEALTH AND SAFETY OF WORKERS

Introduction

For much of this century, as technological advances in industry provided the bedrock for an extraordinary expansion in the wealth and economic vitality of American society, a parallel but grimmer process was also occurring. Industrial workers, as well as those who worked in extractive settings, were suffering the burdens of morbidity and mortality associated with their employment. Sometimes in the form of catastrophic accidents (as in mining), sometimes in the form of acute responses to workplace toxins, on other occasions in the form of chronic disabling diseases, the toll of technological progress was borne by workers.

Throughout this period engineers, scientists, and physicians engaged by private industry helped to fashion, monitor, and preserve a system that produced extraordinary wealth and prosperity as well as illness, suffering, and death. On occasion those who believed the human toll was too great sought to press for modifications; some spoke out in the name of the health and safety of workers. By and large, however, what few critical voices were to be found emerged from settings at some remove from the direct control and influence of private industry—the universities and the newly emerging regulatory bodies at state and federal levels.[1] That those employed in academic settings and by government bodies certainly had greater latitude to speak about occupational diseases and accidents is not surprising. But even such professionals often remained mute, constrained by the sociopolitical, economic, and professional forces at play during the early decades of the twentieth century.

3

What is most striking about the history of the social response to occupational disease is, however, not the effect of socioeconomic forces on the very modest efforts to control or limit the pattern of worker morbidity and mortality, but the way in which the very process of discovering patterns of disease was affected by extrascientific forces. Whatever the brute facts, the diagnosis of occupational disease and its etiological linkage to particular processes of production and mineral extraction often remained as much social as it was clinical.

It was to study the role of scientists, engineers, and physicians in the discovery and control of occupational hazards in the twentieth century that The Hastings Center's Occupational Health Research Group undertook a study entitled "Moral Responsibilities and Moral Decisions in Science and Engineering" in 1983.[2] Our purpose in undertaking this study was, however, not simply descriptive. It was to provide the groundwork for an understanding of the ethical responsibilities of scientists, physicians, and engineers as individuals and as members of professional organizations in dealing with the burdens of technology, in uncovering the human cost of social progress, in proposing changes that might radically reduce those costs, and in fashioning public and private practices and policies that would result in a socially equitable distribution of the burdens of economic and technological progress. In short, to understand how scientists, engineers, and physicians in the workplace ought to behave, we deemed it critical to first understand how they *had* behaved, to understand the social milieu within which their behavior took shape.

To achieve that understanding, The Hastings Center commissioned three lengthy monographs on coal, lead, and asbestos. Each of these substances has played an important role in the development of an advanced industrial civilization. Each has also had a long association with occupational disease. Finally, each has been the focus of a contemporary controversy arising from efforts to establish a regulatory regime designed to protect exposed workers from disease and death.

Coal—the fuel that made possible the development of steam-driven locomotion, power, and the blast furnaces of heavy industry—had long been known to pose hazards to those involved with its extraction from the earth. With the dramatic force of literature, Charles Dickens and Emile Zola sought to awaken attention to these hazards in the last century. Early concern with the dangers of coal mining focused on matters of safety—explosions, cave-ins, and faulty trams were among the prominent hazards that drew the attention of social commentators. Although the diagnosis of health disorders linked to coal dust dates to the mid-nineteenth century, recognition of the respiratory consequences of exposure to coal dust did not become widespread until the twentieth century, when the precise definition of "coal miners' disease" became the focus of intense socio-political as well as medical controversy. Arthur Donovan's study "Health and Safety in Underground Coal Mining, 1900–1969: Professional Conduct in a Peripheral Industry" stresses the ways in which the structure of the industry limited the prospects for reforms in which engineers and physicians in both the public and private sectors might have effectively addressed—had they been so motivated—the toll taken by the mining of coal.

The recognition of lead-related diseases goes back to antiquity. Modern concern dates from the eighteenth century, reflected, for instance, in Bernardino Ramazzini's *Diseases of Workers*. A century later Tanquerel des Planches's *A Treatise on Lead Diseases* documented the hazard of lead exposure. But the use of lead increased dramatically in the nineteenth and twentieth centuries, in the ceramics trades and in paint products but most markedly in the complex of industries that developed around the automobile. In particular, lead began to be used as a fuel additive and in the manufacture of batteries. The rapid rise in the use of lead brought stark medical consequences. Lead-poisoned workers and miners displayed blue-lined gums and wrist drop, and suffered from severe anemia and neurotoxic disorders. William Graebner's study "Private Power, Private Knowledge, and Public Health: Science, Engineering, and Lead Poisoning, 1900–1970" underscores the way in which the scientific understanding of the effects of lead was shaped by the corporate funding of research—the result a paradigm that did not ignore the gross manifestations of lead toxicity but that systematically underestimated the environmental impact of chronic lead exposure. Even though the occupational impact of lead exposure had received greater attention, findings in the 1970s were to demonstrate the extent to which workers remained at increased risk.

The social burden posed by asbestos exposure is clearly the most recently to be understood by the public, government agencies, and workers. Although a 1902 essay by England's inspector of factories included the preparation and weaving of asbestos fibers as among the most injurious processes known,[3] and although the Merewether Report of 1930 prepared by the British Factory Department inspectorate stressed the importance of dust suppression as a response to asbestos-related disease,[4] a full appreciation of the dangers posed by asbestos—of asbestos-related cancers as well as asbestosis—only emerged decades after many thousands of workers and their families had already been exposed. Moreover, the understanding of the hazards posed to millions of individuals exposed to the end products of asbestos has produced a recent public health challenge of enormous proportions. David Ozonoff's narrative, "Knowledge and Its Suppression: Science in the Discovery of Asbestos-Related Disease," is an unsettling tale of how private interests created the circumstances within which a systematic suppression of scientific evidence protected the industry from the threat of the public response that would have attended such revelations.

Each of the three richly documented monographs collected in this book—Donovan's, Graebner's, and Ozonoff's—emphasizes the socioeconomic, institutional, and professional factors that shaped the behavior of those who had, or should have had, firsthand knowledge of the human costs of industrial progress. The roles played and not played by scientists, engineers, and physicians in the discovery of occupational disease as well as in the rudimentary efforts to limit the pattern of morbidity and mortality are set against the pattern of complex interaction of government and the private sector in the first six decades of twentieth-century America.

The social conflicts over occupational health and safety took on a radically different form—an acutely public form—when, as a result of legislation, the federal government assumed direct responsibility for protecting the health and safety of workers. The failure of the private sector to provide adequate standards of protection, as well as the only very limited efforts of government bodies to face the challenge posed by both large and small employers, produced a reformist alliance that resulted first in the passage of the Coal Mine Health and Safety Act of 1969 and then the Occupational Safety and Health Act of 1970. In the case of the Mine Safety Act, Congress provided the forum for dramatic encounters over appropriate safety standards for miners. The enactment of the Occupational Safety and Health Act created an administrative mechanism (The Occupational Safety and Health Administration, OSHA) through which similar encounters with respect to the regulation of workplace hazards would be played out. Here the direct political encounters of the congressional setting would be given a more technocratic form that would only barely mask the conflict of social, economic, and professional interests.[5] Whatever the administrative trappings, the process of decisionmaking would be, in its essential features, every bit as political as that which occurred in the nation's legislative body.

To examine the role played by scientists, engineers, and physicians in the struggle over occupational health policy, the second part of this book has brought together three studies paralleling the longer historical monographs. Curtis Seltzer, in "Moral Dimensions of Occupational Health: The Case of the 1969 Coal Mine Safety and Health Act," analyzes the congressional hearings that preceded the passage of the Act. Studies of the administrative hearings conducted by OSHA during the process of establishing standards of safety for exposure to lead and asbestos are provided in my chapter, "Scientists, Engineers, and the Burdens of Occupational Exposure," and Thomas Murray's "Regulating Asbestos."

While the broad historical monographs seek to provide an overview of the interplay of historical, social, economic, and professional forces in the creation of and response to hazardous occupational settings, the analyses of these three discrete regulatory efforts seek to provide detailed accounts of how differently scientists, physicians, and engineers based in industry, government, and universities viewed the dimensions of the risks to be controlled as well as the prospects for such control. The positivist vision of scientists disinterestedly proferring evidence to policymakers, on the basis of which the latter could make their determinations, was shattered by the bitter encounters surrounding the efforts to regulate workers' exposure to coal, lead, and asbestos—encounters that unveiled the realm of scientific politics. In each of these cases scientists, engineers, and physicians assumed partisan stances definitively marked by the social interests with which they were allied. Empirical evidence, clinical conclusions, and the prospects for rational, affordable, and practical modifications in industrial production processes became the substance of dispute on the contested terrain of occupational health and safety.

As government scientists acknowledged their own uncertainty about the level at which individuals exposed to coal, lead, and asbestos during their working lives would be safe from disease and disability, those individuals identified with trade unions and a maximalist position on health and safety produced evidence demonstrating the potential for pathogenesis, by marshalling evidence of the prospects of long-term consequences, of the prevailing patterns of exposure. Calling upon statistical probabilities underscoring the significance of subclinical changes, these individuals sometimes stressed the effect of chronic exposure, sometimes the effect of even short-term exposure for diseases with extended latencies. All such arguments were put forth to justify the reduction of exposures to ever lower levels. Those who were employed by industry or who spoke on its behalf warned about unwarranted extrapolations based upon what they viewed as scanty evidence and worst-case scenarios. For the defenders of regulatory minimalism politics rather than science motivated the call for what they viewed as extreme demands for overregulation.

As the risks of hazardous exposure were debated, engineers disputed the possibilities of modifying production and extraction processes, retrofitting, and introducing radically innovative but safer technologies. The legitimacy of using costly regulatory requirements as an incentive for forcing technological innovation became a focus of sharp disagreement. Although the "limits of technology" framed such debates, central to the arguments over engineering controls were matters of cost. Would the demands for exposure-reducing changes prove economically ruinous for the coal, lead, and asbestos industries? Would marginal firms be displaced? Would whole sectors of these industries be rendered economically unviable? Alternatively, would the internalization of the social costs of production prove to be both economically rational and socially more equitable?

If the dispute over exposure levels involved at base a conflict over the distribution of the burdens of toxicity, the clash over engineering controls involved a profound disagreement over how the economic costs of preventing illness ought to be borne. In both cases there were disagreements over the distribution of the burdens of uncertainty. Thus, what appeared on the surface to be matters of clinical science, epidemiology, and technology entailed confrontations over what social justice demanded in the context of workplace hazards.

Ultimately, the questions forced upon us by these studies go beyond the descriptions they provide of the scientific politics of three hazardous substances. Can we expect scientists, engineers, and physicians to free themselves from the strictures of the social settings within which they work? In the face of divided loyalties, how will professionals whose work bears on the health and safety of workers respond? Can we expect the articulation of standards of professional responsibility and the establishment of codes of professional ethics to prevent a recapitulation of the conduct revealed in the studies in this volume? Are the prospects for such modification different for engineers, physicians, and scientists?

In the case of engineers, the prospects for changes in professional conduct would appear to be the least sanguine.[6] In part this is so because of the nature of engineering itself. Edwin Layton, in his study of engineers and their professional societies, notes that "engineering is not a lifetime profession, but a stepping stone to more lucrative positions in business management and sales."[7] Despite the changes that have occurred in codes of professional conduct, and despite the efforts to put forth a standard that places the public interest first,[8] Layton argues that "engineering still tacitly accepts the precepts of its first codes, which made loyalty to the employer the engineer's first professional obligation."[9] That this is so is a function not simply of professional culture but of the very definitions of the task placed before the engineer. A. A. Potter made this clear when he baldly stated, "Whatever the numerator is in an engineering equation, the denominator is always a dollar mark,"[10] and that denominator must ultimately be set by those for whom the engineer works.

The professional ethos as well as the career trajectories of scientists and occupational health physicians are not so limiting and suggest at least the theoretical possibly for more independent expressions of concern about how particular production processes might subject workers to hazards. Certainly the existence of academic departments devoted to occupational medicine and the study of occupational toxicity, and the existence of public bodies charged with the responsibility of studying workplace hazards and proposing ameliorative policies, create the prospect for an independent base for the scientific understanding of occupational disease. The evidence of the studies presented in this volume suggests, however, that those who are in the employ of the private sector are not very likely to act publicly to defend the health interests of workers when such action will bring them into conflict with their employers.

There have been and will continue to be "whistle blowers." Their fate within their own professions, however, provides scant ground for optimism. More important, to depend on an ethic of heroism is surely an inadequate social response to the challenge posed by the systemic problem of workplace exposure to hazardous substances. Brian Barry, the political philosopher, has put the point bluntly: "To expect heroic individual action to be repeated on a large enough scale to overcome a framework of decisionmaking that provides fundamentally perverse incentives [in terms of speaking out against risks to workers, consumers, and the general public] is to call upon oneself a strong suspicion of 'bad faith.' "[11] Indeed, to depend on such heroism is to subvert the very prospect of developing social structures and legislatively mandated regimes that would permit scientists, engineers, and occupational health physicians to act on behalf of workers placed at risk by their jobs.

But even were such changes to occur, an irreducible level of controversy would remain over acceptable levels of exposure to workplace toxins—a controversy reflecting different socially grounded conceptions of "acceptable risk."[12] Regulators cannot delay controlling harmful exposures until scientific consensus exists. Decisionmaking under conditions of uncertainty is inevitable. Such conditions require that "considerations of fairness," and concerns about who will suffer and who will benefit, be integrated into any decisionmaking approach, no matter how technically sophisticated.[13] Because matters of distributive justice are involved, the political features of the clash over standards of safety are inevitable.

The papers collected in this book are a contribution to the understanding of why neither appeals to professional ethics alone nor calls for technocratic solutions based on more complete empirical evidence can be an adequate response to the hazards faced by workers.

Notes

1. Morton Corn, "The Role of Health Scientists and Engineers in U.S. Corporate Health Policy," unpublished paper prepared for The Hastings Center Project, "Moral Responsibilities and Moral Decisions in Science and Engineering" (1984).

2. National Science Foundation, Program on Ethics and Values in Science and Technology, grant no. RII 8309869.

3. Adelaide M. Anderson, "Historical Sketch of the Development of Legislation for Injurious and Dangerous Industries in England," in Thomas Oliver (ed.), *Dangerous Trades* (New York: Dutton, 1902), p. 25.

4. Irving J. Selikoff and Douglas H. K. Lee, *Asbestos and Disease* (New York: Academic Press, 1978), p. 23.

5. See for example, Robert W. Crandall and Lester B. Lave (eds.), *The Scientific Bases of Health and Safety Regulation* (Washington, D.C.: The Brookings Institution, 1981).

6. Deborah G. Johnson, "Occupational Health and the Conflicting Loyalties of Engineers," unpublished paper prepared for The Hastings Center Project, "Moral Responsibilities and Moral Decisions in Science and Engineering" (1984).

7. Edwin T. Layton, Jr., "Engineering Ethics: Traditional Concerns, Contemporary Problems and Institutional Constraints," unpublished paper prepared for The Hastings Center Project, "Moral Responsibilities and Moral Decisions in Science and Engineering," p. 22 (1984).

8. Ibid., p. 2.

9. Ibid. See also Edwin T. Layton, Jr., *The Revolt of the Engineers* (Cleveland, Ohio: Case Western University Press, 1971).

10. David F. Noble, *America by Design: Science, Technology and the Rise of Corporate Capitalism* (New York: Knopf, 1977), p. 34.

11. Brian Barry, "Distributing the Burdens of Technology: Reflections on the Case Studies," unpublished paper prepared for The Hastings Center Project, "Moral Responsibilities and Moral Decisions in Science and Engineering," p. 15 (1984).

12. William W. Lowrance, *Of Acceptable Risk: Science and the Determination of Safety* (Los Altos, Calif.: William Kaufman, 1976).

13. James M. Robins, Philip T. Landrigan, Thomas G. Robins, and Lawrence J. Fine, "Decision-Making Under Uncertainty in the Setting of Environmental Health Regulations," *Journal of Public Health Policy* 6, 2 (1985): 322–328.

I

OCCUPATIONAL HAZARDS AND PROFESSIONAL BEHAVIOR

1

Private Power, Private Knowledge, and Public Health: Science, Engineering, and Lead Poisoning, 1900–1970

WILLIAM GRAEBNER

In the late nineteenth century, as lead became an increasingly common component of industrial and commercial processes and products, workers in the lead trades began to experience a variety of lead-related maladies, some of them fatal. In the lead mines and smelters of the West, thousands of workers were hospitalized for the consequences of breathing lead dusts and fumes. The classic symptoms of lead poisoning—blue-lined gums and wrist drop—also appeared among painters, solderers, brass workers, printers, potters, and many others whose labor involved contact with some form of lead.

The twentieth century brought substantial improvements in some industries, including ceramics, mining and smelting, and painting, as well as the rise of new industries—especially the automobile and battery—with lead-related problems of their own. When lead was introduced into fuels in the 1920s as an anti-knock agent, lead poisoning was for the first time briefly perceived as an environmental as opposed to an occupational problem. Not until the 1960s, however, would this understanding of lead's hazardous nature become influential. Federal legislation on lead-related environmental and occupational problems would not emerge until the 1970s.

Scientists, engineers, and physicians were present at almost every stage of this historical process. Chemists created, studied, and modified the technical processes involved in the lead glazing of pottery and labored over the introduction of tetraethyl lead into gasoline, and physiologists studied and debated the effects of lead storage in the body. Engineers designed the smelters and in many factories were responsible for maintenance and supervision of exhaust fans and other equipment designed to reduce dust and fume levels. Physicians encountered the lead hazard as company doctors, as medical scientists engaged in research, or as public health professionals in a variety of occupations and organizations, including the American Public Health Association.

How did these professionals meet the challenge posed by lead? This chapter, based on an examination of the historical record, reveals that with few exceptions, neither scientists nor engineers made any substantial effort—at least no public and easily measured effort, nor one beyond what employers expected of them—on behalf of workers subject to lead poisoning. Engineers served their corporate employers, and for decades, a corporate business perspective shaped the production and dissemination of lead-related scientific knowledge. More striking and troubling, those scientists and engineers from whom we might have expected greater concern for the health-related consequences of lead exposure—university-affiliated researchers and those within the public health services—behaved in much the same way. The United States Public Health Service often acted as if it were a service agency for corporate America, and university scientists were closely linked with the auto, oil, and lead industries.[1]

Despite the dominance of the corporate perspective on lead, it would be a mistake to conclude that the work of scientists, engineers, and physicians who served industry went without challenge. There were those in every age who defended the health interests of working men and women. Alice Hamilton, May Mayers, and, in the modern era, Clair Patterson, all labored to challenge corporate priorities, to bring a measure of humanity to the workplace, or to create a more healthful environment.

That such critics were able to establish a stance of relative independence from the corporate perspective does not mean that those who did not so distance themselves were necessarily morally culpable. To make such a judgment would be to deny the extent to which professional outlooks are profoundly affected by the social and structural setting within which professionals work. Ceramics engineers were little more than technical employees of small industrial corporations; they could hardly have been expected to hold opinions significantly different from those of their employers. Similarly, scientists at General Motors understood the issue of leaded gasoline as a matter of fuel efficiency and the future of the internal combustion engine rather than as one posing serious questions of occupational and environmental health. Physicians who dealt with lead toxicology were also usually corporate employees. Indeed, in most cases it is easier to understand why scientists and engineers acted as they did than to suggest plausible ground for a course critical of dominant interests. Criticism should therefore focus less on moral deficiencies than on the corporate/industrial/scientific "system" that created, enforced, and perpetuated a practice that demonstrated little concern for the health and lives of workers and citizens. What this chapter attempts to develop is a *political economy of knowledge*—an account that attempts to locate the origins of scientific knowledge in political and economic, hence ideological, frameworks.

Historical Background

Unlike many modern hazards to health, lead poisoning has a literally ancient history. The Romans used lead in their aqueducts, a practice that apparently produced no serious health hazard. The Greeks experienced some problems with lead intoxication as a result of the lead produced as a byproduct in their silver mines.[2] By far the most serious pre-industrial health problems occurred when the metal was used to line cooking pots or, worse yet, beverage containers. For two thousand years, a variety of peoples suffered ill health and even epidemics of lead poisoning after drinking wine "sweetened" with acetic acid in lead-lined vessels. The Romans experienced such outbreaks, though without fully understanding the source. Not until the mid-seventeenth century did Samuel Stockhausen and other early occupational physicians link these epidemics of "colic" to lead and to the process of fermentation.[3]

In spite of this discovery, lead continued to be employed in cooking and fermentation. The 50 percent lead content of the pewter utensils used in many households in colonial America was one source of poisoning. Another, more serious, concern was the use of lead worms (lead screws) and still heads in the distillation of rum, a practice prohibited under Massachusetts Bay law in 1723.[4]

The identification of lead as an industrial and work hazard began at least as early as the eighteenth century. Benjamin Franklin's diaries discuss cases of lead poisoning in the printing and plumbing trades, in glass manufacturing and house painting, and among laborers whose task it was to grind colors. In addition, colonial Americans had some awareness that lead intoxication might occur from the red-lead adulteration of pepper; the use of lead salts in the whitening of bread; from wrapping foodstuffs in lead foil; from the manufacture of lead shot, drains, and household gutters; and from the storage in pewter containers of low-pH foods such as lemons and tomatoes.[5] Despite their awareness of these established causes, physicians and scientists were slow to appreciate the disease. Two important studies published in the 1830s—Tanquerel des Planches' clinical observations of over 1,200 cases of plumbism (1838) and Benjamin W. McCready's *The Influence of Trades, Professions and Occupations in the United States in the Production of Diseases* (1837) failed to generate further scholarly inquiry.[6]

Meanwhile, lead poisoning was rapidly becoming a serious problem as the use of lead grew to meet the presumed needs of industrial and urban society. Des Planches' warning of the consequences of the inhalation of lead vapors came home to roost in the lead smelters and refineries of the American West. By 1870, lead dust from carbonate ore (white lead) was a lethal agent in the lead mines of Utah, New Mexico, and Colorado. Other industries and occupations whose workers experienced severe lead-related illnesses included painting, printing, and the manufacture of ceramics and glass.[7]

In the twentieth century, lead use and lead hazards decreased in some industries and increased in others. New glazes made ceramics a reasonably safe industry by 1940. So, too, has the changing technology of printing virtually eliminated the hazardous use of hot lead in that industry. Similarly, today's house painters seldom encounter lead paint, although the removal of old lead paint, especially from bridge spans, remains a dangerous occupation, and the use of spray guns for commercial painting applications has increased hazards for some painters.[8]

The automobile has dramatically changed the shape of the lead hazard in the past half-century. In 1950, storage batteries accounted for about 30 percent of lead consumption in the United States, and tetraethyl lead, used as a gasoline additive, for another 13 percent. By the mid-1960s, more than half of the national consumption of lead by weight was for these two uses.[9] Moreover, the use of lead as a fuel additive had put the general population at risk, creating an environmental risk alongside what had previously been understood as a hazard of occupation. Although most turn-of-the-century lead hazards appear to have been eliminated or substantially reduced, disagreement lingers over the extent to which occupational hazards remain and, especially, over the long-term consequences of airborne lead contamination of the environment.

Science: The Case of Ceramics

The pottery or ceramics industry had been as thoroughly studied by 1940 as any industry in the country. Alice Hamilton had examined the industry in 1910 and 1911, and Emery Hayhurst had focused on Ohio's numerous pottery factories in 1914. The U.S. Public Health Service carried out two studies of the industry, one in 1919 and the other in the late 1930s. In the thirty years covered by these four studies, considerable progress was made in the elimination of lead poisoning. Hamilton found 144 cases of lead poisoning among some 1,500 workers. Hayhurst studied more than 1,000 more workers than Hamilton yet found 35 fewer cases of poisoning.[10] Carried out at the request of the National Brotherhood of Operative Potters—a trade union—the 1919 study found 139 cases of positive lead poisoning, 160 "presumptive" cases, and 168 cases of "suggestive" lead poisoning among 1,809 persons engaged in a variety of pottery trades. Limited to West Virginia, the 1937 study found only one case of lead poisoning among 137 men and women workers. "This reduction in the incidence of lead poisoning in the eighteen years that intervene between the two studies," concluded the Public Health Service, "is a notable example of the successful application of chemical and engineering methods to the problems of industrial hygiene."[11]

The 1919 study managed to combine the rhetoric of Progressive reform with the politics of caution. Although the authors made a point of examining the deficiencies and responsibilities of both workers and operators, they clearly focused on the latter as the critical factor. Workers might well question the existence of hazards, but "the plants have taken no concerted action to teach the hazards in a logical way." Workers were given instructions with regard to "personal hygiene, which if observed would materially reduce the hazard of this occupation," but the thrust of the report was to lay the burden for improvement on plant management. "It seems to the investigators," the report stated, "that those in charge of the plants are either indifferent, or careless, or ignorant in regard to health hazards." "In the last analysis," it concluded, "responsibility for working conditions rests with the management."[12]

Yet the report was circumspect in recommending steps that would bring about a reduction in lead poisoning. For example, although investigators had found that the probability of contracting lead poisoning varied directly with the length of the working day, they failed to recommend a statutory reduction of the working day. In fact, the report did not propose any legislative interference in the pottery industry. Instead, the Public Health Service advocated something akin to laissez-faire. Legislation was unnecessary because "both manufacturers and workers are provided with means through organization, meetings, periodicals, and joint relations, for cooperation to eliminate any and all occupational health hazards arising within the industry."[13]

In the end, however, the service did not want to leave the entire process up to some illusive mechanism of "cooperation." It sought to inform this cooperation, and in doing so, it was entering the realm of management. Its approach was nonetheless both apologetic and consistent with business ideology. The tough, anti-business tone of the body of the report was hedged with disclaimers as the authors introduced their recommendations. "It has been difficult to place the responsibility for these conditions," they wrote, adding, "nor is it deemed best for us to try to place it." Seeking to avoid an antagonistic posture as they introduced a group of recommendations on "plant means and methods," the authors wrote: "It is not our purpose here to dictate a program for plant hygiene which should be accepted in its entirety by each and every pottery."[14]

The Service proceeded to place its recommendations within the only framework acceptable to business: profit. Healthy workers were efficient workers, and healthful working conditions were "vital factors in production cost." Presumably, the potteries would analyze and clean the air, make and enforce a wide variety of regulations, replace sick workers, and even change their production processes because the Service had decided that it was good business to do so.[15] Missing from the report was any notion of an obligation to provide workers with decent working conditions or a healthful worklife.

This ethos of self-interest also informed the report's most important recommendations, which involved reducing or eliminating the lead content in ceramic glazes or modifying the way in which lead was chemically contained within the glaze. The last of these alternatives, called "fritting," was the report's outstanding technical recommendation. (Fritting meant fusing the lead with some other constituent in the glazing process, thereby converting the soluble and dangerous white lead, a lead oxide, into the insoluble and harmless disilicate of lead. Not all fritted glazes were equally safe; some were more soluble, and thus less safe, than others.)[16] According to the report, fritting "seems to be the common ground on which all investigators meet as to the best method of eliminating lead poisoning from the pottery industry." Two decades later, the West Virginia study confirmed the leading role of fritted glazes in virtually eliminating lead poisoning in the pottery industry in that state.[17]

The history of the pottery industry's response to lead poisoning might be read as the history of its response to fritted glazes. Before 1920, potteries did not frit glazes and many workers became poisoned with lead; after 1920, potteries in West Virginia—and, one would assume, elsewhere—gradually adopted fritted glazes, and the incidence of plumbism declined dramatically. In sharp contrast to many other changes recommended in the 1919 report, fritting was at bottom a problem of science and scientific knowledge rather than engineering. A safe pottery industry depended on the development of a science of fritted glazes, on the transmission of that science to engineers, managers, and owners, and on the adoption of fritting within the industry. A review of how and when this was accomplished should provide some insight into the role of the scientific establishment in the pottery industry.

Fritting as an applied science dates at least to the 1890s. English laws passed in 1903 required the fritting of lead in specified processes in pottery making and established limits of solubility for lead glazes. German potters had gone even further and by 1899 had developed formulas for workable glazes that used no lead at all.[18]

Moreover, this knowledge was potentially available to American potters. During the Progressive Era, several scientific, technical, and professional associations existed to transmit and disseminate information considered relevant to the nation's potters. The German work on leadless glazes, for example, was referred to in the first volume of the *Transactions of the American Ceramic Society,* published in 1899.[19] The *Transactions,* filled with the newest in experimental processes, offered a forum for the latest foreign and domestic knowledge on leadless and fritted glazes. The *Journal of the American Ceramic Society,* first published in the late 1910s, was less scientific in orientation. But its readership—engineers, chemists, chemical engineers, ceramic chemists, professors, foremen, managers, and superintendents[20]—would surely have been an ideal one for the dissemination of significant knowledge of advances in glaze science and technology. Even less scientific, but a potential vehicle nonetheless, were journals such as *The New Jersey Ceramist,* a quarterly intended for owners, managers, and supervisory personnel within the New Jersey pottery industry.

These publications reveal an industry—including owners, production managers, and scientists—at most only marginally interested in the health problems of workers and in the fritted and leadless glazes that might have made an enormous difference to those workers. The first volume of the *Ceramist,* published in 1921, contained no mention of health and safety problems, although it did offer an article on glazes that contained some material on fritting.[21] Similarly, the 2,000 members of the American Ceramic Society found little to read on lead poisoning or fritted glazes in their *Journal.* The *Transactions* of the American Ceramic Society, clearly the most scientifically oriented of the industry's publications, was only slightly more likely to print studies on lead poisoning and fritting. Of over 500 papers published in the *Transactions* from 1899 through 1914, several dealt with fritted or leadless glazes. But only one paper, and that by an Englishman from the Staffordshire pottery industry, linked fritting explicitly to a reduced incidence of lead poisoning.[22]

In part, the neglect of the European literature on fritting can be traced to Charles F. Binns, director of the New York State School of Clayworking and Ceramics at Alfred and chairman of the Committee on Ceramic Literature of the American Ceramic Society. It was Binns's task to report to the Society on significant domestic and foreign research. Yet Binns was not sympathetic to the climate of regulation that was developing around the English industry at the turn of the century. Referring to a set of English rules establishing limits on the use of raw lead, Binns held that "if the regulations are enforced the whole pottery industry of England would be killed." "The whole trade," he concluded, "is in revolt owing to this ill-judged and 'grandmother' legislation, from which we in the United States glory that we are free."[23]

But the failures of the scientific community to respond more positively to the hazard of lead poisoning and specifically to the possibilities inherent in fritted glazes cannot be explained in terms of one man's biases. It had much to do with the relationship of chemists and the pottery industry. A large percentage of the nation's ceramic chemists were employed by the pottery companies. In this highly competitive industry, most companies were small, and one would assume, strongly profit-conscious. It seems likely that chemists employed in ceramics and other similarly structured industries were, therefore, as constrained in their thinking and objectives as other management-level employees.

Whatever independence ceramic chemistry had could be found in two places: the United States Bureau of Mines, and the colleges and universities.[24] Yet academic chemists were subject to many of the same pressures facing their colleagues in industrial laboratories. University laboratories and buildings were, in fact, constructed in part with donations from the ceramic industry. The Rutgers University Ceramics Building, opened in 1922, was built with $100,000 from the state government and $25,000 from the state's pottery manufacturers. The dedication of a new ceramic engineering facility on the University of Illinois campus in 1917 was accompanied by much discussion of the growing necessity for intimate cooperation between industry and the academy.[25]

The extent to which the science of ceramic chemistry could be subject to business influence is apparent in the circumstances surrounding the 1937 publication of J. H. Koenig's *Lead Frits and Glazes*,[26] then the most complete statement on the subject. Koenig was not an independent scholar. The study had been commissioned by the United States Potters Association—a trade group—and Koenig was, as a consequence, United States Potters Association Fellow in Ceramics. Koenig remained affiliated with the Engineering Experiment Station at Ohio State University, where the study was carried out and published, but even that affiliation raises certain questions. The station was established in 1913 to make technical investigations that would tend to "increase the economy, efficiency, and safety" of the state's enterprises. But Koenig's study may have been the only one to actually deal with the "safety" component of the legislative mandate. The station was there to serve Ohio's business community.

That this setting influenced the framework within which Koenig's science was placed seems clear. On the first page of his report, Koenig described the pottery industry lead hazard as "not serious." The introduction to his work, by another professor, not only suggests that Koenig's work was designed to make possible the use of lead, that "valuable component of a ceramic glaze," but also emphasized the importance of accomplishing this and other objectives through the private-enterprise system.[27]

Engineering: The Case of Lead Mining and Refining

If turn-of-the-century scientists were beholden to employers and susceptible to business values, engineers were even more likely to hold views consistent with those of their employers. The extent to which this was the case is underscored by an examination of two related industries—lead mining and lead smelting and refining—with a substantial engineering component.

Both industries were exceedingly hazardous. Lead mines in Utah, New Mexico, and Colorado yielded a natural carbonate ore (as opposed to galena, or sulfide ore) that was responsible for a highly toxic dust. After 1870, when Western lead mining began in earnest, poisoning was common. According to one estimate, just three mines produced 5,000 poisoned workers in two decades in the late nineteenth century.[28] Smelters also created a dust problem, for they crushed lead-bearing ore, and some workers were exposed to the toxic fumes that came off the molten ore during smelting.[29]

There does not seem to have been any doubt that plumbism existed in these industries, or any serious disagreement over its basic causes or sources. Alice Hamilton's 1914 study of smelters and refineries confirmed that managers and superintendents understood the dangers of lead dust and fumes, although Hamilton took pains to emphasize the relative importance of inhalation vis-à-vis ingestion. Arthur Murray's 1926 investigation of lead mining added a certain scientific weight to the common knowledge that miners who breathed or ingested lead dust were risking lead poisoning.[30]

It also seems likely that the engineering knowledge necessary for the prevention of lead poisoning was available to operators and engineers at or around the turn of the century. Dust control was a staple of mining technology. Respirators were available. As for smelting and refining, a German engineer had in 1908 laid out a practical program for the management of lead hazards.[31]

Nonetheless, engineers appear to have been largely uninterested in the problems of lead toxicity. Instead, the engineering journals and other publications reveal a profession that was at worst actively hostile to the subject of lead poisoning and at best vaguely sympathetic.

Engineers were interested in production. The annual reviews of lead markets published in the engineering magazines invariably emphasized growth and lamented any declines in the consumption of lead, even in industries known to be dangerous. The hazards posed by lead paint, leaded fuel, and the manufacture of storage batteries apparently were of concern to mining engineers only insofar as they threatened to circumscribe the market for lead.[32]

The prospect of losing 85 percent of the nation's lead market to a prohibition of lead in paints enraged T. A. Rickard, editor of the periodical *Mining and Scientific Press.* Rickard asserted—without foundation—that turpentine, not lead, was the cause of many of the painters' ailments; that lead poisoning had been "abolished" in the pottery industry; and that the substitution of other compounds for lead in paint might well "result only in an aggravation of the trouble."[33] Rickard was less concerned with the health of painters than with the market for lead ore.

The major engineering periodicals carried a mere handful of articles and items dealing with the engineering problems of lead poisoning. Some of these were the briefest announcements or summaries of government publications such as Murray's 1926 study or R. R. Sayers's "Miners' Health and Safety Almanac," published by the United States Bureau of Mines.[34] The most sympathetic article, published in 1912 in *Mining and Scientific Press,* noted that "mining and smelting companies remained indifferent" to lead poisoning and made a few brief suggestions for preventive remedies, including compulsory medical examinations and the wearing of respirators in dusty areas. Its most forthright pronouncement, however, had little to do with engineering. "The most effective protectives against the disease," it said, "are cleanliness and sobriety."[35] Wilbert Slemmons's 1921 article, "The Cause and Control of Lead Poisoning," in *Mining and Scientific Press,* suggested without much technical discussion the use of ventilating hoods. More striking, Slemmons, a bacteriologist for the Carnation Milk Company, concluded that the "best insurance against lead poisoning" was milk![36]

Technical manuals intended for smelter engineers present a more mixed picture. Malvern Iles's *Lead-Smelting: The Construction, Equipment, and Operation of Lead Blast-Furnaces* (1902), was obviously intended for an audience of engineers. While cognizant of the poisonous nature of the fumes produced in the smelting process and of the dangers of inhaling those fumes, Iles did not indicate how such inhalation might be avoided. With his background as assayer, chemist, metallurgist, and superintendent for a variety of Western smelters, Iles was more interested in the fume as a recoverable resource. To its credit, Walter Ingalls's edited collection, *Lead Smelting and Refining* (1906), contained an English translation of a 1905 German essay claiming vastly lower rates of lead toxicity under a new smelting process.[37]

This brief review of the literature of engineering suggests that engineers, no less than owners and managers, were profit- and production-conscious. The acting chief engineer of the Ohio State Board of Health described this engineering stance in 1911, in a reference to the attitude of civil engineers toward sanitation problems:

> The view that the average engineer takes of his profession is a rather prosaic one. He is apt to regard the problems submitted to him for solution as merely involving economic considerations, and is generally well satisfied if his work meets with the approval of his clients and has been done at a minimum cost. Not often does he feel it incumbent on him to demand a higher standard than his clients are satisfied with, nor does he feel called upon to educate the public in matters of health, cleanliness, decency, and justice.[38]

Changing Approaches to "Reform"

In the two decades prior to 1920, what might be called a Progressive approach to lead toxicology took shape. That approach assumed that national and state governments would provide investigatory leadership in the occupational health field. Thus, industrial states such as Illinois and New York conducted extensive inquiries into health and safety conditions in factories and mines operating within their borders. The national government entered the arena in 1912 with the first of several industry studies carried out by the Department of Labor. The assumption was that government could function, at least in some respects, as an independent agency, providing not just data but an alternative perspective to the one then prevailing in the business world. Government would serve as an advocate of the public interest.[39]

Even in the Progressive Era, this model of reform failed to reflect practice. As elaborate and revealing as the federal industry studies were, they stopped short of making legislative recommendations. State investigators were more likely to suggest legislative remedies, but even so, legislative gains appear to have been very limited. Following the 1911 release of the report of the Illinois Commission on Occupational Diseases, six states, including Illinois, passed occupational disease legislation. Pennsylvania followed in 1913 with a law based on the American Association for Labor Legislation's standard bill on occupational disease. In the absence of a thorough study of this legislation, one must be cautious in drawing conclusions with regard to its effectiveness. In the opinion of Alice Hamilton, who carried out many of the federal studies and who was more familiar with lead-related health problems than any other individual, even the best of the state laws, the Illinois statute, was reduced in effectiveness by its reliance on the reports of industrial physicians, whose loyalty to corporate employers often resulted in the reporting of only the most obvious cases of plumbism.[40]

Neither Progressivism nor the Progressive system of occupational health contained within it came to an abrupt end in 1920. In the lead area, the federal government, for example, remained an important source of information. Hamilton, the dominant force in Progressive-Era health reform, remained as active as ever in the 1920s. Yet there is evidence that by the mid-1920s, the Progressive model of reform had been displaced by another, even less likely to produce satisfactory results.

Under this new model, the informal conference replaced the legislature and the study commission. Theoretically pluralist in inspiration and organization, the conference was in fact easily dominated by the very business institutions that were most in need of regulation and control. In the conference process the government was to serve as a facilitator rather than as an advocate of a public perspective. Moreover, while the Progressive-Era system of health regulation had depended for the most part on knowledge produced by federal and state agencies, by the mid-1920s private foundations and laboratories had begun to control the flow of knowledge. The result was an increasingly business-oriented perspective.

Tetraethyl Lead and the Conference System

Henry Ford's automobile assembly line was just a year old in 1914 when scientists at General Motors (GM) began looking for ways to make the internal combustion engine more powerful and efficient. Automotive engineers wanted to manufacture more powerful automobiles, but they were also concerned with possible shortages of fuel. "America does not have an unlimited supply of motor-car fuel," wrote one automotive authority in 1916. "We are already at the point where we have only about two-thirds of it left, and it is getting harder to win each year."[41]

One could easily obtain more power and efficiency from a given quantity of gasoline by increasing engine compression. But this brought on an engine "knock" that was potentially damaging to the engine and unacceptable to consumers. The knock had to go.[42]

During World War I a nontechnical employee of a large copper refining company had suggested the use of tellurium, an unused by-product of copper refining, as an anti-knock agent. GM's tests of the compound showed promise, but tellurium research was discontinued when it became clear that too little of the substance was produced to make it feasible as a gasoline additive. GM turned instead to a relative of tellurium, tetraethyl lead.[43] Although known since 1854, tetraethyl lead had not been tried as a fuel additive. Credit for the "invention" of leaded fuel is usually given to Thomas Midgley, Jr., of the GM laboratory at Dayton, Ohio, who reported his discovery in 1922. Not long thereafter, the Ethyl Gasoline Corporation was founded, with Midgley as its president, to produce and distribute tetraethyl lead.[44] Tetraethyl lead was also produced at Standard Oil of New Jersey's Bayway facility, under a complex arrangement involving Standard, DuPont (which controlled GM), and the Ethyl Corporation; and at Deepwater, New Jersey, where apparently only DuPont had a financial interest.[45]

As word of the research on leaded fuel reached the public, voices were raised in concern and protest. First to be heard from was William Mansfield Clark, a professor of chemistry who confided his anxiety to Assistant Attorney General A. M. Stimson on October 11, 1922. Clark informed Stimson of Midgley's experiments in Dayton and also mentioned that the Dye Works Plant of the DuPont Company was preparing to manufacture tetraethyl lead for distribution by Standard Oil. Clark voiced his fears of serious health dangers involved in both the manufacture of leaded gasoline and in auto emissions produced by the burning of the new fuel. Stimson moved the issue into the lower echelons of the Public Health Service with a letter to R. E. Dyer, acting director of the Service's Hygienic Laboratory. Acknowledging the possibility that a "real health menace" existed, Stimson said the Service ought to have "experimental evidence" on the health effects of tetraethyl lead, and he asked Dyer to develop a proposal to generate such evidence.[46]

By late November, however, these plans had apparently been shelved. The director of the Hygienic Laboratory had "carefully considered" the risk of lead poisoning from the use of tetraethyl lead in gasoline and decided not "to recommend any experimental investigation at the present time." This important decision was justified on three grounds. First, the acquisition of "trustworthy data" would take too much time—"perhaps a year." "This delay," wrote Director G. W. McCoy, "would probably prevent results of an experimental investigation from being of much practical use since the trial of the material under ordinary conditions should show whether there is risk to man." While implying that some portion of the population might serve as guinea pigs for an informal, *ad hoc* experiment on tetraethyl lead toxicity, McCoy added that experimental data derived from animal studies would be difficult to interpret and claimed that experimental results would apply to a "limited set of conditions" that might not normally be encountered. Better, then, not to do an experiment at all. McCoy suggested that companies involved in the manufacture and processing of tetraethyl lead be contacted and asked if health factors had "been given consideration."[47]

At this point the case had reached the federal government's highest official in health matters—Surgeon General E. S. Cumming. Cumming did what McCoy suggested. He wrote to Pierre DuPont, asking if his company had collected data on poisoning dangers related to tetraethyl lead. DuPont routed the inquiry to Midgley, the chief engineer in his Fuel Section, who joined McCoy in offering the American people as guinea pigs. Admitting that "no actual experimental data" had been generated, Midgley nonetheless argued that even under the most extreme conditions—in a vehicular tunnel—the inhalation from leaded gasoline would be harmless. Midgley claimed—from what data one can only imagine—that people exposed to such conditions would absorb only a very small part of one milligram of lead, "while the average congested street will probably be so free from lead that it will be impossible to detect it or its absorption." Midgley then announced the program of human experimentation that McCoy had implicitly condoned. In the near future, he wrote the Surgeon General, DuPont would place a "small quantity" of tetraethyl lead on the market in "some districts." Although doing so was, of course, assumed to be harmless, the company would thoroughly study the toxicity of the compound during this period.[48]

Like DuPont, the Ethyl Corporation sought to prove that tetraethyl lead was harmless without allowing the research process beyond its control. In the spring of 1922, the company asked Yale physiologist Yandell Henderson to undertake an investigation of the health hazards of tetraethyl lead. Henderson later recalled that he and others had "indicated that we would be willing to make an investigation, provided we could do it freely, without any dictation, and simply to find the facts. In practically every case the person addressed intimated—as I did very strongly—that we looked at the matter as one that should be investigated from the standpoint of public safety. Then the Ethyl Gasoline Corporation dropped the matter. They did not have the investigations made."[49]

Rather than undertake its own study of tetraethyl lead, the Public Health Service deferred to an ongoing project of the United States Bureau of Mines.[50] From the moment that the public became aware of it, the Bureau of Mines's research into tetraethyl lead was criticized as biased and flawed. Some critics were disturbed by the study's reliance on animals, others by the death during the study of a large number of those animals (explained by the Bureau on grounds other than lead exposure). Others argued that the study had no bearing on "real" conditions, such as the exposure of garage workers to especially great concentrations of particles over a long period of time.[51]

Most disturbing, however, was the fact that the Bureau's research had been initiated and funded by General Motors, a corporation that obviously had much to gain from a benign report. This relationship was all the more suspect because the Bureau's mission as an institution was not simply one of protecting the public health and safety. From the moment of its creation in 1910, the agency had been charged with the dual responsibility of protecting the public health and safety while promoting the economic needs of business.[52]

Led by Alice Hamilton, critics of the Bureau had a field day. Writing from her office in Harvard University's School of Public Health, Hamilton told Cumming of the unsatisfactory nature of the report. "In the eyes of labor," she emphasized, the participation of GM would "always serve to cast doubt on any negative results obtained by the investigators."[53] By May 1925, even the Public Health Service had joined the hunt, publicly denouncing the influence of GM and the Ethyl Corporation in the fuel studies and criticizing the Bureau of Mines for inadequate explanations of data that had led several states to lift prematurely their bans against public sale of leaded gasoline.[54]

This new, anti-corporate stance was in marked contrast to the Public Health Service's record of acquiescence. For three critical years—from 1922 through late 1924—the Service had done nothing to challenge the adequacy of existing research on tetraethyl lead or to initiate new projects. In this climate, the fuel industry went ahead with its program of *de facto* human experimentation. The Ethyl Gasoline Corporation began marketing ethyl gasoline commercially in February 1923 at Dayton. GM, in other words, did not wait for the results of its own Bureau of Mines research project. At the Standard Oil and DuPont laboratories, potentially hazardous research on tetraethyl lead continued.

In July 1924, in a gesture of social responsibility, Standard Oil, DuPont, and General Motors created a medical committee to study the problem. The committee decided to solicit the "facts" from two "impartial" sources, one of them the Bureau of Mines. Although the committee included eminent scientists, its business origins made it unlikely that it would serve an independent and critical function.[55]

Then, in October 1924, an event took place that changed the tenor of the debate. Five persons were killed and thirty injured as a result of exposure to tetraethyl lead at the Bayway, New Jersey facility of the Standard Oil Company. Headlines such as " 'Looney Gas' Kills Fourth; 11 More Ill," and "Another Man Dies from Insanity Gas" both reflected and fed the public's fears.[56] At least thirteen persons died from lead poisoning at Bayway, at Deepwater, and at Dayton in 1924 and 1925.[57]

Although a New Jersey prosecutor looking into the case claimed the deaths had occurred during the manufacturing process (the mixing of gasoline with tetraethyl lead supplied by the Ethyl Corporation) rather than during experimentation, Standard Oil claimed the opposite. In a prepared statement, the company defined the tragedy as the unfortunate but perhaps inevitable result of a necessary program of "experimental studies, some of which are necessarily attended with danger." The accident had taken place "in the laboratory" (not in commercial production) and in a program guided by the "foremost chemists and engineers" and attended by the "foremost authority in occupational diseases." The company did not explain why the "laboratory" was, like the company's refineries, operating on three shifts.[58]

It is not clear who was killed at Bayway—scientists or workers— or at what facility—a laboratory or a mixing plant. What is clear is that Standard Oil thought it mattered. It was one thing for scientists to die in a risky quest for essential knowledge, another for workers to expire. Apparently others were less concerned. Col. Percy E. Barbour, editor of *Mining and Metallurgy,* a publication of the American Institute of Mining and Metallurgical Engineers, implied that the accident had taken place during commercial manufacture. Barbour praised the endeavor while lamenting the price exacted by progress.

"It is regrettable," he wrote, "that almost every advancement in science is made at the expenditure of considerable human life." For Barbour, science and commerce were on the same continuum, each a part of one larger enterprise of risk.[59]

In a climate of widespread panic, the forces of opposition to tetraethyl lead were captained by Yale physiologist Yandell Henderson. Henderson had begun his career as a chemist interested in respiration. During World War I he took part in Bureau of Mines Studies of poison gas used by American troops in France. Henderson was never fond of this work. Guilty for having plotted "atrocities" and having experimented with "poisoned bullets," Henderson turned against the war and eventually became a pacifist. When Chemical Warfare Services took over the Bureau of Mines gas research, Henderson's conscience rebelled. He refused to enter the army. As the *New York World* reported in 1925, Henderson was quite frank that his experiences with chemical tools of warfare had made him especially sensitive to the issue and possibility of mass poisoning.[60]

Few Americans had actually worked with poison gases during the war, but it was the rare person, indeed, who had not heard about them and did not share some of Henderson's fears. This mindset shaped the public's response to tetraethyl lead. An issue that a decade earlier might have been handled as an occupational problem, one unique to the manufacture of leaded gasoline, was instead defined as a potential environmental catastrophe. Public anxieties focused less on what had happened at Bayway that what might happen on the automobile-congested streets of Manhattan. A single word unified the wartime experiments and the new problem of automotive emissions: gas.

As presented by Henderson, the specter of tetraethyl lead took on the shape of an alien invasion of vehicles from states that, unlike New York, had not temporarily prohibited the use of leaded fuel. "If," worried Henderson, "an automobile from another State using this gas should have engine trouble along Fifth Avenue and release a quantity of gas with the lead mixture, it would be likely to cause gas poisoning and mania to persons along the avenue." Bowing to Henderson's scholarly reputation, the city's chief medical examiner agreed that a potential "menace" existed. "As far as we have been able to ascertain," he told the press, "no automobiles burning gasoline containing this lead have entered New York City."[61]

And there the matter rested, as Henderson and an anxious public, temporarily mollified by state prohibitions on the sale of leaded gasoline and a voluntary cessation of production by the major companies, waited for the Surgeon General to call a conference to consider the matter. By early February 1925, Cumming's failure to do so had left him vulnerable to charges that the lead interests had been influential in his counsels.[62]

The circulation of the overly sanguine Bureau of Mines report on lead in the early months of 1925 only made matters worse from the perspective of the anti-lead forces, for it raised the prospect that the head of steam raised in the aftermath of Bayway might be dissipated. When the New York Public Health Council, acting on the Bureau of Mines report, authorized anew the distribution of tetraethyl lead and the sale of leaded gasoline to the public, Henderson joined hands with the *New York World* in an attempt to recreate the crisis atmosphere of November 1924. Under the *World's* semi-banner headline—"Will Ethyl Gasoline Poison All of Us? Scientists Disagree"—Henderson claimed that the return to the use of leaded fuel could be "the greatest experiment in virtual race suicide ever carried out." As Henderson now defined it, the problem was less one of gas than of lead dust—accumulations of it, tons of it, on every New York City street. The *World,* listening, in a sense, as Henderson and the Ethyl Corporation traded dust estimates, decided that Henderson had the better part of the argument. Its summation brought the issue home to every New Yorker:

> If [ethyl gas is used, and dust accumulates] . . . then when you go out in front of your house or shop when the dust is stirred up, as New York dust always is, and snuff and snuff until you have inhaled from two to three milligrams, and do this every day for a week, then you will be a goner. You will have blue lines close to your gums, and colic, and if you keep up your snuffing, wrist drop and other horrible complications.[63]

Two days later, the Surgeon General temporarily discontinued the distribution of tetraethyl lead and the sale of leaded gasoline, although he had no legal authority to do either.[64]

Then, at long last, Cumming called a conference. Some eighty-five persons attended the late May event, among them the nation's leading authorities in public health, physiology, and occupational disease. Yandell Henderson was there, with a provocative characterization of the participants. "We have in this room," he announced, "two diametrically opposed conceptions. The men engaged in industry, chemists, and engineers, take it as a matter of course that a little thing like industrial poisoning should not be allowed to stand in the way of a great industrial advance. On the other hand, the sanitary experts take it as a matter of course that the first consideration is the health of the people."[65]

Although a large contingent of scientists, many from federal agencies, were in attendance, they remained in the background during the proceedings. R. R. Sayers was there to prevent and defend the Bureau of Mines's controversial report. Several scientists, including Joseph Aub from Harvard, rose to challenge the conclusion of fellow scientist Robert Kehoe that lead was a normal component in the human feces and urine.[66] But this issue, although it perhaps should have been central to the debate, was not fully explored, and the Bureau's report was too weak to become the focus of discussion.

Labor had a mere handful of representatives. One of them, however, was quite vocal. Grace Burnham, director of the Workers' Health Bureau,[67] emphasized the continuing failure of any agency to provide an "authoritative" list of actual deaths and diseases from tetraethyl lead. More important, in calling for an investigation of the lead hazard by a "responsible public agency" and out of "public funds," Burnham leveled an implicit challenge at the institutional and political context in which previous research had been carried out and presented.[68]

The public health contingent was composed of two factions, one critical of industry and cautious about tetraethyl lead, the other ready to allow the production and distribution of ethyl gasoline. The cautious faction came from the universities. David Edsall, dean of Harvard's School of Public Health, found the lead hazard "noteworthy." Arguing that warnings in garages and other public places would be neglected, he raised the possibility of government prohibition. Haven Emerson, a professor of Public Health at Columbia University, called for new and precise studies of people who worked with ethyl gasoline, while expressing his hope that "in the future animal experimentation will precede and not follow human experimentation." Hamilton, also from Harvard, urged the nation's chemists to find a substitute for tetraethyl lead.[69]

Public health officials associated with state and local governments, as well as those linked to the American Public Health Association, were less cautious. Some of these health officials—from Detroit and Ohio, for example—had conducted surveys and studies of their own and had become convinced that tetraethyl lead presented no danger to the general public nor even to those who handled the ethyl fluid and gasoline. Speaking for a committee representing the American Public Health Association, Emery Hayhurst of Ohio State University's College of Medicine defended the sale of leaded fuel.[70]

But business dominated the conference. Numbers alone made the producers and distributors of tetraethyl lead a force to be reckoned with. Oil had thirteen representatives, autos nine, and the Ethyl Corporation alone had six. Business was also granted the opportunity to establish an appropriate framework for the issue. The conference opened with Charles F. Kettering, speaking for the Ethyl Corporation, describing the historical conditions that had given rise to the need for a leaded fuel. The general manager of DuPont spoke next, affirming that leaded fuel could be safely manufactured and marketed and documenting the auto industry's early interest in "impartial" studies of lead's effect. Then Sayers presented the animal study of the Bureau of Mines, and soon thereafter, Robert Kehoe presented the results of his early research for the Ethyl Corporation, emphasizing that lead was relatively nontoxic compared with other heavy metal compounds. When Henderson took the floor as the first person to oppose leaded gasoline, the conference was already hours old.[71] From this point on, Burnham, Hamilton, Edsall, and others were put in the position of having to snipe away at a framework and data base that had been set down by spokesmen from the auto and oil companies and the scientists who served them.

The lead merchants retained this advantage throughout the conference. In the final hour, Frank A. Howard, representing Ethyl Gasoline Corporation, rose to exploit it one more time. In an extraordinary speech, Howard shifted business' defense from the vulnerable ground of the "facts" (i.e., studies demonstrating that leaded gasoline was safe) to the high ground of ethics. From ten years of General Motors research and five years of Standard Oil research, "we have," Howard said, "this apparent gift of God—of three cubic centimeters of tetraethyl lead" that would permit a gallon of gas to take an automobile twice as far as ever before. Standing in the way was "the question of the health hazard. What is our duty under the circumstances? Should we throw this thing aside? . . . Because some animals die and some do not die in some experiments, shall we give this thing up entirely? . . . We cannot justify ourselves in our consciences if we abandon this thing. I think it would be an unheard-of blunder if we should abandon a thing of this kind merely because of our fears." Finally, unable to entirely abandon the "facts," Howard emphasized quite correctly that most of the facts presented at the conference were on the side of tetraethyl lead.[72] He was able to do so, of course, because the Bayway tragedy did not become the focus of the conference; because there was, as Burnham had said, no list of lead-related deaths and disabilities; because labor had little representation; and because no truly independent agency had studied the effect of tetraethyl lead. Howard remained untroubled by the course the conference had taken. How, after all, could one deny a "gift of God"?

In the end, everyone seemed to agree that only the Surgeon General could resolve the matter. The conference passed a resolution calling on the Surgeon General to appoint a committee to prepare for him a statement regarding the health hazard posed by tetraethyl lead. The conference endorsed the Ethyl Corporation's decision to voluntarily discontinue the sale of leaded fuel, and it passed a Burnham amendment calling for a publicly funded investigation, with results to be reported to another public conference at which labor was to be represented.[73]

With the exception of a public health official from Minnesota, the seven-member committee appointed by Cumming was composed entirely of academics representing the fields of physiology, public health, preventive medicine, pharmacology, and chemistry. Of those who had taken a prominent role at the first conference, only Harvard's Edsall was on the new committee. Convinced that "actual experience" provided the only reliable method of evaluating the lead hazard, the committee set off on an unusual course: it conducted its own study. It was able to do so only because the voluntary suspension of production and distribution had left in commercial circulation a small supply of ethyl fluid.[74]

To conduct the study, the committee secured the services of J. P. Leake, a surgeon with the Public Health Service. Leake repaired to Dayton, where leaded fuel was still in use, to study the effect of tetraethyl lead on about 200 garage workers, city drivers, and factory employees who were exposed to lead fumes or lead dust during the working day.[75] The research did not take long, and the committee met in late December 1925 to discuss the study's results and to formulate a statement for Cumming.

Although the sort of anxiety that Henderson had articulated in May was gone, the minutes of this committee's deliberations reveal some continuing suspicions about the risks of tetraethyl lead. One member said it would be "foolish" not to recognize that the fecal record indicated "some source of lead poisoning." Another acknowledged that the study had demonstrated that the use of ethyl gasoline was "accompanied by some increase of storage of lead." Edsall was convinced that the hazard was "not . . . severe," but he believed that there was insufficient evidence to decide whether the hazard was of "any real significance." Still another committee member found the risk "slight" as compared to the risks in occupational lead trades but "sufficiently serious to warrant very careful supervision." Edsall also mentioned the public's need to know that the committee's report was not an attempt to "protect the manufacturers," and he remained convinced that the committee, although helpless from a legal standpoint, had the authority to make the manufacturers do "certain things."[76]

The final report to the Surgeon General smoothed the rough edges of committee deliberations and papered over doubts. Although it included a recommendation for continued investigation in order to measure the effects of "long-term exposure," the report found "no good grounds for prohibiting the use of ethyl gasoline . . . provided that its distribution and use are controlled by proper regulations."[77] When the Surgeon General made the report public, all ambiguity was gone: "No cases have been discovered of lead poisoning or other disease resulting from the use of ethyl gasoline."[78] Left unmentioned were possible long-term health effects, the fact that the scientific investigation had been hastily conducted and was based on a small population studied for only a brief period, the need for an ongoing investigation, and clear evidence of elevated lead levels in study subjects.

Within months, the Ethyl Corporation, DuPont, Standard Oil, and others involved in the production of ethyl fluid and the manufacture and distribution of leaded gasoline had agreed to comply voluntarily with a series of regulations approved by the 1926 Conference of State and Territorial Health Officers. In May 1926 Leake could be seen in Bayway, Dayton, Cincinnati, and other places, inspecting "ethylizing" stations for compliance.[79] And there the matter stood, literally for decades, until in 1958 a new generation of automobile engines forced the manufacturers to reopen the issue with a request to increase the amount of tetraethyl lead added to gasoline.

Whether the program of voluntary adherence to regulations lacking legal sanction was as successful as Cumming would claim in 1928, or as the industry would always assert, is impossible to determine. Clearly the regulations did not eliminate all anxiety. In the early 1930s, rumors circulated in Charleston, South Carolina, of men "losing their arms or legs through the chemical being present in the gasoline." The following year the DuPont company found itself the object of a suit for compensation that looked as if it would be based on a claim of lead poisoning.[80] But these are obviously isolated examples, and there are no historical statistics to help us evaluate the risks of workers engaged in the handling of ethyl fluid or leaded gasoline.

What can be said with some confidence is that the process that began with the 1925 conference and ended with the regulations of early 1926 brought an end to serious controversy over the risks posed by leaded fuel. No less an authority and critic than Hamilton thought that the process had worked to perfection. She was especially pleased with the conference, which she interpreted as the apotheosis of democratic pluralism. "It was to me both surprising and heartening," she later wrote, "to see men of such widely separated backgrounds and interests—manufacturers and their chemists and research workers on one side, trade-union officials, independent physicians, and toxicologists on the other—meet in a spirit of reasonableness and a genuine desire to get at the real facts and deal practically with the problem."[81]

This statement appears in Hamilton's autobiography, published in 1943, and its overly sanguine character might be explained as the product of the nearly two-decade lapse between the event and its recollection. How else might one interpret Hamilton's apparent failure to raise the issue of business dominance of the conference or to broach the conference's disregard of her own plea that a substitute for tetraethyl lead be found? Yet Hamilton's recollection of the events of the 1920s is also consistent with her ardent belief in cooperation and persuasion as problem-solving devices. Hamilton had spent the two decades before 1925 engaged in a personal crusade for occupational health. For permission to observe factory conditions she had had to rely on the voluntary consent of owners, and for results largely on the good will of management. She was accustomed to functioning in a world in which change came less from the law than from persuasion and trust. The conference had not accomplished what she wished, but apparently for Hamilton this was less important than the fact that people assembled, reasoned together amicably, avoided confrontation, and compromised their differences.

The controversy over tetraethyl lead both reflects the climate of the 1920s and prefigures important ingredients in the politics of science through the 1950s. The "conference" emerged as a singularly significant method for managing, if not resolving, controversies over lead toxicity. Although the 1925 conference had at least the appearance of pluralism, many of its successors did not.[82]

The conference method also sanctioned a private and voluntary approach to the solution of social problems. Government played a role in the tetraethyl lead crisis, of course, but it was the role of coordinator, facilitator, and, after the conference and the Committee of Seven had met, of ratifier. Only in a formal sense was the reluctant Surgeon General at the center of the process. The regulations that emerged from the process had no basis in law; compliance was voluntary. According to one public health official, the Ethyl Corporation's statement of intent to manufacture, blend, and market in accordance with those regulations "removed the pressure for State regulations. Subsequently, no State or Federal law has been enacted pertaining to the hygienic aspects of tetraethyl lead."[83]

Although for a time, perhaps a few years, the Surgeon General operated an informal inspection service in order to ascertain compliance with the 1926 regulations, in the long run that function devolved to the Ethyl Corporation. The compliance of distributors such as Standard Oil was secured through a curious semi-contractual relationship with the supplier, the Ethyl Corporation.[84] For Hamilton, this resolution of the tetraethyl lead controversy was a prime example of a "peculiarly American" method of dealing with industrial hazards "which works very well in a country composed of forty-eight independent states, a method without legal compulsion."[85]

Paralleling the private and voluntary approach to regulating lead was the delimiting of the governmental or public role in lead-related scientific research. The tetraethyl lead controversy might have resulted in public financing of lead research, or produced a general commitment to an ongoing program of independent research into the long-term effects of lead emissions, or initiated productive and critical reviews of the contracts, such as that between GM and the Bureau of Mines, whose existence had served only to bring into question the authority of science itself. None of these things happened. Instead, the conclusion of the controversy signaled the beginning of a forty-year period in which research into the health hazards of tetraethyl lead was conducted by scientists who were closely linked to the lead, oil, and automobile industries and who depended for funds on the Charles F. Kettering Foundation and the Mellon Institute. For four crucial decades—decades characterized by geometric growth in automobile traffic—research on lead in the atmosphere remained under the control of vested interests.

Finally, the resolution of the tetraethyl lead controversy represented a victory for an "occupational" as opposed to an "environmental" perspective. Attention to the hazards of particular occupations such as pottery manufacturing and lead mining had been the focus of Progressive-Era efforts. Given the deplorable condition of the turn-of-the-century workplace, this occupational focus was certainly justified. The Bayway tragedy was at first understood in similar terms, as a matter involving either scientists engaged in the occupation of experimentation or workers engaged in the occupation of mixing ethyl fluid with gasoline.

Yet for Henderson and a small group of public health academics, Bayway raised the possibility of environmental genocide. Dangerous as it was, fuel mixing affected only a few persons. The automobile, spewing lethal lead fumes onto congested city streets, affected everyone. It did not help that Henderson had framed the issue in apocalyptic terms, as a battle against imminent catastrophe. But even a less hyperbolic approach would not have won the day for environmentalism. General Motors, Ethyl, and Standard Oil had too much at stake to tolerate the interference with their business that such a view would have—and eventually did—involve.

Hegemony in the Marketplace of Knowledge

The lead industries exerted enormous, indeed hegemonic, influence over the production and dissemination of knowledge about lead poisoning in the four decades after 1925. Hegemony was achieved through a variety of institutions, including the Lead Industries Association, a trade association; the Mellon Institute, a private research organization; the Charles F. Kettering Foundation and the Kettering Laboratory of Applied Physiology; and the American Public Health Association. Through these and other institutions, the lead industry and its allies in the automobile and oil industries underwrote and carried out much of the significant lead-related scientific research in the inter-war years and beyond. Scientists whose work was thereby supported were, in turn, influential in determining how Americans thought about and responded to lead hazards. In addition, the lead industries were able to achieve and maintain this hegemonic control because no significant challenge was mounted to their point of view. Public agencies and professionals, organized in the American Medical Association, the American Association of Industrial Physicians and Surgeons, the American Public Health Association, and the U.S. Public Health Service, failed to provide an alternative perspective or a foundation of scientific knowledge about lead toxicology, free of corporate interest, on which governmental or private actions might be based.

Charles Kettering and Robert Kehoe

The most significant link between the business community and the scientific establishment involved the Kettering Foundation, General Motors, and—at the apex of the pyramid—Robert Kehoe. It would be difficult to overestimate the importance of these ties, because Kehoe was until the mid-1960s the nation's most vocal and influential scientist working on lead hazards. The Surgeon General's 1925 conference on tetraethyl lead was only the first of Kehoe's numerous public appearances. As late as 1966, Senator Edmund Muskie could be seen grappling with Kehoe's science and its implications during hearings on air pollution.[86] Kehoe was by then nearing the end of his career, but he ruled the scientific domain long enough to significantly shape the nation's response to the hazard of lead.

No person was more important in the bonding that occurred between corporate and scientific communities than Charles Kettering. At the age of thirty-three he had left the National Cash Register Company for a position of partial ownership in the Dayton Engineering Laboratories Company, known as Delco. In 1916, Kettering sold his interest in Delco to a company that later became part of General Motors; he remained as an operating head. When GM felt the need for its own research laboratory, Kettering agreed to head it, provided the facility would be located in Dayton. After 1920 Kettering was at the center of GM's scientific and technological efforts. He was involved, for example, in Thomas Midgley, Jr.'s experiments with tetraethyl lead. Kettering also served as a director of the Dayton-based Ethyl Corporation.[87]

Kettering was no less adept at making money than invention, and in 1927 his savings found an outlet in the Charles F. Kettering Foundation. Created to "sponsor and carry out scientific research for the benefit of humanity," the foundation over the years funded programs in photosynthesis, biology, energy conservation, nutrition, and, beginning in 1940, cancer research. The GM connection was enhanced in 1945, when Alfred P. Sloan, Jr., GM's first chairman of the board, provided the funds for what became the Sloan-Kettering Institute for Cancer Research.[88]

The Kettering Foundation's influence over lead research came through the Kettering Laboratory of Applied Physiology, constructed with Kettering Foundation funds at the University of Cincinnati and opened in 1930. Kehoe was the laboratory's first director. Trained as a physician, Kehoe had worked as a hospital pathologist in the early 1920s while holding down his first teaching job as an assistant professor of physiology at the University of Cincinnati. In 1925 he took on the additional post of medical director of the Ethyl Corporation. Kehoe simultaneously held official positions with the laboratory, the University of Cincinnati, and the Ethyl Corporation until 1958, when the relationship with the Ethyl Corporation ended. Kehoe's successor as director of the Kettering Laboratory, Frank Princi, also enjoyed this triple appointment.[89]

Kehoe's education in lead toxicology began in early 1925, when as the Ethyl Corporation's new medical director he investigated 138 cases of poisoning—attributable to tetraethyl lead—in Dayton and Bayway. A year later, Kehoe helped draft the regulations governing the blending of gasoline in refineries.[90]

By 1933 a substantial body of work bearing Kehoe's name or imprint had appeared in the industrial hygiene and medical journals. In these early articles Kehoe laid out the Kettering/Kehoe perspective on lead poisoning. The following arguments were central to that perspective. First, small amounts of lead occurred "naturally" in human tissue, even in persons living in rural areas entirely divorced from modern industrial processes and automobiles. Therefore, to discover the presence of lead in human excreta or tissue was not proof that the subject had encountered some alien source of lead, but only that he had lived "on a lead-bearing planet."[91] Second, this natural accumulation of lead in the body, caused largely by the ingestion of vegetation, did not result in the storage of greater and greater amounts of lead in the tissues. Instead, an "equilibrium" was established between lead intake and lead elimination. Beyond that point of equilibrium, absorption did not occur; the body, it seemed, had a built-in protective mechanism. Third, because lead occurred naturally in human tissue even in primitive societies, and because its storage occurred within an equilibrium, there was no necessary relation between lead absorption and lead intoxication—no necessary connection between lead concentration in the feces, urine, or tissues, and lead poisoning.[92]

For Kehoe, clinical findings were insufficient; one needed to know "that a significant exposure to lead has occurred."[93] In practice, this led directly to a fourth point. Because general, environmental exposures to lead could be measured only clinically, and because clinical findings were inadequate, hygienists should eschew consider-

ation of environmental hazards—such as those potentially attributable to lead emissions—in order to focus on occupational lead poisoning. Although Kehoe acknowledged the possible long-term health
consequences of an increased daily intake of lead (while doing his
best to minimize the relationship of lead poisoning and intake), this
was clearly not the thrust of his work.[94] Thus Kehoe, the Kettering
Foundation, General Motors, and the Ethyl Corporation had joined
hands to create a body of scientific opinion that was ideally suited to
the manufacturers of both tetraethyl lead and automobiles.

Of course, even these arguments obligated the Ethyl Corporation to clean its own house, and it had done so with the 1926 regulations. But this was a small price to pay for insurance against the only
real threat—the threat that lead poisoning might be environmentally
defined and that tetraethyl lead might then be banned.

Kehoe aggressively sought to influence industrial hygiene, public
health, medicine, and science. He served on the 1930 American Public Health Association Committee on Lead Poisoning, whose report
lashed out at legislation and at "arbitrary rules by government agencies" and focused on occupational problems and on diagnosis as a
virtual art form. When the American Public Health Association prepared a report on how to determine the lead content in air and
biological materials, another Kettering employee, Jacob Cholak, did
the work. Kehoe was a member of the American Standards Association committee that developed the 1943 lead standard, and he was
available to testify for companies involved in lead compensation
cases. He had ties to the American Association of Industrial Physicians and Surgeons, the American Medical Association, the American Industrial Hygiene Association (he was a director from 1940 to
1943) and the National Research Council.[95] Kehoe and Cholak were
consultants on the 1952 *Air Pollution Abatement Manual* of the Manufacturing Chemists' Association, a document that described air as a
"natural means of disposing of useless residues" and remarked that
scientific proof of a relation between air contaminants and damage to
health had been "elusive."[96]

Kehoe was still hard at work in the mid-1960s, when airborne
lead again became an issue, this time under the rubric of air pollution.
He could be found at a 1965 Public Health Service symposium on lead
contamination, summarizing and defending a life's work.[97] A year
later he testified before Senator Edmund Muskie. "The situation is in
no sense urgent," he replied when queried about lead contamination
of the atmosphere. When Muskie asked him to comment on the

desirability of a substitute for lead in gasoline, Kehoe avoided the question. Kehoe's three-decade-old repertoire had been fortified with a new, thirty-year Public Health Service/Kettering study of Cincinnati's air and lead pollution, which sought to demonstrate a slight decrease in airborne lead levels. Kehoe had coupled this new data with his forty-year-old emphasis on occupations. One might, he admitted, be concerned about persons who drove trucks or delivery wagons, and who therefore spent considerable time in the proximity of lead emissions. "The point with respect to human exposure," he emphasized, "is that there are really not very many people who spend much of their lifetime on a freeway."[98] Kehoe was vigilant in defense of this occupational perspective—although, as the lead-related patterns of morbidity presented in research in the 1970s were to demonstrate, even this perspective did little to advance the protection of workers from a range of lead-related occupational hazards.

The dominance of the Kettering/Kehoe perspective was a well-known fact within American medical science. At the 1965 Public Health Service symposium, Dr. Harry Heimann, a Harvard physiologist, singled out the Kettering Laboratory. "It is extremely unusual in medical research," he said, "that there is only one small group and one place in the country where research in a specific area of knowledge is exclusively done." The following year the Public Health Service finally acknowledged the heavy industry sponsorship of lead research.[99]

Kehoe did not deny it. He admitted that most of the research on lead and the environment had been financed by the manufacturers and distributors of tetraethyl lead, and that much of it had been carried out in the Kettering Laboratory and in the Department of Preventive Medicine and Industrial Health of the College of Medicine at the University of Cincinnati.[100]

The Mellon Institute

The Kettering Laboratory was unique in the breadth and depth of its influence. But there were other, similar institutions that also shaped the scientific product. The Mellon Institute was founded in 1913 with funds from Andrew W. and Richard B. Mellon, who covered the Institute's operating deficits until 1921, when the Pittsburgh-based facility became "self-supporting" through industry sponsorship. Its first interest in lead surfaced in 1925, when a Mellon Institute representative (who was also a Gulf Refining Company employee) appeared at the Surgeon General's conference on tetraethyl lead. Two years later, the Institute was incorporated for "long-range research in pure and applied science."[101]

The Institute sponsored laboratory research on its premises and also functioned as an umbrella for organizations directly involved in the politics of industrial and environmental health. In the 1950s, for example, the Institute provided office space and other facilities free of charge to the Air Pollution Control Association (APCA).[102]

The APCA dates to the Progressive Era, when it was a smoke control association with a membership of city smoke inspectors. The modern version of the association may be traced to 1936, when R. R. Sayers (responsible for the controversial early-1920s Bureau of Mines research on lead) presented a paper, "Atmospheric Pollution in American Cities," at the annual meeting in Atlanta. Although urban officials and others concerned with smoke abatement remained influential within the organization for many years, by the mid-1950s, when the Mellon Institute offered its support, the APCA was catching up with the rapidly changing science of air pollution, and its membership had come to include some 175 corporations with an interest in pollution. In the early 1960s, the Association's board of directors included technical people from Gulf Oil in Pittsburgh and National Steel Corporation in Weirton, West Virginia, a further indication that the perspective of the APCA was in transition from the urban, regulatory, public-health emphasis of the Progressive Era to a pro-business emphasis on industrial air pollution.[103]

Unlike the Air Pollution Control Association, the Industrial Hygiene Foundation (IHF) was from the beginning linked to the Mellon Institute. Originally called the Air Hygiene Foundation, it was created in 1935 in connection with the Mellon Institute around the issue of silicosis. Some twenty members included Allegheny Ludlum Steel, the Aluminum Company of America, DuPont, Owens-Illinois Glass, the Public Health Service, and the Bureau of Mines. The organization's name was changed to Industrial Hygiene Foundation in 1941. Like the APCA, this research organization was headquartered at the Mellon Institute.[104]

The IHF was described in 1947 as a national, nonprofit research organization for the "advancement of employee health in industry and the improvement of working conditions."[105] But this description conceals the extent to which the organization integrated business and science. The money for IHF programs came from business—more than 335 corporate sponsors in 1947—and the organization's board of trustees, dominated by corporate officers from American Brake Shoe

Company, U.S. Smelting, Refining & Mining Company, and Employers Mutual Liability Insurance Company, reflected these contributions.[106] The foundation's informational and research programs did not offend its business sponsors. Thus the vice-president of the Aluminum Company of America could expound upon the foundation's contributions to free enterprise. "Industry," wrote John D. Harper, "can feel justly proud of the Industrial Hygiene Foundation. It is encouraging to me that in an era when the expansive grasp of government is reaching out to regulate and control more and more phases of economic life, there is a voluntary and nongovernmental research organization to turn to on problems of environmental engineering." Andrew Fletcher, board chairman of the IHF, offered less doctrinaire praise for the foundation's efforts at the November 1955 annual meeting, applauding the organization for its role in stimulating and encouraging health maintenance in industry. Fletcher was president of the St. Joseph Lead Company.[107]

The IHF's credibility as a developer and purveyor of scientific and technical knowledge depended on its maintaining the appearance, at least, of balance and objectivity. This appearance proved not at all difficult to sustain, for the scientific community included many who agreed philosophically with the conservative ideology of the foundation or who were willing to lend their names to its endeavors. Although the board of trustees was dominated by business, it also included Philip Drinker of the Harvard School of Public Health and Dan Harrington of the Bureau of Mines.[108]

In the late 1950s and early 1960s the IHF was as dedicated as ever to a business viewpoint; yet the organization was run by a former government scientist of some reputation, H. H. Schrenk, who had been chief chemist of the Health Division of the Bureau of Mines from 1936 to 1945, and then, briefly, chief of the Environmental Division of the Public Health Service.[109] Schrenk was at once scientist, manager, and advocate of free-enterprise capitalism. He had come to the IHF because it, too, integrated these roles. In 1963 he described his impatience with those who "exaggerate and dramatize accidental occurrences and alleged injurious effects which have not been established." These "attacks" on reasonable industrial practices could be met, Schrenk believed, with "expanded research and education." Through its information services, toxicologic research, and field investigations and seminars, the IHF would contribute to "the positive side of the ledger."[110]

What did the "positive side of the ledger" mean with respect to lead poisoning? First, it meant acceptance and development of Kehoe's work on lead absorption. Schrenk and another IHF scientist agreed that lead was everywhere and that it existed in the human body without any necessarily adverse effects. Second, "the positive side" meant suspicion of "standards"—that is, standards for lead absorption in the body and environmental standards for air quality. Standards served a purpose, but they had to be measured against "the response or lack of response of the worker," and that could be established only by thorough medical surveillance. "Figures," Schrenk concluded, "are not a substitute for sound judgment." This formulation shifted responsibility for the determination of lead poisoning from a standard established by an outside agency to the medical officer in the corporation.[111] It was an argument the IHF's corporate sponsors must have found congenial.

The Lead Industries Association

On the surface, the Lead Industries Association (LIA) was a very different sort of organization from the Industrial Hygiene Foundation. It was a trade association, pure and simple, one unabashedly devoted to telling the story of lead from the perspective of the corporations that produced and used it. As a result, the LIA functioned as a public relations office. Its journal, *Lead,* ran one article after another extolling the virtues of the element. One celebrated the 130 miles of lead pipe that carried the water supply of New Bedford, Massachusetts; another praised the lead paint that protected a bridge over New York's Hudson River; a third triumphantly announced, "Use of Tetraethyl Lead Growing Rapidly."[112] For a time in the late 1930s, the Association ran a series of ads on the back of its journal in which those most likely to be victims of lead poisoning could be found lauding lead's virtues. One of these featured a lead miner, light on his cap, talking about lead paint. "I'm a miner not a painter," he said. "The metal I mine out of the earth is lead. And mister that lead is what gives life and gumption to paint. You think I'm prejudiced? Ask any person who's been at it long enough to see how his work stands weather. He'll tell you the same. . . . So some of the real good painters are boosters for white lead paint. They know that the way a white lead job stands up helps to build their reputation."[113]

On closer examination, however, the aims and methods of the

LIA appear remarkably like those of the IHF. Like the IHF, the LIA realized that the most effective defense of lead was one underpinned by science and presented as science. The Lead Institute, apparently a predecessor organization, had embarked on this course in 1925, when it gave funds to the Harvard Medical School in support of Joseph C. Aub's study of lead.[114]

Although Aub was by no means a mere functionary of the lead industry—indeed, he had spoken up against Kehoe at the 1925 Surgeon General's conference—his work ultimately proved supportive of the industry in several ways. First, while Aub did not argue that lead was present in all human tissues, he did emphasize the importance of determining lead absorption levels for people "living a usual normal life at a given time and place." This implied that a certain level of lead absorption might be "normal," if not "natural." Second, Aub provided an early statement of a notion later more fully developed by Kehoe, that the presence of lead in the excreta was less a sign of poisoning than evidence of a healthy elimination of lead. Third, he observed that much of the lead absorbed by the body was not eliminated but stored in the bones and was, in that state, "apparently harmless."[115] Decades later, Aub's work was being used to support the need for company physicians to distinguish clearly between simple lead absorption and lead intoxication, or "true lead poisoning."[116]

After the LIA was established in 1930, the Association helped finance the Kettering abstracting service and research at Children's Medical Center in Boston, the Harvard Medical School, and the University of Cincinnati.[117] Some of the Cincinnati money most likely found its way to the Kettering Laboratory and to Kehoe.

But the LIA's work did not depend on Kehoe, the Kettering Laboratory, or Aub's 1926 book, *Lead Poisoning*. Plenty of research was being done that buttressed the industry's position; the industry had only to ensure that it received a public hearing and took on an aura of objectivity. This the LIA accomplished through an ongoing series of lead conferences, the stated function of which was to "bring together the qualified minds of the country most likely to reach a consensus as to optimal measures in the prevention, the detection and the therapy of lead poisoning."[118] Invariably, the LIA gatherings assembled those whose work most clearly supported the lead industries. The University of Cincinnati/Kettering Laboratory was always well represented. Another regular speaker was Elston L. Belknap, associate professor of medicine at Marquette University and a consultant to the Globe-Union Company. Belknap could be found, like Kehoe and others, pointing out the dangers of diagnosing lead poisoning purely from laboratory tests. And Harvard's Philip Drinker was only preaching to the converted when he told a 1946 gathering that the dangers of lead paint, lead-painted toys, leaded gasoline, and lead plumbing had virtually ceased to exist, and that "lead poisoning among the population at large is rare."[119]

Ultimately, the LIA was able to wrap itself in a mantle of science not because scientists mistakenly allowed their work to be associated with a trade association, but because the typical scientific product of these years was congenial to the lead industries. From this perspective, the work of Kehoe, Cholak, Drinker, and Aub was no less scientific for having emerged from the political economy of business; it was, quite simply, the shape of science in the decades after 1920.

As was the case with the Industrial Hygiene Foundation, the leadership of the LIA perfectly represented this fusion of industry and science. For many years the association was headed by Felix E. Wormser. An executive with the St. Joseph Lead Company, Wormser had helped organize the LIA in the late 1920s, when public fear of lead poisoning ran high. His approach was pure public relations: replace the bad news with the good. In 1946, reacting to a story that had appeared in the *New York Daily News* with a photo caption "Lead Fume Victims," Wormser described his philosophy of public relations. "Unfortunately," he said, "this is not the type of publicity relished by the lead mining and fabricating industries. They do not mind reading items describing the indispensable tasks performed by lead from day to day in making civilized life comfortable, but they do object to the unfavorable publicity that lead receives occasionally when it is absolutely innocent of any wrongdoing."[120]

Yet Wormser was not just a businessman. He held a degree in mining engineering, was a fellow of the American Association for the Advancement of Science, and served as assistant secretary of the Interior for Mineral Resources under Eisenhower. He also understood that to be effective, lead's defense would have to be based on something more substantial than the unvarnished opinion of the industry that lead was safe. The position of the Association would have to be based on science.[121]

To ensure the viability of this link between the lead industry and science, Wormser's association subvened particular research projects and sponsored scientific conferences. Wormser followed the medical and scientific community closely. He knew which academic and professional committees were likely to be sympathetic to the lead industry's position, and he knew which organizations might be counted on to produce pro-industry reports. He cultivated relations with the University of Cincinnati, the Public Health Service, the American Public Health Association, the United Nations World Health Organization, and the American Medical Association through its Council on Industrial Health.[122]

Although in general the funding of public health by the 1930s was shifting from the private foundations to the federal government,[123] the experience of the Mellon Institute, the Industrial Hygiene Foundation, and the Kettering Foundation suggests that foundations and private corporate wealth maintained a strong position in lead research and policy into the 1960s. Moreover, one should not distinguish between the foundations and other forms of private support for scientific research and its dissemination. Neither the LIA nor the Mellon Institute was a foundation—nor, its name notwithstanding, was the Industrial Hygiene Foundation. Yet each understood the relationship between science and the business community, and each helped the lead industry maintain a formidable presence in the science of public health.

Medical Science and Public Health

At bottom, the failure of the "system" of knowledge occurred less because the corporate sector did what was natural and inevitable than because scientific and medical professionals that could reasonably have been expected to provide an alternative perspective did not do so. The most striking failures in this regard were those of the American Public Health Association, the American Conference of Government Hygienists, and the U.S. Public Health Service. Although one would have expected the American Public Health Association to offer a perspective distinct from the business-oriented American Association of Industrial Physicians and Surgeons (AAIPS), an organization composed largely of physicians who worked for corporations, that was not the case.

Although the Committee on Lead Poisoning of the American Public Health Association included professors, state government officials, and others not eligible for membership in the AAIPS, its ten members in 1930 included the medical director of the DuPont Company and two future directors of the AAIPS, including the ubiquitous Kehoe. The reports of the Committee on Lead Poisoning were, moreover, invariably conservative. Its 1930 report, for example, found "lead poisoning" a "rather unfortunate term" that covered "ideas of extreme distress and dramatic episodes." This report also attacked the "arbitrary rules [laid down by] governmental agencies" and emphasized the commitment of industry, especially the larger companies, to "the economic value of humanitarianism."[124] When the Association called on scientists to study methods for measuring lead content in air, it turned to Cholak and Kehoe of the Kettering Laboratory.[125]

The American Conference of Governmental Industrial Hygienists (ACGIH) performed no better as a source of critical perspectives on lead. Launched in 1938, the ACGIH was an outgrowth of training seminars in industrial hygiene financed by the 1935 Social Security Act. It functioned largely as a coordinating body for fledgling industrial hygiene agencies in the states. Among its objectives were uniform reporting of industrial hygiene activities, uniform collection of occupational disease reports, standard labeling procedures, and uniform state codes—the sorts of activities that had been commonplace within the movement for mine and industrial safety (as opposed to health) some fifty years earlier. The organization also played a major role in the development of threshold limit values. Although the ACGIH was more independent of business and the lead industries than many other organizations, it seems to have accomplished this feat by eschewing any activity—legislative advocacy, for example—that might be considered radical or pro-labor.[126]

Finally, the U.S. Public Health Service must be judged a failure in terms of providing a countervailing force to the hegemony of industry in the system of knowledge regarding lead toxicity. True, early studies of the lead trades by the Public Health Service were not uncritical of industry, but those same studies found the Service reluctant to suggest legislative remedies. Throughout its history, the Service permitted its research agenda to be set by representatives of the lead industry itself. The Service carried out its 1937–1938 study of the lead battery industry, for example, at the request of the National Battery Manufacturers' Association. The Service undertook a 1950 study of water-carrying pipes painted internally with lead for the Lead Industries Association. And apple growers initiated an inquiry by the Service into the health effects of lead-arsenic insecticides.[127]

Although in theory all these studies could have confirmed the worst fears of those who requested them, none of them did. In a conclusion not universally accepted, the Public Health Service virtually dismissed the argument that painted standpipes could affect the public health. Apples sprayed with a lead compound were similarly exonerated, and one official of the Service could be heard commenting on the "long and honorable history" of lead-containing insecticides in modern agriculture.[128] The battery industry study uncovered "no cases of plumbism severe enough to cause disability." Another controversial study, of atmospheric lead, was managed by the Service but actually conducted in cooperation with the automobile industry, fuel producers, and the Kettering Laboratory. The study concluded that levels of airborne lead in 1961 and 1962 were below those of a quarter-century earlier.[129]

Challenges to the Dominant Perspective

More than four decades after the Bayway, New Jersey tragedy caused by tetraethyl lead, Clair Patterson appeared before a 1966 Senate subcommittee. His testimony symbolized a growing appreciation within the academic scientific community of the forces that had delayed the emergence of a cautious environmental approach to lead hazards. Patterson's special contribution to this new awareness would come in locking horns with an institution that was, at least in the public mind, synonymous with scientific objectivity. "The posture of the Public Health Service," Patterson announced, "has been to defend and promote ideas that may be dangerous to the health of all Americans."[130] Patterson had singled out one agency. But, like others who testified before the subcommittee, he understood that the problem went deeper than any single institution.

Despite the dominance of the industrial perspective, dissident voices could be heard. The professional journals—the *Journal of Industrial Hygiene and Toxicology* and the *Journal of the American Medical Association,* for example—printed articles describing hazards in the lead industries in the 1930s and 1940s. May Mayers effectively used the Division of Industrial Hygiene of the New York State Department of Labor as a vehicle for her liberal views. Mayers insisted on the importance of the law in preventing occupational disease, and on the need for physicians to understand a patient's entire occupational history—rather than just the current job—when making a diagnosis.[131] From abroad came warnings that lead poisoning was present at the first pathological sign of the action of lead (1933) and that the system of tolerance values then in use allowed subliminal effects of lead, called "masked" lead poisoning (1960).[132]

But on the whole, the result of the apparatus for the control of knowledge was the suppression of genuine pluralism within the scientific community. So complete was industry domination of research into "knowledge" about the hazards of lead that the central paradigm for understanding lead and its effects remained that pioneered by Kehoe and his associates in the 1920s and 1930s. For the auto industry, the result of this hegemony was almost five decades of unrestricted use of what a corporate spokesman had referred to as the "gift of God" that was tetraethyl lead; for the untold millions who breathed its fumes, it was, of course, something else again.

Accomplishments

Despite its grave limitations, the system that developed around lead—a curious mixture of private and public, of voluntarism and law—was not without its accomplishments. Because the system had brushed aside environmental concerns, those accomplishments were entirely occupational. Major disasters of the sort that visited Bayway in 1924 did not reoccur—at least not until 1960, when eight Americans were killed while cleaning a gasoline storage tank in Japan.[133] More important, the most troubled turn-of-the-century industries—mining, smelting, refining, ceramics, and painting—were by mid-century a great deal less hazardous. Thus the struggle over OSHA's lead standard in the 1970s, described in Chapter 4, would feature debates over subclinical changes, statistics, probabilities, long-term projections, and effects on children, rather than on the poisoned adults that had been the focus of attention in the past.

Because these gains often took place beyond the purview of the state, it is exceedingly difficult to account for them. In painting, printing, and ceramics, technological developments contributed to safer workplace conditions. The Progressive-Era involvement of an investigatory public sector, led by Alice Hamilton, was another factor of importance. Although in succeeding decades the Public Health Service remained unwilling to challenge the private sector in any direct way, its reports on ceramics and other industries at least pointed out continued workplace hazards. The elimination of some of the worst lead hazards perhaps also had something to do with the presentation of the disease of plumbism; blue-lined gums and wrist drop were obvious and unavoidable symptoms of lead-related illness.

Some progress may also have occurred as the result of the establishment of workplace standards of exposure. In September 1943 a national committee of the American Standards Association (ASA) approved a standard allowable concentration of lead in the workplace. Applicable to all places of employment, the standard was 1.5 milligrams of lead for each 10 cubic meters of air. Procedures for air analysis were appended.[134]

Although adherence to the lead standard was entirely voluntary, the mere fact of its promulgation seems remarkable. How could the panoply of different interests be reconciled? How could the views of committee member Alice Hamilton be reconciled with those of fellow committee member Carey McCord, the medical advisor for Chrysler Corporation? What common ground could be found between the American Petroleum Institute, which had two members on the committee, and the several state health officials who served? Could Kehoe, whose research had underpinned the defense of tetraethyl lead, find common cause with the virtually paranoid Yandell Henderson? And why would a committee that included medical officials from General Electric, American Telephone and Telegraph, and General Motors, as well as representatives of the Manufacturing Chemists' Association and the American Association of Industrial Physicians and Surgeons, agree to any standard?

The answer to these questions has less to do with democratic compromise (business wanted a higher figure, labor a lower one) and less to do with inequitable representation (labor was not, in fact, any better represented on this committee than at the 1925 Surgeon General's conference) than with different perceptions of the function of standard setting. A certain ambivalence inhered, in fact, in the idea of a standard. The language under which the lead standard was developed charged the ASA with determining "the allowable concentration limits" of certain substances. That phrase—"allowable concentration limits"—held a paradox. It was at once restrictive ("limits") and enabling ("allowable"). Thus, while Hamilton could rejoice that manufacturers now faced a certain pressure not to pollute the workplace beyond the maximum of the standard, those same manufacturers could rest easier knowing that they had been provided with a license to continue the use of lead—to continue placing workers at risk. The standard also stood as a kind of confirmation of Kehoe's research, for both implied that a little lead—even a little lead absorbed day after day—was not necessarily harmful. Although it probably served as an incentive for a safer workplace, on balance the 1943 lead standard was a victory for the lead industries.[135]

Another possible explanation for the progress made in the lead industries is the spread of workmen's compensation systems. The states of Illinois (1921), New York (1929), and Ohio (1921) either specifically listed lead poisoning as a compensable disease or enumerated various lead trades as "dangerous" and thus injuries sustained while working at those trades as compensable.[136] In 1937 six states— Massachusetts, California, Connecticut, New York, North Dakota, and Wisconsin—left open the possibility for compensation for occupational diseases by using the word "injury" in their statutes rather than "accident." Yet the compensation statutes of fifteen states, including Pennsylvania and Michigan, contained the phrase "injury by accident" or some equivalent. Taken from the English Workmen's Compensation Law of 1897, the phrase had been interpreted by the English courts to exclude occupational diseases—specifically, lead poisoning. Sixteen other state laws expressly excluded all diseases not attributable to an injury by accident.[137] Thus, well into the century the victims of lead-related occupational disease faced obstacles to recovery that no doubt reduced the effect that compensation systems could have had in stimulating employers to create healthier workplaces. Finally, the direct state laws regulating occupational disease, despite their manifest limitations, no doubt contributed to the creation of more healthy working environments. The extent of their contribution, however, awaits detailed study at the state level.

The Politics of Confrontation

The history of lead toxicology entered a new phase in 1958 when the Ethyl Corporation, the nation's only producer of tetraethyl lead, sought the counsel of the Surgeon General on increasing the concentration of lead in gasoline in order to produce a fuel better suited to the big engines of the day. The Surgeon General appointed a committee to evaluate the health consequences of the proposed change. Composed of public health officials, state and local health and air pollution control officials, and industrial representatives, the committee advised the Surgeon General that "the proposed increase in lead apparently would pose no health hazard." The committee also asked for additional research on the health effects of atmospheric lead. In response, the Surgeon General commissioned a study of atmospheric lead in three major urban areas—Cincinnati, Philadelphia, and Los Angeles. The Tri-City study, as it was called, was conducted under the auspices of the Division of Air Pollution and actually carried out by the Public Health Service in conjunction with the auto industry, gasoline manufacturers, and the Kettering Laboratory. The study became the focus of an intensive national debate over atmospheric lead.[138]

These events signaled the end of an era in which occupational concerns had been the only focus of lead hygiene inquiries. Additional progress toward an environmental perspective occurred in 1966, when Senate hearings on air pollution moved the issue of lead hygiene into the national legislative arena for the first time in decades. Nonetheless, through the mid-1960s the problem of atmospheric lead was handled in much the same way as it had been forty years before. The new debate involved many of the same political processes and many of the same institutions—and even some of the same people—as had its earlier counterpart.

As in the 1920s, the Surgeon General and the Public Health Service were at the center of the modern inquiry. But the agency remained legally powerless. As Surgeon General William H. Stewart lamented in 1966, "the Public Health Service has never had, does not have, and in all likelihood will never have the power to directly insure a completely safe, sane, and wholesome environment for all Americans."[139] Specifically, the Surgeon General could not legally prevent the Ethyl Corporation from adding more lead to gasoline. At most, the office could create an informational and moral climate in which such an act would become unlikely.

No matter what the goal, the mechanisms for achieving it were the same as they had been in the 1920s: commission a study and call a conference. Under what one Public Health Service official described as "tremendous pressure . . . to move forward" toward a solution of a problem that industry defined as economic, the Surgeon General asked the auto industry, the gasoline producers, and the Public Health Service to conduct the urban atmospheric lead survey. Published in early 1965, the study seemed to confirm the industry's position. Of 2,300 persons studied, only 11 were found to be in ill health because of exposure to lead emissions.[140]

The December 1965 Public Health Service Symposium on Environmental Lead Contamination followed the format of its 1925 predecessor—or very nearly so. Public Health Service officials were more in evidence than they had been four decades before, but they invariably spoke for business interests. One praised the work of Kehoe and defended the use of lead-containing insecticides. Another, Herbert Stokinger, the chief of the Toxicology Section of the

Division of Occupational Health at Cincinnati, examined the Tri-City study and concluded that "exposure to air-borne lead, dust and fume is less by a factor of several magnitudes in all industrial categories since 1934." Kehoe followed Stokinger with a summary of his life's work, and Kehoe was in turn followed by the deputy director of the Kettering Laboratory. The technical director of the Ethyl Corporation made a presentation, as did a spokesman from the Universal Oil Products Company, a manufacturer of refining equipment and developer of a catalytic converter for the control of auto emissions. The American Petroleum Institute (API) also presented its points of view.[141]

This coalition of institutions appeared invincible in the early 1960s, and it remained a major influence in the politics of lead as Senator Muskie mounted his hearings on air pollution in 1966. From the API Committee for Air and Water Conservation, P. N. Gammelgard described the Institute's contracts with the Bureau of Mines and private engineering firms and interpreted the Tri-City study in a positive light. The Lead Industries Association had a spokesman in Felix Wormser, who waxed eloquent over a new study released by the United Nations World Health Organization. "I can positively assert," Wormser said, "that lead constitutes no public health hazard in America today."[142] And again, it was Kehoe whose science was the center of attention. Near the end of a long and influential career, Kehoe led the Senate subcommittee through his 1933 studies on lead absorption. He frankly and proudly described the dominance of the Kettering Laboratory, the University of Cincinnati, and the distributors and manufacturers of leaded gasoline in the science of lead absorption. He found nothing but optimism in the Tri-City study, going so far as to suggest that the 11 cases of lead poisoning represented "pure chance phenomena." In hearings that focused on the environment, Kehoe insisted on the primacy of occupation.[143] More important than the content of Kehoe's remarks, however, is the fact that Kehoe was a prominent figure at these hearings, presenting a body of scientific conclusions that had been originally published in the first year of Franklin Roosevelt's presidency.

Yet there were winds of change blowing over the nation in the early 1960s, and they did not bypass the political economy of lead hygiene. One sign of a new scientific and social climate was the publication of the Philadelphia lead-poisoning study. Carried out from 1955 to 1960, this study concluded that lead poisoning among children was most likely to be found in poor and minority areas where the housing stock was old, likely to have been painted with lead-based paint, and dilapidated, so that the lead paint was peeling and "edible." In contrast to most previous work on lead poisoning, the Philadelphia study was environmental rather than occupational in inspiration and epidemiological rather than clinical in diagnostic approach.[144] By the early 1960s the Aub interpretation of skeletal lead storage as harmless was under attack from medical scientists and others who believed that metabolic changes might release stored lead and cause poisoning. And in 1964 a British physician described for an American audience the "spectacular results of legislative interference" in Great Britain's lead industry. He insisted on the need for U.S. legislation if employers failed to move leaded workers to nontoxic jobs.[145]

This new spirit of confrontation—this new willingness to challenge the old authorities—was especially obvious by 1965 and 1966. Several aspects of the political economy of lead hygiene came under direct attack at the Public Health Service symposium. Harriet Hardy, assistant medical director in charge of occupational medical service at the Massachusetts Institute of Technology, questioned the occupational focus of previous lead hygiene efforts while imputing a kind of sexism to that occupational perspective. Calling for a new approach that involved examining special population groups such as small children and retarded children (an approach suggested by the Philadelphia study), Hardy announced that "prevention of diagnosable lead poisoning in healthy male workers is important but not enough in our society."[146] Melvin First, from Harvard's program in applied industrial hygiene, challenged Stokinger's benign interpretation of the Tri-City data. But it was Harry Heimann, a senior research associate in Harvard's Department of Physiology, who most directly challenged the old guard. "There has been no evidence that has ever come to my attention," Heimann wryly began, "that a little lead is good for you. I say this because I believe there are some persons who imply that this is so." He went on to indict the Kettering Laboratory for its exclusive control over research on lead absorption, and he implied that the Kettering/Kehoe studies on equilibrium ought either to be repeated for verification or thrown out.[147]

It was the threat of airborne lead that focused the opposition to the old guard in 1966. Leadership came, appropriately, from California, whose Los Angeles basin had for decades suffered some of the nation's worst air pollution. Clair Patterson, a geochemist from the California Institute of Technology, testified before Senator Muskie's

Subcommittee on Air and Water Pollution in June 1966. The year before, Patterson had authored an electrifying essay on "Contaminated and Natural Lead Environments of Man," only to have the article labeled "science fiction" and its author—disparagingly—a "second Rachel Carson" by the Public Health Service's Stokinger.[148]

In his testimony Patterson presented a broad critique of the science and ethics of lead hygiene as it had been practiced in the past. He labeled the Tri-City study a "whitewash" and raised the possibility that persons living near California freeways, especially children, might well be endangering their health. Far from decreasing since the mid-1930s, lead levels in American cities had, claimed Patterson, increased some one hundred times. Patterson found the Public Health Service, the California State Department of Public Health, and academics in occupational medicine and environmental health engineering guilty of failure to distinguish clearly between "typical" and "natural" concentrations of lead in food and human tissues. "On the contrary," said Patterson, these organizations "have implied in various reports and publications that typical values are natural and therefore safe and harmless." Patterson directly challenged Kehoe's analysis of the Tri-City findings and called Wormser's summary of the World Health Organization study "false and fallacious."[149]

He did not stop there. Patterson found the source of this misinformation in an unfortunate alliance between American science and "material" influences. The Department of Agriculture had been too solicitous of the apple industry in setting its limits on lead arsenic; the Public Health Service had acted inappropriately in utilizing the lead industries in carrying out the Tri-City studies. For Patterson the material world and the scientific world were not compatible. "It is not just a mistake," he told the Senate subcommittee, "for public health agencies to cooperate and collaborate with industries in investigating and deciding whether public health is endangered—it is a direct abrogation and violation of the duties and responsibilities of those public health organizations."[150]

As the 1960s ended, it was not clear whether these attacks would have permanent and meaningful consequences. The old system of reform, with its occupational focus, had handled the most obvious workplace problems while allowing the automobile industry freedom from potentially damaging environmental regulations. This approach continued to make sense for the industry. But as the significance of airborne lead became apparent, many Americans who had no interest in workplace reform became committed to regulation of airborne tetraethyl lead. This constituency, now concerned for its own health as it had not been in the controversy over emissions in 1924 and 1925, appeared to provide a source of ongoing support for efforts to eliminate lead from gasoline. Whether this new constituency would also stand up for continued improvements in the workplace, and whether it could resist the inevitable attempts to recreate the old political economy of lead, remained to be seen.

Notes

This study was undertaken while I was a participating member of The Hastings Center's Occupational Health Research Project, funded by a grant from the National Science Foundation's Program in Ethics and Values in Science and Technology. The work has benefited at every stage from the charged atmosphere of Hastings Center meetings. I am especially grateful to project members Arthur Donovan, Vilma Hunt, and Ronald Bayer for their comments on earlier drafts of this essay. I would also like to thank the Cincinnati branch of the National Institute of Occupational Safety and Health for an extensive computer search of the literature back to 1925. The computerized collection of secondary materials at the National Library of Medicine in Bethesda, Maryland, also proved invaluable. Most of the research for the study was carried out at the National Library of Medicine and the Library of Congress.

1. Vicente Navarro, "Work, Ideology, and Science: The Case of Medicine," *International Journal of Health Services* 10 (1980): 537. For a perceptive historical introduction to the problem, see David A. Hollinger, "Inquiry and Uplift: Late Nineteenth-Century American Academics and the Moral Efficacy of Scientific Practice," in Thomas L. Haskell (ed.), *The Authority of Experts: Studies in History and Theory* (Bloomington, Ind.: Indiana University Press, 1984), pp. 142–156.

2. H. A. Waldron, "Lead Poisoning in the Ancient World," *Medical History* 17 (1973): 393; Stanley M. Aronson, "Lead and the Demon Rum in Colonial America," *Rhode Island Medical Journal* 66 (January 1983): 37–38. For a good general history of lead and associated health problems, see Jacqueline K. Corn, "Historical Perspective to a Current Controversy on the Clinical Spectrum of Plumbism," *Milbank Memorial Fund Quarterly: Health and Society* 53 (Winter 1975): 93–114.

3. Josef Eisinger, "Lead and Wine: Eberhard Gockel and the *Colica Pictonum*," *Medical History* 26 (1982): 295; Alice Hamilton, *Hamilton and Hardy's Industrial Toxicology,* 49th Ed., rev. Asher J. Finkel ed. (Boston: John Wright, 1983), p. 62.

4. Carey P. McCord, "Lead and Lead Poisoning in Early America,"

Michigan Medical Center, Institute of Industrial Health, pamphlet no. 6 (Ann Arbor, Michigan, n.d.), pp. 17, 4; Aronson, "Lead and Demon Rum," p. 38.

5. Aronson, "Lead and Demon Rum," pp. 38–40; McCord, "Lead and Lead Poisoning," pp. 30–31, 5.

6. Eisinger, "Lead and Wine," pp. 300–301; Hamilton, *Industrial Toxicology,* p. 62; Ludwig Teleky, *History of Factory and Mine Hygiene* (New York: Columbia University Press, 1948), p. 52.

7. McCord, "Lead and Lead Poisoning," pp. 11–15; U.S. Department of Commerce, Bureau of Mines, "Lead Poisoning in the Mining of Lead in Utah," by Arthur L. Murray, technical paper 389 (Washington, D.C.: GPO, 1926), p. 1.

8. Hamilton, *Industrial Toxicology,* p. 64.

9. U.S. Department of Health, Education and Welfare, Public Health Service, "Symposium on Environmental Lead Contamination," 13–15 December 1965, sponsored by the Public Health Service, U.S. Public Health Service publication no. 1440 (Washington, D.C.: GPO, 1966), pp. 8, 11.

10. U.S. Public Health Service, "Lead Poisoning in the Pottery Trades," Public Health Bulletin no. 116, by Bernard J. Newman, William J. McConnell, Octavius M. Spencer, and Frank M. Phillips (Washington, D.C.: GPO, 1921), p. 13.

11. U.S. Public Health Service, "Silicosis and Lead Poisoning Among Pottery Workers," Public Health Bulletin no. 244, by Robert H. Flinn, Waldemar C. Dreessen, Thomas I. Edwards, Edward C. Riley, J. J. Bloomfield, R. R. Sayers, John F. Cadden, and S. C. Rothman (Washington, D.C.: GPO, 1939), pp. 40, 49, 54 (quotation).

12. U.S. Public Health Service, "Lead Poisoning in the Pottery Trades," pp. 54, 15, 169, 177.

13. Ibid., pp. 128, 22 (quotation).

14. Ibid., pp. 171, 173.

15. Ibid., pp. 173 (quotation), 175–178.

16. D. J. Evans and A. E. Jones, "The Development of Statutory Safeguards Against Pneumoconiosis and Lead Poisoning in the North Staffordshire Pottery Industry," *Annals of Occupational Hygiene* 17 (August 1974): 9.

17. Ibid., pp. 177, 180 (quotation); U.S. Public Health Service, "Silicosis," p. 41.

18. Ibid., p. 9; J. H. Koenig and W. H. Earhart, *Literature Abstracts of Ceramic Glazes* (Philadelphia: College Offset Press, 1951), p. 170.

19. Koenig and Earhart, *Literature Abstracts,* p. 170.

20. See *Journal of the American Ceramic Society* 4 (June 1921), pt. II: *Yearbook,* pp. 80–130.

21. J. B. Shaw, "Preparation of Glazes and Enamels," *The New Jersey Ceramist* 1 (March 1921): 52–57.

22. American Ceramic Society, *Lists of Papers and Discussions Contained in the Transactions of the American Ceramic Society, Volumes I to XVI* (*inclusive*) (Columbus, Ohio: Edward Orton, 1915); Wilton P. Rix, "Lead Fritts and Their Adaptation to Pottery Glazes," *Transactions of the American Ceramic Society* 4 (1902): 200–207.

23. See Binns's report in *Transactions of the American Ceramic Society* 7 (1905): 274; Rix, "Lead Fritts," p. 207 (quotation).

24. U.S. Public Health Service, "Lead Poisoning in the Pottery Trades," p. 180.

25. *Ceramist,* June 2, 1922, pp. 123–28; *Journal of Industrial and Engineering Chemistry* 9 (January 1917): 84–86; "The Universities and the Industries," *Journal of Industrial and Engineering Chemistry* 8 (January 1916): 59–66.

26. J. H. Koenig, "Lead Frits and Fritted Glazes," The Ohio State University, Engineering Experiment Station, Bulletin no. 95, July 1937 (Columbus, Ohio: Ohio State University, 1937).

27. Ibid., title page, pp. iii, 1, 2, inside back cover.

28. McCord, "Lead and Lead Poisoning," pp. 11–15.

29. James O. Clifford, "Industrial Lead Poisoning," *Mining and Scientific Press* 105 (6 July 1912): 10.

30. U.S. Department of Labor, Bureau of Labor Statistics, "Lead Poisoning in the Smelting and Refining of Lead," by Alice Hamilton, BLS Bulletin no. 141 (Washington, D.C.: GPO, 1914), pp. 10, 50; Bureau of Mines, "Lead Poisoning in the Mining of Lead in Utah," pp. 5–8.

31. Bureau of Labor Statistics, "Lead Poisoning in Smelting," p. 14.

32. "The Production of Lead and Spelter in 1909," *Engineering and Mining Journal* 89 (8 January 1910): 67; Clinton H. Crane, "Lead," *Engineering and Mining World* 1 (February 1930): 62–63.

33. *Mining and Scientific Press* 123 (8 October 1921): 491–92, editorial.

34. *Engineering and Mining Journal* 123 (28 May 1927): 904; *Mining and Scientific Press* 122 (29 January 1921): 162, editorial. See also "Preventing Lead Poisoning in Mining," *Engineering and Mining Journal* 123 (19 March 1927): 493.

35. Clifford, "Industrial Lead Poisoning," pp. 9, 10.

36. Wilbert S. Slemmons, "The Cause and Control of Lead Poisoning," *Mining and Scientific Press* 122 (26 March 1921): 427–429.

37. Malvern Wells Iles, *Lead-Smelting: The Construction, Equipment, and Operation of Lead Blast-Furnaces* (New York: John Wiley, 1902), pp. 139, 179–180, title page; Walter Renton Ingalls (ed.), *Lead Smelting and Refining* (New York: The Engineering and Mining Journal, 1906), pp. iii, 160–162.

38. Paul Hansen, "The Civil Engineer as Sanitarian," *Ohio State Board of Health Monthly Bulletin* 1 (July 1911): 212.

39. This model of Progressive-Era reform is used to explain the federal

government's role in eliminating the use of white phosphorus in matches in R. Alton Lee, "The Eradication of Phossy Jaw: A Unique Development of Federal Police Power," *The Historian* 29 (November 1966): 1–21.

40. See Pennsylvania, Department of Labor and Industry, *Labor Laws of Pennsylvania* (Harrisburg, Pennsylvania: William Stanley Ray, 1914), pp. 30–34; Ohio, *Revised Labor Laws of Ohio,* Columbus Edition (n.p., 1928), pp. 59, 69; Bureau of Labor Statistics, "Lead Poisoning in the Smelting and Refining of Lead," Appendix II, pp. 85–87; Barry L. Johnson and Robert W. Mason, "A Review of Public Health Regulations on Lead," paper presented at the Symposium on the Neurotoxicity of Lead, 20–22 September 1982, Chicago, Illinois; Barbara Sicherman, *Alice Hamilton: A Life in Letters* (Cambridge, Massachusetts: Harvard University Press, 1984), pp. 158, 170, 177, 179; John R. Commons and John B. Andrews, *Principles of Labor Legislation,* 4th ed., rev. (orig. 1916; New York: Harper & Brothers, 1936), pp. 189–191, 195.

41. The Society of Automotive Engineers, *Transactions* 11 (1916), pt. 1, p. 322; S. W. Sparrow and J. O. Eisinger, "Recent Cooperative Fuel Research," *SAE Transactions* 20 (1925), pt. 1, pp. 1–2; *New York World,* 3 May 1925, in Records of the United States Public Health Service, in Record Group 90, NIH Materials, box 22, file "Tetra-Ethyl Lead"; U.S. Treasury Department, Public Health Service, *Proceedings of a Conference to Determine Whether or Not There is a Public Health Question in the Manufacture, Distribution, or Use of Tetraethyl Lead Gasoline,* Public Health Bulletin no. 158 (Washington, D.C.: GPO, 1925), p. 4 (hereafter referred to as Public Health Service, Conference on Tetraethyl Lead).

The controversy over tetraethyl lead in the 1920s is traced in David Rosner and Gerald E. Markowitz, "A Gift of God? The Public Health Controversy over Leaded Gasoline During the 1920s," *American Journal of Public Health* 75 (April 1985): 344–352.

42. Public Health Service, Conference on Tetraethyl Lead, pp. 4, 5; Stuart Leslie, "Thomas Midgley and the Politics of Industrial Research," *Business History Review* 54 (Winter 1980): 482–484.

43. "Bureau's Experiments Indicate Tetra-Ethyl Lead Fairly Safe," Record Group 90, NIH Materials, box 22, file "Tetra-Ethyl Lead."

44. Frederic J. Haskin, "Is Ethyl Gas Deadly," *Washington Post,* 17 May 1925, in Record Group 90, NIH Materials, box 22, file "Tetra-Ethyl Lead"; John E. Mitchell, "Will Ethyl Gasoline Poison All of Us? Scientists Disagree," *New York World,* 3 May 1925, in Record Group 90, NIH Materials, box 22, file "Tetra-Ethyl Lead"; Joseph C. Robert, *Ethyl: A History of the Corporation and the People Who Made It* (Charlottesville, Va.: University Press of Virginia, 1983), pp. 117–119.

45. Public Health Service, Conference on Tetraethyl Lead, pp. 4–5; Haskin and Mitchell, cited n. 44; Silas Bent, "Deep Water Runs Still," *The Nation* 121 (8 July 1925): 62–64.

46. Memorandum, William Mansfield Clark to Assistant Attorney General A. M. Stimson, 11 October 1922; Stimson to R. E. Dyer, Acting Director, Hygienic Laboratory, 13 October 1922, both in Record Group 90, NIH Materials, box 22, file "Tetra-Ethyl Lead."

47. Memo to file, G. W. McCoy, 23 November 1922, in Record Group 90, NIH Materials, box 22, file "Tetra-Ethyl Lead."

48. Letter E. S. Cumming to P. S. DuPont, 20 December 1922; letter Thomas Midgley, Jr., to H. S. Cumming, 30 December 1922, in Record Group 90, NIH Materials, box 22, file "Tetra-Ethyl Lead."

49. Public Health Service, Conference on Tetraethyl Lead, p. 108.

50. Letter Surgeon General to Alice Hamilton, 14 February 1925, Record Group 90, Public Health Service, General Files 1924–1935, box 109, file "Tetra-Ethyl Lead Poison."

51. Mitchell, n. 44; letter Yandell Henderson to Mrs. Grace M. Burnham, 10 February 1925, in Record Group 90, Public Health Service, General Files 1924–1925, box 109, file "Tetra-Ethyl Lead Poison."

52. "Agreement Between the Department of the Interior and General Motors Research Corporation, Dayton, Ohio," 19 October 1925, Record Group 70, Records of the United States Bureau of Mines, National Record Center, Suitland, Maryland, 101869.725; file memo, "The Toxic Effects on Animals of Ethyl Gasoline and Its Combustion Products," n.d., Record Group 90, Public Health Service, General Files 1924–1935, box 109, file "Tetra-Ethyl Lead Poison"; William Graebner, *Coal-Mining Safety in the Progressive Period: The Political Economy of Reform* (Lexington, Ky.: University Press of Kentucky, 1976), ch. 1, 2.

53. Letter Alice Hamilton to E. S. Cumming, 12 February 1925, Record Group 90, Public Health Service, General Files 1924–1935, box 109, file "Tetra-Ethyl Lead Poison."

54. "Mines Bureau Hit By Health Service for Partial O.K. of Ethyl Gasoline," *New York World,* 3 May 1925, in Record Group 90, NIH Materials, box 22, file "Tetra-Ethyl Lead."

55. Public Health Service, Conference on Tetraethyl Lead, pp. 23–25; letter Hamilton to Cumming, 12 February 1925, cited n. 53.

56. " 'Looney Gas' Kills Fourth; 11 More Ill," dateline 29 October 1924; "Another Man Dies from Insanity Gas," *New York Times,* 20 November 1924, edition M; "Bureau's Experiments Indicate Tetra-Ethyl Lead Fairly Safe," [1924], Record Group 90, NIH Materials, box 22, file "Tetra-Ethyl Lead."

57. Willard F. Machle, "Tetra Ethyl Lead Intoxication and Poisoning by Related Compounds of Lead," *Journal of the American Medical Association* 105 (24 August 1935): 578–585, republished in a collection of the University of Cincinnati, College of Medicine, Kettering Laboratory of Applied Physiology, *Experimental Studies on Lead Absorption and Excretion* (Cincinnati, Ohio, 1936), p. 2 of Machle. This collection is hereafter referred to as Ketter-

ing Laboratory, *Experimental Studies.* See also Bent, "Deep Water Runs Still," pp. 62–64.

58. "Another Man," cited n. 56.

59. "Bureau's Experiments," cited n. 56.

60. "Mitchell," cited n. 44.

61. "Another Man," cited n. 56.

62. Letter Haven Emerson to H. S. Cumming, 9 February 1925; letters 28 and 29 November 1924, Cumming to GM, Ethyl, and others, both Record Group 90, Public Health Service, General Files 1924–1925, box 109, file "Tetra-Ethyl Lead Poison."

63. Letter Yandell Henderson to H. S. Cumming, 10 February 1925, in Record Group 90, Public Health Service, General Files 1924–1925, box 109, file "Tetra-Ethyl Lead"; "Mines Bureau Hit By Health Service," cited n. 54; Mitchell, cited n. 44 (long quotation). See also Haskin, cited n. 44.

64. U.S. Congress, Senate Committee on Public Works, "Air Pollution—1966," Hearings before a Subcommittee on Air and Water Pollution of the Committee on Public Works, on S. 3112, a bill to amend the Clean Air Act, and S. 3400, 7, 8, 9, 14, and 15 June 1966, 89th Cong., 2d Sess. (Washington, D. C.: GPO, 1966), pp. 127–128.

65. Public Health Service, Conference on Tetraethyl Lead, p. 63.

66. Ibid., pp. 30, 71, 74.

67. See David Rosner and Gerald Markowitz, "Safety and Health on the Job as a Class Issue: The Workers' Health Bureau of America in the 1920s," *Science & Society* 48 (Winter 1984–1985): 466–482.

68. Public Health Service, Conference on Tetraethyl Lead, p. 95.

69. Ibid., pp. 76–78, 83–84 (quotation p. 84), 99. Edsall and Cecil Drinker had attacked the Bureau of Mines study in the *Journal of Industrial Hygiene.* See letter Alice Hamilton to H. S. Cumming, 12 February 1925, cited n. 53.

70. Public Health Service, Conference on Tetraethyl Lead, pp. 86, 90, 101.

71. Ibid., pp. v–vii, 4–8, 11, 30, 49; Senate Committee on Public Works, "Air Pollution—1966," *Hearings,* p. 204.

72. Public Health Service, Conference on Tetraethyl Lead, pp. 106–107.

73. Ibid., 115–116.

74. Surgeon General, statement making public the report of the committee, 19 January 1926; letter, Committee to Cumming (its report), 17 January 1926, both in Record Group 90, Public Health Service, General Files 1924–1935, box 109, file "Tetra-Ethyl Lead Poison."

75. Letter Committee to Cumming, 17 January 1926, cited n. 74.

76. "Conference of Tetraethyl Lead Gasoline Committee of Experts," minutes, 22 December 1925, in Record Group 90, Public Health Service, General Files 1924–1935, box 109, file "Tetra-Ethyl Lead Poison," pp. 4–5, 8.

77. Letter committee to Cumming, 17 January 1926, cited n. 74; Alice Hamilton, *Exploring the Dangerous Trades* (Boston: Little, Brown, 1943), p. 416.

78. Surgeon General, statement 19 January 1926, cited n. 74.

79. Letter S. B. Grubbs to Surgeon J. P. Leake, 4 May 1926; letter J. P. Leake to Surgeon General, 12 March 1926, both in Record Group 90, Public Health Service, General Files 1924–1935, box 109, file "Tetra-Ethyl Lead Poison"; Senate Committee on Public Works, "Air Pollution—1966," Hearings, p. 128.

80. Senate Committee on Public Works, "Air Pollution—1966," Hearings, p. 129; letter, Cumming to David L. Edsall, 25 October 1928; C. O. Thompson, "Poison in Gasoline," 8 September 1933, statement that appeared in the Charleston, S.C., *News and Courier;* and letter G. H. Gehrmann, Medical Director, E. I. DuPont, to L. R. Thompson, Assistant Surgeon General, 29 May 1934, all in Record Group 90, Public Health Service, General Files 1924–1935, box 109, file "Tetra-Ethyl Lead Poison." The Gehrmann item is in the first file in the box, the other two in file 0875–132 General. See also E. Elbridge Morrill, Jr., "Tetraethyl Lead Poisoning Incident with Eight Deaths," *American Industrial Hygiene Association Journal* 21 (December 1960): 515–517.

81. Hamilton, *Exploring the Dangerous Trades,* p. 416.

82. Sherry Lee Baron, "Watches, Workers, and the Awakening World: A Case Study in the History of Occupational Health in America," B.A. thesis, Harvard University, December 1977, p. 63. My thanks to Vilma Hunt for bringing this essay to my attention.

83. Senate Committee on Public Works, "Air Pollution—1966," Hearings, p. 129.

84. Robert A. Kehoe and Willard F. Machle, "The Occupational Lead Exposure of Men Engaged in Mixing Tetra-ethyl Lead (Ethyl Fluid) with Gasoline," pp. 1–2, and "Regulations for Handling and Mixing of Ethyl Fluid by Means of Barrel Equipment," both in Kettering Laboratory, *Experimental Studies.*

85. Hamilton, *Exploring the Dangerous Trades,* p. 415.

86. Senate Committee on Public Works, "Air Pollution—1966," Hearings, pp. 204–208.

87. Zay Jeffries, "Charles Franklin Kettering," National Academy of Sciences, *Biographical Memoirs,* vol. 34 (New York: Columbia University Press, 1960), pp. 107–113.

88. Charles F. Kettering Foundation, *Report for 1961* (Dayton, Ohio, n.d.), pp. 1 (quotation), 3–5.

89. *Industrial Medicine* 12 (September 1943): 572; Senate Committee on Public Works, "Air Pollution—1966," Hearings, p. 204; "Symposium on Lead," *Archives of Environmental Health* 8 (February 1964): 13.

90. Willard F. Machle, "Tetra Ethyl Lead Intoxication and Poisoning by Related Compounds of Lead," *Journal of the American Medical Associa-*

tion 105 (24 August 1935): 578–585, in Kettering Laboratory, *Experimental Studies*, p. 2.

91. Robert A. Kehoe, Frederick Thamann, and Jacob Cholak, "On the Normal Absorption and Excretion of Lead," *Journal of Industrial Hygiene* 15 (September 1933): 257, 258, 271 (last quotation), reprinted in Kettering Laboratory, *Experimental Studies*. The Kehoe perspective could be interpreted as a "paradigm," in the sense in which Thomas S. Kuhn uses the word in *The Structure of Scientific Revolutions* (Chicago: University of Chicago Press, 1962).

92. Robert A. Kehoe, Frederick Thamann, and Jacob Cholak, "On the Normal Absorption and Excretion of Lead, II: Lead Absorption and Lead Excretion in Modern American Life," *Journal of Industrial Hygiene* 15 (September 1933): 282, reprinted in Kettering Laboratory, *Experimental Studies*.

93. Robert A. Kehoe, Frederick Thamann, and Jacob Cholak, "On the Normal Absorption and Excretion of Lead, III: Lead Absorption and Lead Excretion in Modern American Life," *Journal of Industrial Hygiene* 15 (September 1933): 296, reprinted in Kettering Laboratory, *Experimental Studies*.

94. Robert A. Kehoe, "Problems in Handling Ethyl Fluid and Ethyl Gasoline," *National Safety News* 29 (January 1934): 19–20, reprinted in Kettering Laboratory, *Experimental Studies*.

95. American Public Health Association, Committee on Lead Poisoning, "Lead Poisoning" (New York: American Public Health Association, 1930), pp. 29, 17, 3; American Public Health Association, Industrial Hygiene Section, "Methods for Determining Lead in Air and in Biological Materials," a report prepared by the Subcommittee on Chemical Methods of the Committee on Ventilation and Atmospheric Pollution of the Industrial Hygiene Section of the APHA, 1944 (New York: APHA, n.d.); American Standards Association, "American Standard Allowable Concentration of Lead and Certain of Its Inorganic Compounds," approved 16 September 1943 (New York: ASA, 1943); Letter G. H. Gehrmann, Medical Director, E. I. DuPont, to L. R. Thompson, Assistant Surgeon General, 29 May 1934, in Record Group 90, Public Health Service, General Files 1924–1935, first file in box; and biographical sketch in *Industrial Medicine* 12 (September 1943): 572.

96. Manufacturing Chemists' Association, Air Pollution Abatement Manual (Washington, D.C.: Manufacturing Chemists' Association, 1952) ch. 1, p. 4, and ch. 4, p. 3.

97. Public Health Service, "Symposium on Environmental Lead Contamination," 1965, pp. 155–157.

98. Senate Committee on Public Works, "Air Pollution—1966," Hearings, pp. 205 (quotation), 206, 212, 207, 216 (quotation).

99. Public Health Service, "Symposium on Environmental Lead Contamination," 1965, p. 147 (quotation); Senate Committee on Public Works, "Air Pollution—1966," Hearings, p. 130.

100. Senate Committee on Public Works, "Air Pollution—1966," Hearings, p. 207.

101. Henry B. Selleck in collaboration with Alfred H. Whittaker, *Occupational Health in America* (Detroit, Mich.: Wayne State University Press, 1962), p. 290; Public Health Service, Conference on Tetraethyl Lead; Mellon Institute, "Welcome to Mellon Institute" (Pittsburgh, 1969).

102. William G. Christy, "History of the Air Pollution Control Association," *Journal of the Air Pollution Control Association* 10 (April 1960): 135.

103. Ibid., pp. 131, 135; *Journal of the Air Pollution Control Association* 11 (June 1961): 300.

104. Ludwig Teleky, *History of Factory and Mine Hygiene* (New York: Columbia University Press, 1948), p. 92; Foreword, *Archives of Environmental Health* 6 (March 1963): 308.

105. *Occupational Medicine* 3 (March 1947): 318–319.

106. Ibid.; Industrial Hygiene Foundation, "History of Industrial Hygiene Foundation" (Pittsburgh: Mellon Institute, 1956), p. 4.

107. John D. Harper, "The Growing Importance of Industrial Hygiene," *Archives of Environmental Health* 6 (March 1963): 315; Industrial Hygiene Foundation, "History of Industrial Hygiene Foundation," p. 19.

108. *Occupational Medicine* 3 (March 1947): 318–319. Others who lent their talents and names to the IHF include Dr. A. J. Lanza, formerly medical director at Metropolitan Life, and C. O. Sappington, a past president of the American Association of Industrial Physicians and Surgeons and the medical director of Montgomery Ward & Company in the mid-1920s. See Industrial Hygiene Foundation, "History of Industrial Hygiene Foundation," p. 7, and *Industrial Medicine* 1 (November 1932): 75.

109. *Archives of Environmental Health* 6 (March 1963): 445.

110. Ibid., p. 308.

111. Robert T. P. de Treville, "Natural Occurrence of Lead," in "Symposium on Lead," *Archives of Environmental Health* 8 (February 1964): 212–221; H. H. Schrenk, "Hygienic Lead Standards," *Industrial Medicine and Surgery* 28 (March 1959): 109, 106.

112. "Lead Pipe's Great Record for New Bedford's Water Supply," *Lead* 1 (November 1930): 8; "Use of Tetraethyl Lead Growing Rapidly," Ibid.; "Lead Paints Protect Mighty Hudson River Span," *Lead* 1 (January 1931): 4.

113. *Lead* 9 (May 1939): back cover.

114. Joseph C. Aub, Lawrence T. Fairhall, A. S. Minot, and Paul Reznikoff, *Lead Poisoning* (Baltimore: William & Wilkins, 1926), p. x; Senate Committee on Public Works, "Air Pollution—1966," *Hearings,* p. 234.

115. Aub et al., *Lead Poisoning,* pp. 55 (first quotation), 42, 76 (last quotation).

116. Elston L. Belknap, "Differential Diagnosis of Lead Poisoning," *Journal of the American Medical Association* 139 (March 26, 1949): 818–819.

117. Senate Committee on Public Works, "Air Pollution—1966," Hearings, pp. 234—235.

118. *Industrial Medicine and Surgery* 28 (March 1959): 93.

119. Lead Industries Association, *Proceedings of the Lead Hygiene Conference,* Bismarck Hotel, Chicago, 15–16 November 1948 (New York: Lead Industries Association, n.d.), pp. 47–48, 53; Philip Drinker, "Public Exposure to Lead," in "Conference on Lead Poisoning," papers presented in a Conference on Lead Poisoning at the Seventh Annual Congress on Industrial Health, Boston, 30 September 1946, printed in *Occupational Medicine* 3 (February 1947): 145–149 (quotation on p. 149).

120. Felix E. Wormser, "Facts and Fallacies Concerning Exposure to Lead," in "Conference on Lead Poisoning," 1946, p. 135.

121. Senate Committee on Public Works, "Air Pollution—1966," Hearings, p. 233.

122. Ibid., p. 238; Wormser, "Facts and Fallacies," p. 138; Lead Industries Association, *Proceedings of the Lead Hygiene Conference,* 1948, p. 8.

123. George Rosen, "Patterns of Health Research in the United States, 1900–1960," *Bulletin of the History of Medicine* 39 (May/June 1965): 201–221. See also Richard H. Shryock, *American Medical Research: Past and Present* (New York: The Commonwealth Fund, 1947), esp. pp. 98–102.

124. APHA, Committee on Lead Poisoning, "Lead Poisoning," 1930, pp. 5, 29 (quotations).

125. APHA, Industrial Hygiene Section, "Methods for Determining Lead," p. 1, cited n. 95.

126. John J. Bloomfield, "What the ACGIH Has Done for Industrial Hygiene," *Annals of the American Conference of Industrial Hygiene* 9 (1984): 3–9; William G. Fredrick, "The Birth of the ACGIH Threshold Limit Values Committee and Its Influence on the Development of Industrial Hygiene," *Annals* 9 (1984): 11–13; Morton Lippmann, "ACGIH: Its Background, Membership, and Activities," *Annals* 5 (1983): 5–11; Jacqueline K. Corn, "Historical Review of Industrial Hygiene," *Annals* 5 (1983): 13–17. My thanks to Morton Corn for directing me to these materials.

128. Public Health Service, "The Control of the Lead Hazard in the Storage Battery Industry," from the Division of Industrial Hygiene, National Institute of Health, Public Health Bulletin no. 262, by Waldemar C. Dreessen, Thomas I. Edwards, Warren H. Reinhart, Richard T. Page, Stewart H. Webster, David W. Armstrong, and R. R. Sayers (Washington, D.C.: GPO, 1941), p. 1; Hervey B. Elkins, "The Lead Content of Water from Red-Lead Painted Tanks," *Industrial Medicine and Surgery* 28 (March 1959): 112; Lead Industries Association, *Proceedings of the Lead Hygiene Conference,* 1948, p. 7. At least one study was done for a trade union.

128. Elkins, "Lead Content," pp. 114–115; Public Health Service, "Symposium on Environmental Lead Contamination," p. 19.

129. Public Health Service, "Control of Lead Hazard," pp. vii, 124 (on the storage battery industry); Public Health Service, "Symposium on Environmental Lead Contamination," pp. 30–31; Senate Committee on Public Works, "Air Pollution—1966," Hearings, pp. 130–131.

130. Senate Committee on Public Works, "Air Pollution—1966," Hear-

ings, pp. 312–313. The enigmatic role of the Public Health Service in the area of asbestos-related illness is described in Paul Brodeur, *Expendable Americans* (New York: Viking, 1973), pp. 18–28.

131. May Mayers and M. N. McMahon, "Lead Poisoning in Industry and Its Prevention," New York State Department of Labor, Division of Industrial Hygiene, Special Bulletin no. 195 (1938), abstracted in NIOSH computer survey, described in material preceding n. 1; M. R. Mayers, "Occupational Disease Diagnosis," *New York State Journal of Medicine* 52 (1952): 2381–2385, abstracted in NIOSH computer survey.

132. C. Badham, "Basophilia and Lead Excretion in Lead Poisoning," *Medical Journal of Australia,* 16 December 1933, pp. 816–821, abstracted in NIOSH computer survey; D. Stofen, "The Prevention of Hazards Associated with Lead Additives in Petrol—Criteria and Consequences," *Stadtehygiene* 21 (1960); 94–97, abstracted in NIOSH computer survey. See also Harriet L. Hardy, *Challenging Man-Made Disease: The Memoirs of Harriet L. Hardy, M.D.* (New York: Praeger, 1983), pp. 116–124.

133. Morrill, "Tetraethyl Lead Poisoning Incident," 515–517.

134. American Standards Association, "Allowable Concentration of Lead," p. 5, cited n. 95. The American Conference of Governmental Industrial Hygienists created its own set of standards during the war years, through its Committee on Technical Standards. See Fredrick, "Birth of ACGIH Threshold Limit Values Committee," n. 126.

135. Public Health Service, "Control of Lead Hazard," pp. 124–125.

136. "History of Occupational Disease Legislation in Illinois with a Review of Leading Cases," *John Marshall Law Quarterly* 3 (1937–1938): 240–257; "Workmen's Compensation—Injury Arising Out of the Employment—Occupational Disease," *Oregon Law Review* 16 (1937): 84–91; George E. Beers, "Compensation of Occupational Diseases," *Yale Law Journal* 37 (1927–1929): 579–594. Other sources on lead legislation include Johnson and Mason, "A Review of Public Health Regulations on Lead," weak on early state regulations; *Revised Labor Laws,* pp. 59, 61, 69; Bureau of Labor Statistics, "Lead Poisoning in the Smelting and Refining of Lead," Appendix II; and Pennsylvania Department of Labor and Industry, "Labor Laws of Pennsylvania," pp. 30–34, all cited n. 40. See also American Association for Labor Legislation, "Prevention of Occupational Diseases with Special Reference to Lead Poisoning," leaflet no. 9 (n.p., [1912]); International Association for Labour Legislation, British Section, *The World's Labour Laws* 3 (August 1913): 22–29.

137. William W. Rabinowitz, "Compensation of Occupational Diseases from a Legal Viewpoint," *Wisconsin Law Review* 12 (1936–37): 198–218.

138. Senate Committee on Public Works, "Air Pollution—1966," Hearings, pp. 129–131 (quotation p. 129).

139. Ibid., p. 155.

140. Ibid., pp. 130 (quotation), 131. See also Corn, "Historical Perspective," pp. 104–105.

141. Public Health Service, "Symposium on Environmental Lead Contamination," 1965, pp. 18–19, 31 (quotation), 51–62, 123ff.

142. Senate Committee on Public Works, "Air Pollution—1966," Hearings, pp. 246–248, 238, 239 (quotation).

143. Ibid., pp. 222, 212, 207–208, 216.

144. Theodore H. Ingalls, Emil A. Tiboni, and Milton Werrin, "Lead Poisoning in Philadelphia, 1955–1960," *Archives of Environmental Health* 3 (November 1961): 577–579.

145. Ethel Browning, "The Latent Period in Industrial Disease," *The Transactions of the Association of Industrial Medical Officers* 11 (January 1962): 161–163; Ronald E. Lane, "Health Control in Inorganic Lead Industries," in "Symposium on Lead," *Archives of Environmental Health* 8 (February 1964): 250.

146. Public Health Service, "Symposium on Environmental Lead Contamination," 1965, p. 80.

147. Ibid., pp. 91 (First), 147 (Heimann), 155–157 (Kehoe).

148. Senate Committee on Public Works, "Air Pollution—1966," Hearings, pp. 318–319.

149. Ibid., pp. 32 (quotation), 314, 313 (quotation), 312, 322 (quotation).

150. Ibid., pp. 324, 313, 315 (quotation).

2

Health and Safety in Underground Coal Mining, 1900–1969: Professional Conduct in a Peripheral Industry

ARTHUR L. DONOVAN

Everyone seriously concerned with problems of occupational health and safety agrees that underground coal mining is an industry that commands attention. The dangers associated with underground mining, the size and importance of the coal industry, and its dolorous record of death and disablement are too well-known to require additional demonstration. Health and safety problems are therefore matters of inescapable and pressing concern to all those associated with coal mining. But the industry's response to these problems has by and large been informed by a strategy that is quite different from that followed by modern science-based professionals in their campaigns to reduce the health and safety risks of industrial labor. This chapter examines the perceptions and modes of understanding that gave rise to and continue to sustain these distinct and in many ways opposed strategies of reform.

The examination of these two strategies of reform is more than an exercise in abstract comparison. The coal industry, an enterprise that both makes use of and supplies energy for a wide range of industrial technologies, employs thousands of highly trained individuals, people whose expertise and sense of professionalism is based on their command of scientific and technical knowledge. As employees working in and for the coal industry, these technically informed specialists are obliged to respond to the industry's health and safety problems in ways that accord with the industry's strategy for dealing with these problems. But because they are professionals as well as employees, we expect these specialists to bring to their engagements with the industry's problems certain modes of analysis and levels of concern that may not be strongly represented elsewhere in the industry. And because we think of the engineers, scientists, and physicians who serve the industry as working in a state of tension created by the differences between the values of the industry and the values of professionalism, we expect that their historical experiences in the industry will reveal how these two sets of values have been reconciled in practice.

This is not an unreasonable expectation; nonetheless, a reading of this particular history in fact teaches quite a different lesson. The first task facing those who believe that professional values have a bearing on the conduct of professionals in industry is to reexamine how they define professionalism and how they conceptualize relations between professionals and the institutions they serve. Although many individuals who consider themselves professionals have worked in the coal industry, they have experienced little of the conflict of values anticipated by those professionals who contemplate the problems of the industry from afar. Thus, although conceptually the conflict between industrial values and professional values remains, historically those employees of the coal industry who would normally be classed as professionals have largely conformed to the industry's view of how one should respond to health and safety problems. This finding appears to render problematic the historical utility of the received notion of professionalism.

The period examined in this chapter runs from 1900 to 1969. The beginning date can be taken as representing the point at which bituminous coal displaced anthracite as the dominant source of industrial energy in the United States; the closing date is the year in which the industry's responsibility for health and safety problems was redefined by the passage of landmark federal legislation. The first section contains an historical account of the concerns and values that dominated the industry during this period. The industry can be characterized as peripheral not because it was unimportant, which was certainly not the case, but because in its technical and organizational structure it remained marginal within the larger world of American business. Dispersed, unconsolidated, intensely competitive, and trapped in a boom-and-bust cycle, the coal industry remained institutionally backward while those industries which occupied the center of the American economy found ways to eliminate crippling structural liabilities. And it was the institutional structure of the coal industry that gave rise to and sustained the social values that have long been associated with this especially unenlightened sector of the American economy.

The second, third, and fourth sections offer brief descriptions of the settings in which engineers, scientists, and physicians connected with the coal industry worked. In practice these professionals were well integrated into the industry and had little reason or inclination to feel that a serious conflict in values existed between their responsibilities as professionals and the ways in which they served the industry. These accounts are not meant to convey moral judgments of the conduct of those who worked in the coal industry. Historians have no warrant for doing so, and introducing an external ethical standard would only undermine the attempt to characterize the contexts within which the individuals in question worked. Nor does this chapter represent an attempt to assess the various justifications that were and still are offered for actions taken by those working in the coal industry, for they too lie outside the concerns of this chapter.

This chapter will have served its main purpose if, by providing an historical account of the institutional structure of the coal industry, it renders more intelligible the social attitudes of those involved with underground coal mining and if, by describing the contexts within which members of certain professions served the industry, it makes more intelligible as well their attitudes and actions as practitioners. A related aim, as indicated earlier, is to question the received definition of what it means to be a professional, and the final section suggests one way in which that definition might be reconceptualized.

It is especially important that we come to realize that certain assumptions about how professionals interact with the larger world are radically at odds with the historical experience of the coal industry. Consider, for instance, the common assumption that the proper way for science-based professionals to engage problems of occupational health and safety is to discover causes and control their effects. This image of the autonomous professional improving the lot of working people by using scientific methods to analyze and alter physical circumstances is highly appealing to certain social reformers, but it hardly accords with the ways in which engineers, scientists, and physicians have actually engaged the health and safety problems of underground coal mining. Rather than a "discover and control" model of professional intervention, it would be more accurate in the coal industry to speak of a "disaster and response" model. This latter model, while less flattering to professionals who pride themselves on the predictive and beneficial powers of their cognitive resources, is more descriptive of the way the coal industry and the professionals who work in it have come to grips with the very difficult and all too frequently disastrous health and safety problems of underground mining.

Coal Mining as a Peripheral Industry

It may seem odd, given coal's importance in the industrialization of America, to call coal mining a peripheral industry, and yet there is a sense in which the term is appropriate. The context in which such a characterization is justified is not that defined by aggregate economic parameters such as percentage of the energy market supplied, total labor force, and value of total sales; it is rather the evolving institutional structure of American industry. To understand in what way the coal industry was and in many ways still is peripheral, one must compare its institutional history to that of the more advanced sectors of American industry. Such a comparison can be undertaken with some confidence by making use of the historical analysis that informs Alfred D. Chandler, Jr.'s magisterial *The Visible Hand—The Managerial Revolution in American Business.*[1]

Chandler presents his history of "the rise of modern business enterprise and the brand of managerial capitalism that accompanied it" as a contribution to the "new institutionalism" that in recent years has emerged as a major theme in American history.[2] He concentrates on the years between the 1840s and the 1920s and describes how the modern multiunit business enterprise replaced smaller traditional businesses by creating forms of administrative coordination that made possible greater productivity, lower costs, and higher profits than could be realized by coordination through market mechanisms. The institutional revolution he describes was achieved in three stages. The first involved a revolution in transportation and communication, with the railroads emerging in the 1850s and 1860s as the first modern business enterprises. The second phase saw revolutions in distribution and production with the creation of mass marketing and mass production. The third phase involved the combination of mass production and mass distribution, a fusion carried out by the modern, vertically integrated industrial corporations that established control over major sectors of the economy and have subsequently grown into multinational enterprises. Chandler tells his story with verve, and his subject is obviously one of surpassing importance.

As Chandler makes clear, not all commercial enterprises evolved into modern businesses. Coal mining was one of those enterprises which did not; and so by the mid-1920s, because the traditional structure of the coal industry had not changed dramatically, that industry then appeared institutionally backward when compared to more advanced enterprises. This was so even though coal production and employment increased tremendously up until the end of World War I.[3] By the mid-1920s, however, the coal industry was experiencing the kind of depression the rest of the country would know in the 1930s, and most observers agreed that the industry had become "sick." Although this medical analogy was not especially informative, the specific cause of the industry's ills was widely and correctly perceived to be excess capacity—"too many mines and too many miners." What was lacking, therefore, was not an understanding of the industry's problems but rather a willingness to prescribe a course of treatment that would either eliminate the cause of illness or mitigate its more dire effects. Explaining the failure to modernize the industry when its institutional backwardness was beyond dispute therefore stands as the central problem in the history of the American coal industry. It is also a question of general interest as well, for it reveals a great deal about who won and who lost during the triumphal era of American business.[4]

Before addressing this problem, however, we need to understand why the coal industry did not evolve into a modern business enterprise during the era in which it served as the preeminent source of energy for American industry. As Chandler points out, traditional businesses depended on the market for coordination of the supply of raw materials, integration of production, and distribution of the goods produced. The allocating and coordinating function of the market is nicely described by Adam Smith's enduring image of the "invisible hand," but merchants and manufacturers knew from experience that when performing these functions, the market frequently operates inefficiently and ineffectively. They therefore sought to minimize their exposure to what Joseph Schumpeter later called the "creative destruction" of capitalism by internalizing within their enterprises as many of the market functions as possible. This could be done in a variety of ways, but not all strategic options were equally available to all industries. The railroads were able to gain and exercise administrative control over rail traffic by making use of the possibilities presented by new technologies of transportation and communication, new financial arrangements, and new hierarchical organizations of management. The pioneers of modern enterprise used these means to establish extensive rail networks that provided high-volume, high-speed transportation at relatively low cost. As rail traffic was brought under the control of monopolies and oligopolies, the market played less and less of a role in transportation. The allocation and coordination of traffic was internalized and subjected to administrative control; the "visible hand" of management displaced the invisible hand of the market.

During the nineteenth century the coal industry, like commercial agriculture, was denied relief from the rigors of unfettered competition by a variety of circumstances. Although the United States' deposits of minable anthracite coal are confined to a relatively restricted region in northeastern Pennsylvania, bituminous coal, which claimed an ever-increasing share of the coal market as the rail network expanded, occurs in minable formations in many parts of the country; this fact made it practically impossible to control the amounts of coal brought to market by limiting access to the natural resource. Coal mining also was until recently a low-technology and low-cost-of-entry industry, and these features made it difficult to limit the amount of coal brought to market by restricting access to the technology needed to mine it or to the capital required to open a mine. Because the coal industry lacked the physical and technical characteristics needed to restructure itself so as to avoid the frequently destructive effects of market coordination, it continued to be plagued by excess capacity, intense competition, low wages and profits, and a boom-and-bust cycle of production. When all businesses suffered together, such hardships could be tolerated. But when some enterprises, such as the railroads, found means to avoid the harsh discipline of the market, and especially when these consolidated enterprises used their new-found power to exploit such traditional producers as coal miners and farmers who were dependent upon their services, such conditions appeared intolerable. But as an institution the coal industry was simply incapable of modernizing itself in a way that would remedy its many problems, among which were those of health and safety.

The advent of mass production brought no relief. Although the coal industry produces in high volume and employs masses of workers, it lacks certain key attributes that enabled selected other industries, such as the automobile industry and the petroleum industry, to develop new techniques of mass production during the early years of

the twentieth century and thereby restrict their exposure to the inefficiencies of the competitive market. Chandler characterizes modern
mass production in terms of the new technologies employed and the
organization of production. Technologically, mass production was
achieved by "the development of more efficient machinery and equipment, the use of higher quality raw materials, and an intensified
application of energy." Organizationally, mass production involved
"improved design of manufacturing or processing plants and innovations in managerial practices and procedures required to synchronize
flows and supervise the workforce." When brought together in a
single industry, these innovations resulted in "a sharp decrease in the
number of workers required to produce a specific unit of output."
The industries that successfully made the transition to mass production had the common characteristics of being "capital-intensive,
energy-intensive, and manager-intensive."[5]
    Mining was not one of the industries that made this transition.
As Chandler explains,

> the working of mines involved little more than having small teams of
> men doing much the same thing in different parts of the mine. Until the
> twentieth century the workers . . . relied largely on hand tools. Here, as
> in agriculture, there was little opportunity to speed up the processes of
> production by more intense application of energy. There was little need
> to build a complex organization to coordinate the flow of goods from
> one process to another. These industries long remained labor-
> intensive.[6]

    The coal industry was therefore obliged to stand aside during the
second phase of the managerial revolution in American business, as it
had during the first phase as well. Not having reconstructed itself as a
mass production industry, it slipped even further into institutional
marginality and backwardness. As long as the demand for coal continued to grow, the structural problems of the industry could be ignored,
especially while the high wages and prices paid during World War I
cast an aura of robust health over the industry. But by the mid-1920s
the consequences of the coal industry's failure to achieve consolidation could no longer be denied. The only question, then, was how to
find a socially acceptable way to preserve an economically essential
industry that had remained structurally unchanged as new forms of
industrial enterprise had evolved around it.
    Two strategies were considered.[7] The option favored by the coal

operators and by John L. Lewis, who in 1920 began a 40-year reign as president of the United Mine Workers of America (UMWA), called upon the coal industry to reconstruct itself through mechanization. Another option, occasionally but always timorously advanced by federal and state commissions created to examine this "sick" industry, was to relieve the industry's problems by adapting federal regulations so as to shield the industry from the most destructive aspects of the market. The institutional history of the coal industry from the 1920s through the 1960s was shaped by those two strategies, even though neither of them succeeded in moving the coal industry from the periphery to the center of corporate life in America.

So far, this chapter has used "the coal industry" taxonomically, in the same sense in which a natural historian refers to genera of animals or species of plants. The industry was in fact composed of numerous geographically dispersed individual companies, most of them quite small; and although they shared many characteristics, they were not united by allegiance to any overarching institution, as would have been the case had they been owned by a single holding company or governed by a powerful industrial council. The owners and operators of coal mines therefore lacked the institutional cohesion needed to act in concert so as to fulfill agreed-upon goals, and it was precisely this lack of collective control over their own destinies that exposed the individual members of the coal industry to the rigors of an over-supplied market. But within the industry there was one institution that spoke for at least one segment of the entire industry, and that was the UMWA. Founded in 1890 and dedicated to the ideals of business unionism, the UMWA claimed to represent all coal miners and consistently sought to bring all miners under a national contract. And while the UMWA leaders had no desire to operate the mines, they did feel compelled to point out what needed to be done within the industry so that miners could be paid a decent wage. This is what John L. Lewis did in 1925 when he published *The Miners Fight for American Standards*.[8]

The American standards for which Lewis said the miners were fighting were the wage levels being paid in those industries which, by mastering the techniques of mechanization, had created "the new industrialism" of the first quarter of the twentieth century. However, until production was coordinated with demand and productivity was raised through mechanization, coal companies could not afford to pay miners according to the new American standard. It was management's job to bring the industry under economic control, yet Lewis realized that without some outside pressure, the coal operators were incapable of doing what needed to be done. He therefore pledged union support for mechanization, a pledge he stood by throughout his career, and committed the union to do all it could to encourage the rationalization of the industry. As he said in his book,

> in insisting on the maintenance of an American wage standard in the coal fields the United Mine Workers is . . . doing its part, probably more than its part, to force a reorganization of the basic industry of the country upon scientific and efficient lines. The maintenance of these [wage] rates will accelerate the operation of natural economic laws, which will in time eliminate uneconomic mines, obsolete equipment and incompetent management.[9]

What assumptions were implicit in this strategy? One was that the union, by insisting on a national contract, could force the industry to modernize in ways that it was incapable of achieving on its own. Coal operators and coal engineers were well aware of the many advantages of mechanization, and they were constantly exhorting one another to turn the mines into factories underground. Not only would such a development increase the productivity of each worker and thus reduce labor costs and increase profits, but it would also enable the operators to "deskill" coal mining and get rid of the independent-minded hand miners.

But the mechanization of underground mining has proved to be a difficult task, one that has still been only partially achieved. A coal mine differs from a factory in that neither the raw material, the workplace, nor the routine of production can be completely subordinated to engineering specifications. It is possible, of course, to force the pace of technological change in coal mining, as did the health and safety legislation of 1969, and this is clearly what Lewis expected a national labor contract requiring high wages would do. But there are technical and economic limits to the extent to which the rate and direction of technological change can be forced, and mechanization of the coal industry has in fact turned out to be a much more difficult undertaking than either Lewis or the coal operators appear to have anticipated. We should not, however, assume that their dreams of mechanization were based entirely on rational assessments of the task itself. Surely they knew that had it not been such a daunting technical undertaking, the coal industry would have transformed itself into a mass production industry on the Chandler model without being forced to do so. Lewis's assumption that the union could force the industry to do what it had not done on its own therefore appears on close examination to be more an ideologically constrained hope than an objectively and pragmatically determined policy.

Another basic assumption in Lewis's strategy was that the industry—that is, the operators and miners—could salvage the coal industry within the existing political context without federal intervention. Anyone familiar with John L. Lewis's career knows how effectively he used a variety of federal agents and agencies to consolidate his control of the UMWA and gain a better deal for coal miners; but throughout his presidency of the union, which ended in 1960, and indeed throughout his life, which ended nine years later, he remained convinced that management should be left in the hands of managers.[10] He believed the government should protect the rights of workers, just as it protects the property rights of owners, but that it should not play a role in the operations of the industry. As Curtis Seltzer has put it, "Lewis and the industry feared government more than they feared each other."[11]

A third assumption, closely allied with the second, was that all the problems associated with coal mining are fundamentally economic. Lewis understood that mechanization would lead to a tremendous reduction in the number of miners, but he accepted this consequence as an inevitable trade-off for bringing the wages of those still employed in the industry up to acceptable levels. He felt confident that once the industry was economically healthy, the union would be able to gain through contract negotiation the authority within the workplace and the funds needed to make mining an adequately safe and healthy activity. He also believed that only those in the industry could address the problems of the industry and that those problems could not be resolved until the industry itself had been placed on a firm economic footing. And at this point the circle of assumptions closed, for he believed that mechanization provided the key to the future economic health of the coal industry.

Underground coal mining has indeed become more mechanized since 1925, but the pace of change has been governed more by technical and economic factors than by union pressure or managerial strategy. The introduction of mechanical coal-loading equipment in the 1930s and of continuous mining machinery in the late 1940s resulted in steady increases in productivity. The rapid decline in the demand for coal following the end of World War II, when combined with these gains in productivity, then led to a rapid reduction of employment in the coal industry, known as "the great shakeout." The social consequences of these changes were dramatic and appalling, as John Kennedy discovered when he campaigned in West Virginia in 1960.[12]

By 1950 it appeared that Lewis's strategy was succeeding. Changes in the technology of underground coal mining and in the market for coal, which had become more concentrated as large electric power plants began taking an increasing share of the coal produced, finally convinced the operators that they should meet Lewis on his own ground. They therefore formed an industry-wide association, the Bituminous Coal Operators' Association (BCOA), to represent management in negotiations with the UMWA. Organized and headed by George Love, president of Pittsburgh Consolidation Coal Company, the nation's largest, the BCOA was designed to be the operators' counterpart to the union. Its job was to organize and discipline the coal operators as Lewis had organized and disciplined the miners. Lewis, not surprisingly, took full credit for these developments, saying in 1952 that

> the American coal operators never could have mechanized their mines and increased per-man-day productivity unless they were compelled to do so by the pressure of the organization of the mineworkers. . . . We want participation. We ask for it. We ask for it . . . to compel him to modernize. Otherwise, he wouldn't move.[13]

Whether Lewis's crowing should be accepted as history is another question. While it now appears that the formation of the BCOA marks a turning point in the history of the industry, one need not accept that it was union pressure that finally brought about the kind of institutional concentration that at last enabled the coal industry to begin internalizing and administratively controlling the allocation of resources and the coordination of production and marketing. If in fact underground coal mining is at last being transformed by a long-delayed "Chandlerian" revolution—and the transformation has to date been only partially realized—it is primarily because coal mining's means of production and its markets have changed in ways that now allow us to conceive of the industry as capital intensive, energy intensive, and manager intensive.[14] We can now see that Lewis's strategy for salvaging the coal industry contained several serious flaws and inadequacies. (We need not linger over the effects of his presidency upon the internal governance of the UMWA, a subject that does not directly impinge upon either Chandler's analysis of the evolution of American management or the account developed here.) In any case, the reconstruction of the UMWA following Lewis's departure, and the defeat of his chosen successor, did not begin in earnest until 1970. Historically, however, it is indisputable that Lewis was never able to exercise effective control over the production of coal by bringing all miners under a single national contract, and as long as this goal eluded him, he could not force mechanization and eliminate marginal producers by requiring all operators to pay high wages. One may regret this failure, even if it seems inevitable given the technological and geographical characteristics of the coal industry, but one should not ignore it when evaluating the degree to which a single labor organization was capable of altering the structure of an entire industry.

From the point of view of worker's rights and welfare, Lewis's strategy made the improvement of health, safety, and community life entirely dependent on the coal companies' ability to fund such improvements. He believed that mine safety was a management responsibility and that miners should have the right, guaranteed by contract, to stop work and leave a mine they considered unsafe. But safety costs money, and as long as the union was unable to close down marginal operations that scrimped on safety, Lewis could not mount a vigorous and effective safety campaign. Health programs cost money too, especially those designed to reduce worker exposure to potentially damaging conditions. Lewis in fact never made the prevention of occupational diseases an issue, and it is easy to see why. But immediately after World War II he did force the industry to finance a health care program that was for many years a model for the nation and that succeeded in providing vastly improved health care for miners and their families. Yet this program too was vulnerable to being undermined by competition from nonunionized mines.

Lewis's insistence that the operators and miners manage their own affairs without outside interference not only excluded the participation of independent experts (except for those retained by one side or the other), but also delayed until 1969 the use of the power of the federal government to ensure that consideration of health and safety issues was not held hostage to the corporate structure of the industry. Lewis knew that the industry was peripheral in institutional terms, and he had a clear strategy for modernizing it; but given the ineffectiveness of that strategy and the many decades it has taken the industry to modernize through technological and organizational evolution, it is now clear that with regard to health and safety, Lewis's strategy was in fact one that prolonged the agony of the miners he meant to serve. Indeed, it seems fair to conclude that his entire career as a labor leader, like his strategy for the modernization of the coal industry, was more constrained by ideology than guided by practicality.

The alternative to Lewis's strategy of mechanization was to utilize the regulatory power of the federal government to cure the coal industry. During the 1920s and throughout the New Deal there were many attempts to use the means available to federal regulators to get the coal industry back on its feet, none of which were notably successful or long lived. But like Lewis's strategy of mechanization, these attempts to regulate the industry back to health are revealing, for they tell us a good deal about the ways in which industries have been regulated in the United States and the limits imposed on the uses of this remedy.

It will be helpful at the outset to distinguish between prescriptive regulation and proscriptive regulation. The first establishes standards of performance that must be met in the activity being regulated; an example in the coal industry would be regulations stipulating that in working mines the concentration of methane gas is not to exceed a certain level and that gas levels are to be monitored in a certain manner. A proscriptive regulation prohibits certain activities; an example of relevance to the coal industry is a regulation stipulating that coal operators are not to engage in business practices that restrain trade and elevate the price of coal. As these examples suggest, in the coal industry prescriptive regulation has normally been concerned with safety, whereas proscriptive regulation has been concerned with business practices. Historically, the federal government has been extraordinarily reluctant to impose prescriptive regulation upon the coal industry, but through the courts the government has vigorously upheld the proscriptive regulations of the antitrust laws. The two forms of regulation therefore must be examined separately.

The coal industry, like other forms of production and commerce that flourished prior to the Civil War, was organized into several state industries long before it became a national industry. Regulation of the industry therefore lay originally with the separate states and remained a state responsibility long after the industry had become national in scope. States with significant mining activity acknowledged their responsibilities in this regard by passing legislation that prescribed certain standards and practices designed to ensure the safety of underground mining. Compliance with such legislation was seldom

rigorously enforced, the expectation usually being that the mine foreman would ensure that the safety code was followed. Such a system
was obviously less than adequate for a national industry, and the
dolorous record of fatalities—according to one calculation, between
1839 and 1977 121,209 men died in the mines—is stark testimony to
its failure as a method for managing the safety problems of this particular industry.[15] And yet the reluctance to pass and enforce effective
safety legislation is quite understandable, if hardly excusable. Prescriptive regulation legally mandates expenditures of capital and labor that do not contribute to productivity. As long as profits and
market shares remained marginal and insecure, operators had a
strong inducement to minimize such expenditures. Because different
states stipulated and enforced different safety codes, competition
tended to force down the demand for and effectiveness of prescriptive
safety regulation.[16]

The federal government had good reason to avoid becoming
involved in prescriptive safety regulation. As with wage rates, the
establishment of national standards would in theory have stabilized
safety costs, but since mines differ greatly in the hazards they pose,
the actual effect would have been a significant restructuring of the
industry. A more important historical factor was the absence of a
powerful group within the industry that favored federal intervention.
The operators of locally and regionally based coal companies certainly did not want the federal government inspecting their mines,
and the UMWA argued that the best way to achieve safety in the
mines was through union recognition and the establishment of safety
committees with contractually guaranteed rights. It is true that during
the 1930s Lewis called upon the federal government, then preoccupied with reviving American industry, to strengthen federal laws and
enforcement procedures pertaining to mine safety. His efforts were
unavailing, however, for the federal officials involved considered
safety regulation to be a state function. Yet Lewis persisted even
when he knew no response would be forthcoming, his purpose being
to speak out on safety issues so as to build up a record that would
protect him from rank-and-file wrath on this front.[17]

As long as the coal industry remained unconsolidated, establishing effective federal regulation for safety and health appeared too
daunting a task to even consider. Big government could deal effectively only with big business and big labor, so once again action
designed to remedy the ills of the coal industry was made to wait on
institutional reconstruction. President Harry Truman rightly de-

nounced as a "sham" the federal safety bill he signed into law in 1952. The federal standards it contained applied only to mines employing fifteen or more workers, thereby exempting the small mines that were frequently the most dangerous, and it still left primary responsibility for safety with the states and contained no effective enforcement procedures.[18] Later in the decade, however, the big operators, acting through the BCOA, began cooperating with Lewis in using the safety issue to work toward their common goal of industrial concentration. Together they agitated for a stricter mine safety law, but as Lewis's biographers observe, "here was a classic case of 'corporate liberalism,' for although the overt purpose of the law was to save miners' lives, the covert aim was to force small companies out of business by imposing on them the same expensive safety standards required of larger producers."[19] Following another decade of "study," and then only in response to the worst mine disaster since 1952, federal legislation requiring the development of detailed and effective health and safety regulations was finally passed in 1969, nearly two decades after the industry had begun the long process of consolidation that made possible prescriptive regulation on the national level.

The story of proscriptive regulation is very different, for throughout the twentieth century federal courts have intervened vigorously to prevent the formation of trusts and other forms of institutional cooperation that would have exempted certain sectors of the coal industry from full exposure to the free market. In doing so the courts have not singled out the coal industry; rather, they have simply applied existing antitrust statutes to the various cases brought before them. And there has been no lack of cases, for the coal operators have tried again and again to devise ways of transforming ruinous competition into stable cooperation. As George Love, president of the Pittsburgh Consolidation Coal Company and the industry's leading spokesman, declared in 1955, "we can see all through the history of the constituent companies [of Pittsburgh Consolidation] and their predecessors, an overwhelming urge to consolidate, not to get larger but as an attempt to meet the drastic competition always present in a natural resource industry with excess capacity."[20] The UMWA regularly supported these moves and during the New Deal even took the lead in securing legislation designed to shield the coal industry from the vigilence of the trustbusters. Why the industry has repeatedly attempted to achieve consolidation in this way and why it has been consistently denied this form of relief are fascinating and revealing questions. A recent essay by Thomas McCraw, "Rethinking the Trust Question," offers a fresh approach to these questions, and his ideas inform the analysis that follows.[21]

McCraw begins by emphasizing that the Industrial Revolution was above all else a revolution in productivity and that in economic terms its most dramatic and disruptive consequence was chronic overcapacity in the industries it transformed. Societies that through historical experience had learned how to distribute scarce goods, however inequitably, suddenly found themselves facing a flood of cheap industrial products. The ability to produce manufactured goods advanced rapidly while the economic and institutional rearrangements needed to expand markets for them and coordinate supply and demand lagged far behind. As a result, nineteenth-century industrialists found themselves being buffeted by the economic storms of a boom-and-bust business environment. They responded by forming associations and mergers designed to harness the new productive capacities to the available markets, a move they had good reason to believe would help stabilize the turbulent worlds of industry and commerce. The primary motive behind the formation of trusts was thus the need to bring the new productive forces under control; the primary goal was to stabilize the institutional structure of business.[22]

This characterization of the movement toward consolidation that transformed much of American industry during the final decades of the nineteenth century flies in the face of the popular "Robber Baron" image of the gilded-age captains of industry. Taught by three generations of Progressive social critics to see industrial capitalists as greedy and self-serving malefactors, Americans have looked with satisfaction on a variety of legal instruments, beginning with the Sherman Anti-Trust Act of 1890, designed to thwart the monopolization of wealth and power by the new leaders of industry. These barriers, far from being creations of the law alone, reflect deeply held popular notions about the nature of trusts and their political and economic implications. Not only are trusts seen as the offspring of evil desires, they are considered unnatural. They constrain or eliminate access to markets and thereby restrict participation in economic life to those who control the trusts or who are subject to their control. They also reduce competition, thereby perverting relations best governed by the invisible hand of the market, and they create artificial shortages and high prices, thereby depriving the common person of goods he or she might otherwise enjoy. It is this venerable and still powerful hostility toward industrial consolidation that McCraw argues needs to be subjected to dispassionate reevaluation.

Before beginning this reevaluation, McCraw introduces several analytic terms that are especially relevant to the institutional description of the coal industry. "Vertical integration" he defines as a means of improving a company's efficiency by reducing the transaction costs of production.

> One approach to the problem of transaction costs was for a company to minimize its market relationships with intermediates and instead to do all its business operations itself, from the derivation of raw materials to the selling of finished manufactured products at retail. Such a company is said to have achieved complete "vertical integration."[23]

Although the concept of vertical integration is hardly novel, McCraw's insistence that the motive that led to this form of integration was rooted in the search for business efficiency rather than in the lust for monopoly power deserves attention. "Within the framework of the trust question," McCraw maintains, "the important point is that the chief purpose of vertical integration historically has been to promote productive efficiency, even though it can also serve as a competitive weapon to preempt supplies or markets." While the objectionable consequences of vertical integration obviously must be attended to, they should not be used to condemn in entirety a form of industrial organization that offers real economic advantages.

Another form of industrial organization McCraw discusses is "horizontal combination." This type of combination involves agreements among producers either to limit production or to keep prices up, or both, the larger purpose being to smooth out supply-and-demand fluctuations and ensure stability in production and profitability. Unlike vertical integration, horizontal combination does not directly reduce transaction costs or increase productive efficiency, but historically it has often contributed to these ends by creating the conditions in which vertical integration could be carried out. But these longer-term effects have not been universally realized, nor are the links between horizontal and vertical integration easily perceived; and the more immediate effects of horizontal combination—namely, the maintaining of prices above the levels they would otherwise fall to—is popularly seen as an unwarranted exploitation of the ultimate consumer. This highly visible consequence of horizontal combination has long fueled antitrust fires even though, as McCraw rightly insists, "the fundamental strategy of these companies categorically emphasized the constancy of production far more than it did the fleecing of consumers or the building of monopolies."[24]

McCraw also distinguishes between business firms at the center and those at the periphery. As Alfred Chandler's historical studies have demonstrated, "the industry structure characteristic of the American center economy evolved largely during the forty-year period between 1880 and 1920."[25] Firms at the center, such as Standard Oil, American Tobacco, and Carnegie Steel, had the characteristics of being technologically advanced, enjoying economies of scale, being vertically integrated, having a long-range perspective, and being capital intensive. Those firms on the periphery tended to be "small, labor intensive, managerially thin, and bereft of economies of either scale or speed." Forced to concentrate on survival in the short term, peripheral firms competed in a relatively free market, and they still "form the backbone of small business in all capitalist economies." Lacking the characteristics needed to achieve vertical integration, they frequently seek shelter from the vagaries of the market through the formation of local price-fixing arrangements, but such efforts are easily detected and dismantled by antitrust regulators. Thus, for several generations there have in fact been two different systems of business operating side by side in a dual economy, one composed of center firms and the other of firms on the periphery. Clearly the coal industry is in these terms peripheral.[26]

Whereas Chandler celebrates the success of center firms, McCraw directs our attention to those which fell by the wayside. And as he rightly emphasizes, the inherent institutional and technological features of the peripheral industries, and not the individual failings of their leaders, doomed them from the outset.

> Try as they might, businessmen in peripheral industries simply could not make their combinations work, precisely because of the nature of those industries. Their experience—an experience of failure unrelated to talent, entrepreneurship, or dedication—is one of the forgotten aspects of the trust movement, unfortunately for subsequent understanding of the issue.[27]

Indeed, in the United States powerful antitrust sentiment compounded the problems faced by peripheral firms, for although antitrust legislation failed to thwart the consolidation of center firms, as a glance around the corporate landscape today will confirm, it was effective in preventing the kinds of loose horizontal combination that might have started peripheral firms down the road to vertical integration and the real gains in efficiency it makes possible.

McCraw's analysis helps explain why the coal industry, which time and again attempted to create institutional arrangements that would bring about production and price stability, was forced to remain on the periphery of the American economy while many of the industries it served waxed fat and powerful at the center. The anthracite coal industry had the great advantage of geographic concentration and thus could be fairly easily dominated by the railroads that hauled its coal to market. The bituminous coal industry, being widely dispersed, posed a more difficult problem. If it could in some way be brought under administrative control, then those participating in the industry could look forward to stable prices and production. But every arrangement proposed inevitably excluded some producers, usually among those located on the edge of the industry in the more remote coalfields of West Virginia and eastern Kentucky. Thus, those who opposed the formation of horizontal combinations in coal could always find someone in the industry to file a suit charging that the merger, marketing association, sales agency, or trade association that excluded them from the market or obliged them to conform to certain terms of entry was an undue restraint of trade. In fact, it did not take especially vigorous antitrust prosecution to keep the coal industry divided against itself.

From the 1880s until the beginning of World War I, the coal industry struggled to achieve stability and some form of consolidation, but to no avail.[28] The coal barons, as the leading operators came to be known, were beset by intense competiton within their industry, the challenge of the UMWA, and the need to find some way to organize the coal industry so that it would not be completely subordinated to the gigantic corporations that were consolidating other industries. Embattled and fiercely independent, these exemplars of individualistic capitalism had little talent for conciliation and compromise. As captains in an industry that extracted and marketed a natural resource consumed directly by a large part of the citizenry, the coal operators provided a perfect target for the Progressive trustbusters. The demands of war made what appeared to be selfishness even less defensible, especially after federal attempts to arrange cooperation in production and marketing during the early stages of World War I dissolved into acrimonious chaos. By 1917, when the Lever Act gave President Woodrow

Wilson broad authority to organize the nation's industries for war, the coal industry had become a scapegoat. Astonishing as it now seems, Wilson actually spent hours going over Federal Trade Commission cost sheets before personally setting the prices to be charged for coal in various markets. Predictably, and justifiably, the operators were appalled and outraged.[29]

Despite the dreadful public image of the coal barons, however, their understanding of the fundamental problem of their industry should not pass unnoted. In 1917 Francis S. Peabody, president of the Peabody Coal Company (now one of the largest coal-mining companies in the United States), read a paper on "coal wastage" to a meeting of the American Institute of Mining Engineers.[30] Although not himself an engineer, Peabody had been in the coal mining and marketing business for thirty years. Like others in the coal industry, he responded to the outbreak of war and the conservation movement of the Progressive era by deploring the use of mining methods that left roughly 50 percent of the coal unrecovered. But Peabody was concerned with other forms of waste as well: "The coal industry is beset by all manner of waste, waste of natural resources, waste of the human element, and waste of capital, and we do not seem to realize how dearly future generations must pay for it." The chief causes of this wastage, he believed, were excess productive capacity and ruinous competition, which were themselves caused by the ease with which small operators could enter the industry. As Peabody said, "the coal business is not a business for small capital; that is one of its greatest difficulties today." Unfortunately, the industry had been prevented from organizing itself so as to limit production and market competition. Although both the English and the Americans had in place laws designed to prevent "unreasonable" restraint of trade, they differed in their interpretations of what was reasonable. As Peabody noted, "consumers will lose in the long run if the mine operators do not make a fair profit or the miners do not receive a fair wage." The English Privy Council understood this point and therefore decided that "the mere intention of an agreement [among coal producers] to raise prices does not always prove the intention to injure the public." But in the United States no such legal precedent for reasonable restraints of trade has been established.

Although Peabody would have preferred a revision of American antitrust law so as to permit reasonable restraints of trade, he believed that the wastage endemic in the industry in fact could be alleviated only by immediate and thorough federal regulation.

It would be far better if a situation could be created in the near future with strong governmental control, preferably through the medium of the Federal Trade Commission, so that the bituminous coal industry could be thoroughly regulated with respect to the operation of present properties, so that all may operate on a reasonable basis, returning a fair percentage of recovery, with regulations that will insure the best conditions for the safety of life and limb, and so founded that the operator will be assured of a reasonable return on his capital invested.

Such regulation of the coal industry when it does come must begin at the bottom; the industry must be regulated from every standpoint.[31]

Caught between an industry that operated in a socially unacceptable manner and a law that prevented it from reforming itself, Peabody turned to federal regulation for relief. He realized that such a proposal would generate considerable opposition, but he remained convinced it was the only available avenue to the desired end, the elimination of the undercapitalized operator:

All this regulation would necessarily involve much time and study and would gradually be revised as new conditions were met. Objections would be raised; no doubt many attempts would be made to prove the early acts unconstitutional; no doubt claims would be made, that only those controlling large amounts of capital could enter the business, and such would undoubtedly be a fact.[32]

It was a bold strategy based on an analysis that some of Peabody's contemporaries challenged and calling for actions that many operators found unacceptable.[33] Although not implemented, it nevertheless had the virtue of addressing directly and comprehensively the structural problems that have dogged the American coal industry for well over a century. It was not ignorance but a lack of will that perpetuated the wastage Peabody so surprisingly and forcefully deplored.

Soon after the end of World War I, the coal industry entered a prolonged period of depression. Subsequent attempts to revive it in the 1920s and in the New Deal involved considerable leadership on the part of the federal government and the UMWA, yet the industry continued to suffer from being internally divided and from continued judicial opposition to horizontal combination, even when sanctioned by legislation.[34] The tempestuous courtship of Lewis and Roosevelt and the rise and fall of the National Recovery Act (NRA) are oft-told tales that provide many moments of high drama for students of American labor history and of American public policy, yet in the end the coal industry was not granted effective relief from the legal impediments that prevented horizontal combination. Failing that, and failing nationalization, the industry was obliged to manage as best it could with a declining share of the American energy market. The coal industry, like much of American industry, really recovered only when the nation again went to war.

Were we to end our examination of the effect of antitrust sentiment on the coal industry at this point, we would be accepting the notion that with regard to the organization of industry, Americans have been so captivated by antitrust ideology that they are incapable of learning from experience. The truth is, however, that lessons were learned and attempts were made to put into practice what had been learned. Yet in the end all attempts to reorganize the coal industry by means of legislation failed. It is therefore the failure of actions taken, rather than inaction, that must be explained.

Although the statutes used to bar horizontal combinations had been put in place well before the 1920s, legislation designed to create and legitimate such combinations in the coal industry was introduced again and again throughout the New Deal.[35] When tested in court, however, these legislative initiatives were invariably thrown out as unconstitutional. Surely something more than an unbending fidelity to the statutes of an earlier generation sustained this judicial denial of legislative will. What lay behind the government's persistent inability to reconstruct the economic circumstances in which an indispensable but sick industry was forced to operate? Why was the federal government incapable of putting into effect a policy that would successfully compensate for the "natural" characteristics that kept the coal industry and those who worked in it in such socially unacceptable conditions? The answer can be found by digging more deeply in the ideological soil that nourished political and legal resistance to the formation of trusts and infused that resistance with an overwhelming moral fervor.

Let us begin by distinguishing between consumer values and producer values. The values people honor when acting as consumers emphasize fair trade and maximization of utilities. Consumers of coal want to have available an adequate supply of good-quality coal at a reasonable price, the reasonableness of the price being determined by the prices charged by alternative vendors and the cost of turning to other sources of energy. Yet while the interests of consumers are real and important, they hardly provide an adequate basis for denying an industry the right to organize in a way that will enable it to function in a socially acceptable manner. Throughout the industrial era in the United States, as in England, coal miners have supported the idea of limiting output to maintain prices so that coal operators will be able to pay decent wages.[36] It seems unlikely that the public at large, the ultimate consumers of coal and the goods produced with it, is unwilling to pay the price required to achieve this goal. Consumer values are central to economic calculations, but the cost advantages realized by denying the coal industry legislative relief simply were not great enough to sustain the political fervor that defeated all attempts to reform the coal industry during the New Deal.

Producer values, as they have been articulated in the United States, were capable of generating such fervor. Personal freedom and social utility merge in the American conception of work, and we are especially inclined to honor the independent and enterprising producer of such basic goods as food, fuel, and shelter. The Jeffersonian farmer, like the small businessman in commerce and industry, is popularly regarded as a man of virtue contending with malign social and natural forces that threaten to crush his spirit and defeat him in his struggle to attain personal fulfillment by contributing materially to his society. When the small businessman prevails against these forces, it is a confirmation of all that the United States stands for; when they defeat him, we are all diminished. This heroic image of the producer has not been without effect in the coal industry, even though it is clearly an inadequate representation of how that industry has actually functioned in the twentieth century.[37]

Within the coal industry one must make two distinctions that complicate somewhat the definition of who produces coal. The first is between those who own and manage the mines and those who work in them; the second is between the large firms that mine coal and the small operators. Although coal mining and farming are similar in many ways—both are rural enterprises, labor intensive, widely distributed geographically, and make use of natural resources—they differ in that the coal miner is the archetypical industrial laborer, whereas the farmer is the embodiment of agrarian independence. Throughout the history of American labor, and especially during the rise of industrial unionism in the 1930s, the coal miner has symbolized the ideals of solidarity, toughness, determination, and militancy. Whether or not this is in fact an accurate representation of miners as a whole, the perception has exacerbated the undeniable polarization of management and labor within the industry. As a consequence, coal miners are commonly thought of as workers who take up tools provided by others and do tasks set for them, not as initiators of new enterprises, contributors to a vital economy, and members of civil society. When it comes to identifying those members of society who as virtuous producers of useful goods deserve to be protected from both ruinous competition and the depredations of the powerful, coal miners simply do not seem to fit the part. Although they actually are the producers of an essential source of energy, they are thought of as tough and contentious men who can be left to look out for themselves.[38]

At the other end of the spectrum of producers stand the big corporations that mine coal. Like the miners, the big corporations simply do not fit the image of the productive individual; hence, the legitimacy associated with the production of useful goods does not extend to them. As one defender of the coal operators complained in 1917, "somehow the liberties of the consumer always seem so big and those of the producer always seem so small."[39] The coal industry is, however, the most unconcentrated of the major energy industries, an unwelcome and troublesome characteristic that is the source of most of its social problems.[40] The social consequences of this lack of concentration have not been widely appreciated, however, and it is the small operator who is popularly portrayed as the beleaguered defender of individuality and free enterprise—a yeoman entrepreneur who is constantly being threatened with extinction by the vast resources and monopolistic cravings of the major corporations. It is thus the small operator who in the coal industry emerges as the archetypical producer and the representative of those producer values which Americans generally regard as virtuous. It is his access to markets and right to sell at any price that have been so assiduously protected by antitrust legislation. The small operator manipulates and in turn is possessed by a powerful image, whatever the real consequences of its defense, and this image has continued to provide a rationale for opposition to horizontal combinations in the coal industry long after the destructive effects of unfettered competition have been made obvious to all.

The historical force of these perceptions and of the producer values that inform them has distorted the institutional history of the coal industry throughout this century. Although antitrust sentiment continues to be refreshed by popular faith in the efficacy of the market and popular sympathy for the rights of small producers, the coal industry is held responsible for providing a steady supply of fuel, even while being denied an opportunity to reconstruct itself in a way that would enable it to meet its responsibilities in a rational and reliable manner. Consider, for example, the way in which those responsible for the production of coal are characterized when the possibility of a scarcity arises. Because market forces are almost always effective in keeping the price of coal to a minimum, fluctuations in price have seldom created a demand for public intervention, even when, following the energy crisis of 1973, coal prices trailed oil prices and more than doubled. But should difficulties within the industry raise the possibility of a shortage, then the politicians begin the search for scapegoats. In 1902 a skillfully led strike in the anthracite coal industry made it appear that there would be severe fuel shortages in the Eastern cities during the coming winter. Teddy Roosevelt conjured up visions of a freezing, rioting public and called the crisis "only less serious than that of the Civil War."[41] Such a calamity must have been caused by a villain, and in that Progressive age "the coal barons offered a perfect target for antitrust emotions, and a great many took this opportunity to unload."[42] George F. Baer, the imperious president of the largest anthracite railroad, unwittingly but marvelously played the role of chief antagonist. Labor historians will be forever grateful to him for saying in a letter to a stockholder that

> the rights and interests of the laboring man will be protected and cared for—not by the labor agitators, but by the Christian gentlemen to whom God has given control of the property rights of the country and upon the successful management of which so much depends.[43]

And yet, although he was clearly a man one could love to hate, Baer spoke the truth when rejecting a proposal, made by union president John Mitchell, that would have had members of the clergy arbitrating the dispute: "Anthracite mining," Baer reminded him, "is a business, not a religious, sentimental, or academic proposition."[44] The coal operators may have had terrible public relations, but they knew their business as it existed, not as others wished it to be. Roosevelt, however, had a political problem to solve, and rather than addressing the underlying problems of the industry, he responded to the crisis by using the office of the presidency to force the dispute into arbitration. It was a response that many of his successors would be driven to as well.[45]

The federal government never did develop a policy that effectively helped the coal industry reform those institutional characteristics which made it peripheral; and at the end of World War II the industry and all its problems, including those concerning health and safety, were left to await whatever salvation the slow evolution of mining technology and changes in the market for coal might provide. From the late 1940s to the late 1960s the industry did manage, however, to achieve a notable but far from complete mechanization and consolidation. Thus, by the time a variety of historical forces converged in 1969 to bring about the passage of federal health and safety legislation, a major segment of the coal industry had already developed institutional structures that partially shielded it from the inefficiencies of the unfettered marketplace. As we can now see, the federal government's attempts, both prescriptive and proscriptive, to regulate this peripheral industry during the first seven decades of this century were radically inadequate both with regard to health and safety and to stabilization. These efforts do not add up to one of the more enlightened chapters in the history of American public policy.

Engineers as Supervisors of Production

The coal in America's bituminous regions lies below the surface in nearly horizontal seams of varying thickness. Although the coal in any one seam is usually fairly uniform in character, miners extracting it routinely encounter unpredictable difficulties. Not only are the seams themselves frequently fractured and mixed with other rocks, but the strata bounding them are often structurally unstable as well. Therefore, no matter how highly mechanized coal mining may become, and by 1969 it was only partially mechanized, it can never be transformed into an entirely controlled process. Coal mining, like seafaring and farming, requires experience, constant attention, and human judgment of a sort that has been largely eliminated in intensely engineered industries such as automobile production. Coal mining may seem to be brutish work, and in many ways it is, but it is not work that can be fully planned in the engineering office and then carried out by robots. Miners know this, and so do mining engineers. A coal mine is not an underground factory, whatever the level of capital investment and mechanical assistance involved; it is a workshop in which the constantly varying materials presented by nature are processed in a changing and threatening environment.

How have mining engineers responded to the health and safety problems associated with underground coal mining, and why have they responded as they have? The answer to the latter question is not to be found in certain types of special knowledge they acquired while preparing to enter the profession of engineering. The answer lies rather in the organization of coal-mining companies and the engineer's place and function within that order. And because the normal career path for successful engineers involves a rather rapid move from positions that require technical expertise to positions that call for managerial skills, one must also keep in mind the goals and duties associated with the managerial positions to which most mining engineers have aspired.

As W. P. Tams, Jr., a prominent West Virginia coal baron, noted in a memoir published in 1963, "the development of today's vast army of executives and administrators has been a comparatively recent phenomenon in the coal industry. By present standards, the internal organization of the early coal company was simplicity itself."[46] The person in charge of the company was called the operator, a position that in small companies was and frequently still is filled by the owner. Salaried employees might include a mine foreman, who would be in charge of all underground operations; a superintendent, who would be in overall charge of operations at a single mine; a manager for the company store; and clerks for payroll and the store. A company that operated several mines might have its own mining engineer and assistants, whereas individual mines generally employed the services of an engineering firm as needed.

As this description makes clear, the line between management and labor put the superintendent and the foreman on one side and the miners on the other. The foreman gained his position by rising through the ranks of miners, and he represented management in supervising the underground operations of mining. As state and later federal safety regulations became more detailed, he was increasingly burdened with the often conflicting responsibilities of maximizing production while ensuring the safety of the miners. As a coal company safety director wrote in 1954, it is the foreman's job to train his men in safe work habits and then to see that they in fact work safely: "Day after day he must supplement his instructions by constantly policing his section to make sure that his men are performing their work as safely as they can. . . . Here, then, is where the safety program will either stand or fall."[47]

The superintendent is the overall mine manager who carries out the policies set by the owners of the company. It is, of course, not unknown for individuals to rise from the ranks of miners to the position of superintendent, but as Keith Dix has pointed out, early in this century it became increasingly common to recruit engineers as superintendents.

Civil and mining engineering were the fields of study

> most commonly sought after by the mining companies as qualified persons were hired from the railroad, construction and other industries. As states established schools of mines, mining engineers who showed a talent for administration were much in demand and education became a substitute for experience for the mine superintendent's job.[48]

Superintendents necessarily identified with the operators and other professionals in the mining community, and successful superintendents quickly learned that their foremost responsibility was to ship coal from the mine at the lowest possible cost. As mine owner Justus Collins told a newly appointed superintendent in a long letter of instruction: "Never lose sight of the fact that the sole purpose of the organization is to make money for [its] stockholders."[49]

When mining companies became large enough and sufficiently concerned to appoint safety engineers, those so designated were given staff rather than line positions within the management structure. Responsibilty for the supervision of production remained with the superintendent and his foremen, and the safety engineer did what he could to encourage conformance with the existing safety codes and the utilization of safe practices. The safety director for the Hanna Coal Company, a major Pittsburgh firm, described the duties of the safety engineer in the following terms:

> The foreman is aided by the safety engineer, who accompanies him periodically on inspection of his portion of the mine, pointing out to him where he has violated company safety policy, State mine law, and Federal law or code, watching closely the work habits of the men and bringing to his attention any sub-standard performances he observes. His report is made to the mine superintendent, and copies are sent to the general safety director and the vice president. The safety engineer leaves notes of his findings with the mine foreman and the section foreman concerned.[50]

However effective individual safety engineers may have been, and however much authority they may have been given in particular circumstances, it is clear that in organizational terms safety remained a matter of secondary, if nonetheless real, importance within the management structure of coal companies. It therefore seems unreasonable to expect that an engineer concerned with safety and working in such a setting would insist that his opinion as a technical expert be considered of overriding importance. Professional autonomy that created value conflicts within management was not what the coal industry was looking for in its engineers.

In light of this overwhelming economic imperative, which was unquestioned among those who controlled advancement within the industry, the mining engineer was compelled to subordinate whatever technical considerations might create conflicts to more comprehensive and commanding economic considerations. The social structure of the industry prevented him from making common cause with the miners who suffered the consequences of unsafe and unhealthy working conditions, especially as neither state nor federal governments enforced the technical regulations they mandated to improve safety. But it would be wrong to presume that many mining engineers found this to be a particularly stressful situation, for in the past, as at present, they largely accepted the industry on its own terms. When asked why he did not provide more roof supports to prevent the rock falls that routinely killed his immigrant miners, an operator is said to have replied that "wops are cheaper than props." The same point was made in less odious terms by an outraged state mining commissioner in 1912:

> Newly arrived immigrants are very cheap. While it would cost something, say one per cent per ton of coal mined, to make conditions comparatively safe, the present system is perhaps cheaper. It is doubtful if the average miner killed during the last twenty years has cost his employer $50 in damages paid to his dependents. If these men were slaves worth about $2,000 apiece, as in ante bellum days, they would not have killed 30,000 of them in twenty years, bringing upon themselves a loss of $60,000,000. They would have made their mines as safe as those in Europe, or else have gone out of business.[51]

Given such attitudes, we should not be too quick to judge the engineers who served the industry as it existed. If we feel compelled to castigate them for failing to discharge their duties in a professional manner, this is perhaps because we have projected onto the mining engineers attitudes and concerns they would have found quite foreign or at best of secondary importance to the practice of their craft.

To better understand how mining engineers could accept the harsh economic imperatives of a peripheral industry while still thinking of themselves as professionals, we need to examine the values and attitudes held by those who founded the profession of mining engineering. This line of investigation requires a temporary detour away from the coal industry, for the most prominent early spokesmen for mining engineering, men such as Herbert Hoover, worked primarily in metal mining rather than coal mining. Nevertheless, the attitudes they championed largely reflected the thinking of mining engineers of all sorts. Whether in the end we will want to call those attitudes professional remains an open question.

Edwin Layton has described the early history and guiding ideology of the mining engineers in sharp and revealing detail. Their professional organization, the American Institute of Mining and Metallurgical Engineers (AIME), was the second of the four "founder" engineering societies established. From its inception in 1871 this society distinguished itself from the older Society of Civil Engineers by emphasizing industrial issues rather than the concerns of independent professionals. The AIME was prepared to admit to membership anyone "practically engaged in mining, metallurgy, or metallurgical engineering."[52] Rossiter W. Raymond, who dominated the AIME from its founding until 1921, thought of the engineer as a businessman, and he successfully opposed all attempts to develop a code of ethics for the society. Later events were to reveal that his opposition to a code of ethics was not unrepresentative of mining engineering in general. In 1908 a group of mining engineers who wished to set more stringent admission standards for membership in their professional association formed a rival organization, the Mining and Metallurgical Society of America. While they succeeded in drawing attention to the special kinds of knowledge that professionals command, they too were unwilling to commit themselves or their society to a code of professional ethics.[53]

Whether or not mining engineers are, in some all-embracing sense of the term, professionals, it can hardly be doubted that the society they created reflects the predominant view of their duties as mining engineers. According to this view, loyalty to management must be unstinting—a commitment that was of great importance in the polarized society of mining camps. As one mining engineer told a group of younger colleagues in 1931, "we as employees owe the company our best efforts not only while at work but at all times, promoting always the company's interests by representing them favorably.

This we can best do by active, harmonious participation in the community social, civil, and spiritual activity."[54] Furthermore, because the preferred career path for engineers led to management, a move that did not, however, entail abandoning one's identity as an engineer, the AIME soon contained a large proportion of members who, having once served as engineers, were no longer practicing as such. As the editor of *Mining and Metallurgy* observed with satisfaction, "naturally such men are highly influential in establishing the policies of engineering societies."[55] Attention to coal company interests in AIME affairs was also assured by the practice of having employers pay employee dues, and it was widely understood that the society's publications were edited so as to avoid making public reports that might embarrass members who worked in industry.

Perhaps in the end one should emphasize the engineers' collective longing to belong to a profession rather than evaluate the degree to which every engineer conducted his affairs in a professional manner. No one expressed this longing more eloquently than the Great Engineer himself, Herbert Hoover. His *Principles of Mining,* first delivered as a series of lectures at Stanford and Columbia and then published in 1909, concludes with a chapter on "The Character, Training, and Obligations of the Mining Engineering Profession." Its first eight pages develop the point Hoover considers to be of overriding importance, that "the most dominant characteristic of the mining engineering profession is the vast preponderance of the commercial over the technical in the daily work of the engineer."[56] Then, in the final pages,, he turns to those other aspects of the profession which he says are "of no less moment." What follows is general in the extreme and, although well-intentioned and high-minded, dwells primarily on the etiquette of engineering practice rather than on the more difficult issue of the engineer's responsibilities to those he serves. Mining engineers wrapped themselves in the cloak of professionalism, as did a great many of their contemporaries, but the realities of their employment meant that they could be professional only in a highly restricted sense. It is thus hardly surprising that mining engineers seldom took positions on health and safety issues that were at odds with company policy.

Company policies do change, however, and when the coal operators were obliged to pay greater attention to safety in underground mining, the engineers they employed responded promptly. The passage of workmen's compensation laws, beginning in 1910, provided a powerful incentive to reduce the loss of life and limb in the mines. This recasting of the liability law was designed to make the incentive for reducing accidents one that employers could not ignore, for they could not minimize their operating costs unless they met the new standards of safety. As an engineer remarked in 1917 when describing the various lamps employed by coal miners, "the passage of the recent Employer's Liability Act in Pennsylvania has made it necessary for many coal-mining companies to take out liability insurance, and the companies underwriting such insurance have made it desirable for the insured to permit the use of none but illuminants of established worth."[57] It thus appeared that the legal requirement to carry liability insurance would make allies of the insurance companies and the engineers in the battle for greater safety in coal mines.[58]

Although this is not the place to undertake an assessment of the effectiveness of the workmen's compensation laws, it should be pointed out that specific new institutional arrangements were developed to satisfy their requirements. The "no-fault" features of the laws were designed to prevent the use of litigation to avoid payment of legitimate claims, and the requirement that liability insurance be carried was intended to ensure that the companies involved would be able to pay legitimate claims. The insurance industry responded to this new demand for services by forming a group called The Associated Companies, which included the 10 largest insurers of coal mines. The Associated Companies had two purposes: first, to spread as broadly as possible the risk of insuring mines against disastrous losses, and second, to reduce as much as possible the occurrence of accidents. To meet this second goal, The Associated Companies established a safety engineering service that assisted in the setting of insurance rates for individual mines by determining the causes of accidents, rating these causes as to seriousness, and then inspecting mines to see to what extent the conditions in which these causes take effect were present.[59] As the chief inspector of The Associated Companies noted, the persuasive power of this system, which was immediate and financial, was not lost on the economically pressed coal operators:

> The inspection of a mine by the engineer or inspector of an insurance company, with the fixing of numerical values for relative safety of each of the elements which may produce accidents, has a marked influence in drawing the attention of mine officials to the hazards of their operations, the existence of which may not have occurred to them. Even State inspection, with its police powers, is not so influential in pressing home

the nature of the risk and the value of preventive measures as is an increased insurance rate or a reduction in insurance premium under workmen's compensation legislation.[60]

Indeed, the Mine Safety Standards set by The Associated Companies acquired police power as well when these standards were sanctioned by state insurance departments, as soon occurred in many of the coal-producing states, and they generated a newfound interest in safety engineering in major coal companies. If the workmen's compensation program did not fulfill all the expectations of its most fervent proponents, it did mark a real step forward in the struggle to make safety a matter of concern to the coal operators.

It should be remembered, however, that in underground coal mining, safety engineering was believed to be primarily a management problem rather than a technical problem. It was widely agreed among mining engineers that up to 90 percent of all accidents were the result of careless work practices and that the only effective solutions were increased education and closer supervision.[61] The problem, therefore, was not one that made much use of the special knowledge possessed by engineers. Howard N. Eavenson, chairman of the AIME Committee on Safety and Sanitation in 1917, reported that at U.S. Steel's model company town in Gary, West Virginia, a system of cash bonuses had been very effective in improving the safety record of the mine, and a year later he again insisted that at Gary they were convinced that worker welfare was the key to safety: "There is no question at all in my mind that . . . welfare work is one of the largest points in accident prevention."[62] The safety engineers deserve credit for engaging the question before them on its own terms, but whether in doing so they were acting as professionals depends in large part on how one defines what it means to be a professional—a question to which we will return in the last section of this chapter.

Scientists and the Politics of Natural Knowledge

Scientists bring to the problems they address knowledge of natural substances and natural laws and, in addition, the ability to use certain methods of investigation to expand that knowledge. When free to choose, they take up theoretically interesting questions they can answer by using the techniques of investigation and interpretation available to them. In their day-to-day work, however, scientists pursue their research in social institutions of varying degrees of complexity, and these institutions are subject to multiple and frequently conflicting claims on their resources. Thus, very few scientists have in practice the kind of autonomy in research that is held up as an ideal of pure science. But we should not therefore jump to the conclusion that scientists limited to working on research problems not entirely of their own choosing are not in fact doing science, for the work undertaken in all but a relatively few scientific research institutions always represents a compromise between the demand that certain practical ends be served and the desire to concentrate on theoretically interesting problems. As long as those engaged in research continue to consider themselves scientists and make use of the methods and techniques of science, our understanding of the institutional pressures that help shape their work will not be advanced by forcing a distinction between "pure" science, conceived of as essentially disinterested inquiry, and "applied" science.

These preliminary observations are relevant to a discussion of scientists' involvement in the coal industry because that industry's problems, and more particularly its health and safety problems, have in very few cases possessed theoretical implications of such intrinsic interest that they have attracted scientists free to set their own research agendas. While it is true that geologists have long been interested in explaining how coal is formed and how coal seams were laid down in the formations in which they occur, these problems are hardly of immediate importance to those involved in digging coal out of the ground and getting it to market. But many scientists have in fact wrestled with problems of direct interest to the coal industry, and they have done so because they and those who employed them believed that bringing scientific expertise to bear on the industry's problems was a reasonable and potentially beneficial way to go about solving those problems. Why was this strategy thought to be reasonable, and how was it implemented during the historical period we are examining? These are the questions examined in this section. Approaching the subject in this way may seem unnecessarily indirect, yet it has the advantage of leaving open the question of whether it is a good idea to recast as scientific problems such practical problems as the excess productive capacity of the coal industry or the safety hazards associated with underground mining.

Underground coal mining has always been an exceptionally dangerous and unhealthy occupation. Where new hazards have been created by innovations based on science, such as occured when coal haulage was electrified, it has seemed reasonable to insist that techno-logical means be found to reduce or eliminate the specific new dangers created. But traditionally and statistically the greatest hazards in-volved in underground mining are caused by natural conditions that become apparent only in the process of extracting coal. Roof falls, the greatest single cause of fatalities year in and year out, are the result of rock faults and ground pressures that are specific to the formation being mined and exceedingly complex in nature. Should one address problems of this type by attempting to apply the techniques of science, or should one concentrate on establishing work routines that incorpo-rate the lessons of experience? One can, of course, do both, but it should be evident that attacking the problem scientifically is not neces-sarily either more rational or more efficacious—there is, in other words, no general reason for treating the resources of science as privi-leged when addressing the problems of coal mining. It is therefore a valid and interesting historical question to ask why these resources were applied to the industry's problems in certain specific situations. Furthermore, only when we have a better idea of why certain members of the industry turned to science will we be able to estimate the extent to which the scientists' involvements with this industry were shaped by the institutions that employed them.

There are basically two types of institutions that have directed the attention of scientists to the problems of the coal industry: agen-cies of the federal government and large corporations involved in coal mining. Of these two, the federal government has been by far the more active and important. But before looking at several instances in which the federal government tried to help the coal industry by orga-nizing and supporting scientific research, we should take a moment to reflect on its failure to adapt what appears at first glance to be the most appropriate model for federal assistance through science: the system developed to support agriculture.

Throughout the first half of the twentieth century, both commer-cial agriculture and bituminous coal mining functioned as peripheral industries operating in the unconsolidated sector of the American economy. Composed largely of highly dispersed small producers, both industries have experienced intense market pressures and wide fluctuations in levels of production, and the graphically portrayed hardships of farmers and miners have posed some of the most intracta-ble problems of equity and social welfare that federal policy experts have had to address. But if the problems raised by these industries have much in common, the federal response, especially with regard to relief through science, has been very different.

Ever since the passage of the Morrill Act in 1862, which authorized the establishment of federally endowed land-grant colleges, the federal government has initiated and underwritten a variety of programs designed to develop and disseminate useful knowledge for American farmers. The establishment and growth of the Department of Agriculture, and especially the achievements of its research centers and its federal-state programs for agricultural experiment stations and agricultural extension services, represents America's oldest, most extensive, most successful, and most emulated federal effort to bring the resources of science to the aid and relief of an essential but economically vulnerable industry. Yet it is a model that has never seriously been considered by those who have sought federal support for scientific research that would be useful to the coal industry.[63] Certainly there are points of disanalogy between farming and coal mining that would have made it difficult to apply the agricultural model directly to the problems of the coal industry, but the absence of any serious attempt to adapt such a prominent model at the very least prompts us to ask why the possibilities were not explored. Despite the similarities between the economic and institutional structures of these two industries, one might argue that the symbolic contrast between the family farmer and the prolitarian coal miner is so great that the claims to public welfare made by spokesmen for these two peripheral industries have been viewed as politically incommensurable. If this is so, then political ideology, and especially the agrarian notion of citizenship that informed the dominant American conception of republican virtue, once again compounded the difficulties faced by those who worked in the coal industry.

There have been two sorts of federally supported scientific programs designed to alleviate the problems of the coal industry, but only one of these has dealt directly with health and safety issues. Twice in this century, disasters in underground coal mines have triggered significant responses in Congress. The first of these responses led to the creation of the Bureau of Mines in 1910; the second, to the passage of the Federal Coal Mine Health and Safety Act of 1969. In both cases a convergence of earlier developments prepared the ground for federal intervention, and the disasters provided the political boost needed to turn bureaucratic proposals into legislative action. The second type of federal scientific program has sought to encourage modernization of the coal industry by stimulating science-based innovation. As with Lewis's strategy of mechanization, it was thought that such an effort would help make the mines safer by concentrating the mining of coal in the hands of those companies capable of using the new techniques and dominating the markets they would create. In the 1950s and 1960s federal support for coal-related scientific research followed this second strategy, most notably in the funding of the Office for Coal Research.

When one turns to the industry itself, one finds very little investment in science-based research, especially on the part of the mining companies. Whether a greater investment in research and development would have been beneficial remains a moot point, for as long as the coal industry remained structurally fragmented and only marginally profitable, it could hardly afford to make such an investment. Perhaps in no other area of corporate activity is there such a striking difference between firms at the center and those on the periphery:

> In 1953, the chemical industry's R&D budget of $361 million was 30 times larger than the coal industry's net earnings of $12 million. Of the $17 million spent on coal research in 1955, coal producers (excluding captive operators owned by steel and utility companies) contributed only $2.4 million. The rest came from government sources, equipment manufacturers, and other industrial firms.[64]

Although the coal industry, unlike the science-based industries at the center of the American economy, did not establish a coordinated industrial research program, there was a period during the early decades of this century when certain industrialists with interests in coal mining believed that the newly developed social sciences could help them solve the labor relations problems plaguing the industry. If the marginal character of the industry made it impossible to emulate those industries which were investing heavily in applying the knowledge made available by the physical sciences, perhaps the coal industry could achieve greater stability by making use of the knowledge available in the social sciences. It was a hope that John D. Rockefeller, Jr., found congenial, especially when faced with a violent attempt to unionize the Colorado coal company he owned.

In 1907, 361 miners were killed when a coal mine in Monongah, West Virginia, exploded. Disasters of this magnitude were widely reported and brought the nation as a whole face to face with the agonies that awaited those who mine coal. Although the day-to-day hazards of roof falls and the other dangers associated with working underground killed more miners than did such disasters, these disasters had a dramatic appeal that the press exploited and that created political pressures for federal action. It was felt that something had to be done, and there were plenty of Progressive bureaucrats in Washington eager to seize the moment and use the resources of the federal government to ensure that such outrages would not occur again. The Monongah disaster thus helped create the political conditions that made federal action possible.

Prior to the Monongah explosion, a modest federal research program devoted to the problems of mining had been started within the United States Geological Survey. Thus, when Congress, reacting to the Monongah disaster, authorized a federal program of scientific research and education designed to prevent coal mine disasters, funds were sent first to the Technologic Branch of the Geological survey. It soon became evident, however, that a new agency would have to be created, for the Geological Survey had been established to support scientific geology and was very reluctant to expand its involvement in the practical problems associated with coal mining. Congress therefore authorized the creation of a new Bureau of Mines within the Department of the Interior and approved the appointment of Joseph A. Holmes, the former head of the Technological Branch, as its first director.[65]

The Bureau of Mines had all the features of a child of politics. Its emphasis on scientific investigation reflected the Progressives' faith in the ability of science to provide solutions to the social problems associated with modern industry. It was charged with preventing disasters, even though they were not the chief cause of death in the mines. It was not given any powers of inspection, these being left with the states, and it had no way of ensuring that the steps it recommended to prevent disasters would be followed. It was to investigate the "natural," that is to say the physical, causes of underground explosions and not probe into the social factors and legal responsibilities involved, a limitation that led the *Journal* of the UMWA to complain about turning the new Bureau over to "long-haired theorists." Concentration on "natural" causes also steered the Bureau away from areas of proprietary interest, thereby ensuring that its efforts would not intrude on engineering practice and that its results would be equally applicable to all mines. The mine operators, in general opposed to federal intervention, welcomed a program committed to searching for the causes of disasters, for such an effort would serve to delay and perhaps prevent passage of legislation that might prescribe performance standards and thereby alter the competitive structure of the industry. Clearly, then, the political advantages of a response that stressed scientific research into the causes and prevention of disasters were considerable, whatever the practical utility of such a response.

During its first few years of operation, the Bureau of Mines continued the research and education programs begun under its predecessor, the Technologic Branch of the Geological Survey. These consisted of research into the causes of mine explosions, the development of safer explosives for use underground, and the establishing of mine rescue stations and training programs—all these undertakings being acceptable under the Bureau's mandate. On the question of the causes of mine explosions, European investigators were far in advance of their American colleagues. Their attention had been focused on this problem by the 1906 Courrières explosion in France, in which 1,230 miners had been killed. That mine, like the Monongah mine, was relatively gas free, and subsequent study revealed that the disastrous explosion had been caused by coal dust. The Bureau therefore concentrated on finding ways to alleviate this danger and by 1914 had identified a variety of techniques that were effective, the most important being rock dusting. But getting the industry to use these techniques was not something the Bureau was equipped to do. In the words of William Graebner, "the Bureau could only cajole and reason, and such methods proved inadequate; the nation's operators would not act on available scientific and technological information."[66] Scientific knowledge, when not coupled with immediate economic advantage or prescriptive regulation, proved to have little effect on the practices of the industry.

Attempts to encourage the use of safer explosives developed by the Bureau, called permissibles, encountered similar resistance. Miners traditionally purchased their own explosives, and permissibles were more expensive than those they were designed to replace. Attempts were made at the state level to require their use, but the miners resisted, and as late as 1922, over a dozen years after the first list of permissibles had been published, they still accounted for only 18 percent of the explosives used. As Graebner points out, "experience did not bear out [the] optimistic prediction that the mere existence of a permissible list would have a 'moral effect' almost as great as statutory law."[67] Here, too, the Progressives had overestimated the power and efficacy of scientific knowledge and rational self-interest.

The one Bureau initiative that was taken up with enthusiasm by the industry was the equipping of mine-safety stations and the training of miners in rescue techniques. Organizing and aiding in rescue efforts evidently struck nearly everyone involved as a proper federal response to disasters that were popularly understood to be acts of God. It should be noted, however, that the UMWA was outspoken in insisting that the Bureau spend more of its resources on investigating and preventing disasters and less on rescue. The mine operators, however, were quite happy to have the federal government assume the costs of equipping rescue stations and instructing the miners in rescue techniques. Eager to exploit whatever opportunities were available to mitigate the effects of mine disasters, the Bureau encouraged the growth of rescue-team meets and competitions, events that became and remain popular activities at miner's conventions. Like coastal life-saving stations, volunteer fire departments, and emergency medical services, mine rescue teams provide an institutional focus for community response and hope during periods of "natural" disaster. They also provide a valuable social service, but one that depends only slightly on the involvement of scientifically trained professionals.

By 1915 the Bureau of Mines's concern with coal-mining safety, the concern that had led to its creation, was largely spent. The Bureau's research into the causes of disasters and its efforts to reduce the loss of life in underground explosions were considerable and commendable, but for reasons that had little to do with the Bureau's programs, the incidence of mine disasters declined temporarily. Meanwhile, the carnage of coal mining was displaced in the press by the carnage of battle as the nation geared up to enter World War I. More important, however, was the fact that the coal industry, being notoriously divided and preoccupied with short-range prospects, had failed to develop the kind of constituency pressure needed to ensure a steady flow of federal funds to support research of interest to it. In the absence of public pressure, therefore, Congress and the federal bureaucracy did not feel compelled to concern themselves further with the problems of the coal industry.[68] Meanwhile, other problems requiring federal intervention were arising in the metallurgical industries and in the booming oil industry. Furthermore, these industries were developing the industrial councils and coordinated political programs needed to ensure continued support for the agencies that served them. The coal industry, again handicapped by being peripheral, soon drifted to the periphery of the Bureau of Mines as well.

As the federal commitment to solving the safety problems of the coal industry receded, a very different attempt to use social science to solve the problems of labor relations was underway within the industry. This effort was part of a larger development known to historians as welfare capitalism, a response to the social problems of industrialism that emerged in the 1880s and finally faded into insignificance in the 1930s. Welfare capitalism has been defined as the practice of having the company provide services for the comfort or improvement of employees that are neither necessary for the functioning of the industry nor required by law.[69] While it is comparatively easy to distinguish between productive services and welfare services in some industries, it is seldom evident where this line should be drawn when one is looking at the company towns created to support miners and mining communities in rural settings. Certainly the apologists of welfare capitalism in the coal industry were eager to demonstrate that happy workers were more efficient workers. As the sociological director of the Ellsworth Collieries Company of western Pennsylvania wrote in 1918,

> sociological work, under whatever name, should be of such a character as to influence the life of a workman in such a manner as to establish a cooperative interest in his work, foster within him a spirit of contentment in his home, lead him so to employ his leisure time that he will not lower his efficiency as a workman, destroy his domestic happiness, or endanger his standing in the community as a citizen.[70]

One of the most important goals of welfare capitalism in unorganized companies was to prevent unionization. The strategy for doing so consisted of having the company establish forums for employee representation and provide benefits that would anticipate and neutralize the appeal of unionization. Naturally no one expected the workers to get everything they wanted. The challenge, enlightened capitalists believed, was to convince the workers that they were more likely to secure reasonable wages, acceptable working conditions, and additional benefits by engaging in cooperative negotiation rather than militant confrontation. To do this, channels of communication had to be opened and new forms of representation devised. For advice on these matters, the capitalists turned to social scientists.

In 1913 the United Mineworkers of America struck the Colorado Fuel and Iron Company, which at the time was controlled by the Rockefeller family. As the strike dragged on, it became increasingly embittered and violent. Several members of strikers' families that had been evicted from company housing and were living in a tent colony were killed, an event that was immediately labeled the Ludlow Massacre, and the nation once again watched in dismay as the social antagonisms of modern industrialism raged unchecked.[71] John D. Rockefeller, Jr., was particularly distressed by this strife in one of his companies, and he turned to his young friend Mackenzie King for advice. King, making the best of an opportunity that fit his interests exactly, conducted a thorough study of the problem and then devised the famous Rockefeller Plan for employee representation. Announced in 1915, it became the prototype for innumerable other company unions. Among the many committees to be established under the plan was one on wages and working conditions.

Canadian born and educated, William Lyon Mackenzie King had recently completed a doctorate in economics at Harvard. Deeply impressed by Jane Addams's work with immigrants at Hull House in Chicago, he had made industrial relations the subject of his dissertation. After accepting Rockefeller's request for assistance, he wrote that he intended to use Colorado Fuel and Iron "as a laboratory in which to demonstrate what could be done as a result of applying certain principles in which I firmly [believe].[72] He intended to be scientific, and his research was adorned with the trappings of scientific objectivity, but the assumptions he brought to his study were hardly unprejudiced. He conceived his task to be to construct a system of industrial relations that would encourage negotiation while never allowing evil to dominate good.[73] In the great struggle with the union, the main issues were recognition and collective bargaining, but King believed that working conditions was the real issue. He therefore designed a structure for negotiation that would allow workers to address this more fundamental problem without raising the issue of union recognition. Rockefeller was convinced the strategy had merit and supported its implementation. The hope was that this plan would replace the strife of industrial conflict with a scientifically grounded system of harmonious consultation.

There is no need to linger over the later history of the Rockefeller Plan. The formation of a company union at Colorado Fuel and Iron may have led to some improvements in health and safety, but it did not provide a long-range solution to the problems of the industry.

The sources of contention that made union recognition so essential to the miners were not dispelled by the veneer of scientific reasonableness. An immigrant miner summarized the inadequacy of the company union precisely:

> Company officials good, smart educated men. The representative, he only one man, he got no backing, he got to fight everybody. . . . Under union, miners have educated men who no work for company, but give all their time to take up grievances. Pretty hard for man who works for the company to take up grievances because he afraid that if make the boss mad, maybe he be fired, or given bad place [to work].[74]

In the 1930s, as the UMWA led a massive expansion of industrial unionization, it became clear to everyone that the concept of industrial relations embodied in company unions and the modes of science it drew on could no longer command center stage in the American labor movement. However honest and well-intentioned the architects of the Rockefeller Plan may have been, they had built on sand.

In the 1950s the coal industry faced a bleak future. Production was down although productivity had been rising, and coal's major markets were being lost to other sources of energy. The railroads had been dieselized, oil and gas had captured most of the home heating market, and atomic power, spurred on by extraordinary federal subsidies, was threatening to take over much of the electrical generating market. Spokesmen for the coal industry therefore once again turned to the federal government for relief. In a statement submitted to the Eisenhower administration, a group of coal-company executives pleaded for "changes in administration policies and in the antitrust laws, which would have the effect of encouraging physical consolidations and mergers."[75] What they got, after six long years of political give-and-take, was the Coal Research and Development Act of 1960, which created the Office of Coal Research (OCR) within the Department of the Interior.

How, one wonders, did members of Congress come to be convinced that the structural problems of the industry could be remedied by investing federal funds in research and development? To answer this question, one must recall that for nearly a full generation following the end of World War II, R&D was regarded as a panacea that could be successfully applied to social problems of all sorts. There were, however, more specific reasons as well. In the post-war period the federal government established the Atomic Energy Commission (AEC), one of whose missions was to develop atomic power for an already abundantly supplied energy market. This policy, motivated above all by anxiety over atomic diplomacy and world trade,[76] created a federally subsidized competitor for coal, a consequence that even the most obtuse had to admit was unfair. Because the AEC was politically untouchable, the best way to offset the unwanted consequences of its activities appeared to be to provide comparable support for the coal industry. Surely no one could fault an investment in research and development, even if it was a highly indirect way to achieve the ends sought. Thus, once again the coal industry was offered a form of relief shaped more by political ideology than by the basic needs of the industry.

The short career of OCR and its ultimate demise in the mud of pork-barrel politics need not detain us.[77] Had it managed to revitalize the coal industry by expanding its markets, OCR might have helped lay the economic groundwork for improvements in health and safety. What it did, in fact, was initiate a series of increasingly expensive engineering projects designed to test various processes for turning coal into liquid fuels or synthetic gas. Coal-state congressional leaders competed to have these projects located in their states, and those who captured them then argued annually for increased appropriations. The mining industry, meanwhile, once again demonstrated that it was incapable of developing industrial councils and legislative pressure groups like those which served the petroleum and atomic energy industries so well. As the projects supported by OCR became increasingly expensive and less and less plausible in market terms, resistance to further funding began to build. Because the industry was incapable of sustaining the flow of funds for coal research, the demise of OCR, which began in 1970, also signaled the end of this round of federal support for the coal industry. Overall, the industry was not well served by this particular venture in federally funded science.

In November 1968, seventy-eight miners were killed when a supposedly safe mine in Farmington, West Virginia, located only ten miles from Monongah, exploded. In responding to this disaster the federal government at last accepted responsibility for ensuring that underground coal mining is conducted in a reasonably safe manner. The Coal Mine Health and Safety Act, signed into law in 1969, mandated a broad attack on the problems of underground mining and required a new level of scientific commitment to solving the hazards of the industry. The history of the contemporary era in coal mine health and safety begins with the passage of that act. The politics involved in its passage are discussed in Chapter 5.

Physicians to a Hazardous Industry

The medical profession has a long history of serving those who mine coal. Coal mining is a large, labor-intensive industry. Coal miners for the most part live in geographically isolated settings, a circumstance that places them and their families beyond the reach of medical services located in cities and commercial towns. Among the most dangerous of industries, underground coal mining produces an inordinate number of cases that challenge the physician's ability to preserve life, repair injured bodies, and rehabilitate the disabled. Finally, the mining of coal causes a variety of occupational diseases that require medical attention. The provision of professional medical care to coal miners has therefore long been an activity of considerable scope and importance.

The way in which health care has been organized and provided within the coal industry reflects the social and institutional structure of the industry itself. Like the industry's engineers, doctors whose practices lie entirely within the industry—and this has been the norm rather than the exception—have been obliged to adapt their attitudes and practices as professionals to the circumstances in which they work. Once this organizational accommodation has been made, physicians have found that the level of medical care they can offer depends directly upon the economic fortunes of the community in which they work.

Although physicians working in the coal fields are by the nature of their work constantly being reminded of the health and safety hazards of coal mining, in practice they have been able to do little more than repair the miners' broken bodies after damage has been done. It would certainly be cynical to suggest that these doctors and other health professionals, committed as they are to the preservation of health, have been insensitive to the pain and suffering of those in their care. It would, however, be equally naive to assume that the disparity between their goals as professionals and their experience with this industry has inevitably fueled an intense if suppressed outrage over the circumstances in which those in their care have labored. This kind of outrage has, to be sure, been expressed by certain medi-

cal professionals ever since coal mining has been a significant industry, and it has frequently inspired campaigns to reform the industry;
but such a response to the health and safety problems of coal mining
has almost always been championed by physicians and others who are
not themselves directly involved with (or, more tellingly, dependent
upon) the industry itself.

The organization of medical care in mining communities has long
been structured in a way that reflects both the distinctive traditions of
mining and the fundamental polarization of the industry. While several state-funded hospitals for miners were established in Pennsylvania during the nineteenth century, miners have in general looked to
the industry itself for the funds needed to support adequate medical
care facilities.[78] Until the end of World War II, these funds were
provided by the miners themselves through prepayment plans administered by the coal companies.[79] One of John L. Lewis's proudest
achievements was transfering the cost of the miners' prepaid health
plans to the operators while capturing control of the administration of
the funds for the union. Under both arrangements, however, physicians were paid by the funds to provide medical care on a prepaid and
fixed-fee basis.

The first of these health funds was established in the early 1860s
by Cornish miners working in the Michigan copper fields. Each
month the mining companies deducted a fixed sum, arbitrarily set at a
dollar a month for married men and 50 cents for bachelors, from the
wages of the miner, in return for which a company doctor treated the
miner and his family. This system, in which the company employed
the physician and administered the funds contributed by the workers,
soon became widespread, and by the beginning of the present century, miners from the coal fields of West Virginia to the iron fields of
Minnesota were paying the same fees.[80]

During the early decades of the twentieth century, when the
medical arts were less highly specialized than they are today, the
prepayment plans established by miners were evidently capable of
providing an acceptable level of health services—at least such was the
conclusion of a 1923 Department of Labor survey of health care in
West Virginia:

> The check-off had risen by then to $.75–$1.25 for single men and $1.50–
> $2.00 for married men, with an additional charge of $7–$25 for maternal
> care. Each physician usually covered an area of riverbed homes from

one to three miles long housing fewer than 200 families. In one section of eleven company towns there were three hospitals and two of the towns were served by a public health nurse. More than 90 percent of the mothers had a doctor in attendance at births, and infant mortality figures (ninety-four deaths per thousand live births before age one) were in line with contemporary rates.[81]

The persistence of this way of organizing medical care in the coal fields was amply documented in the famous Boone Report of 1947.[82] In 1946 Lewis, who had by then been head of the UMWA for over twenty-five years, led the coal miners out on what turned out to be a long strike. When it became apparent that certain industries, most notably steel and electric power, that were essential for post-war reconstruction soon would have to shut down, President Truman seized the mines by executive order and told the miners to go back to work. Lewis welcomed the order, for he knew he could negotiate a better contract with the government than he could win from the operators and that the operators would have to accept the terms of the federal settlement to regain control of the mines. Lewis also recognized in this federal intervention an opportunity to transfer the cost of health to the operators. He therefore insisted that the new contract commit the government to making a survey of medical conditions in the bituminous coal fields. "The purpose of this survey," the contract declared, "will be to determine the character and scope of improvements which should be made to provide the mine workers of the Nation with medical, housing and sanitary facilities conforming to recognized American standards."[83] Admiral Boone of the Navy Medical Corps was told to organize and conduct the survey, and the report he prepared became a landmark in the history of the coal industry and in the history of American public health.

The Boone survey found that despite vast changes in American society and in the practice of medicine elsewhere, medical care in the coal fields continued to be organized around the prepayment system.

> Tradition and custom have perpetuated the system; and today, even in areas where many coal-mining communities are near urban centers, camp doctors still are found. There are long valleys and hollows in the Appalachians and broad canyons in the western Rockies dotted with mines and populated heavily enough to make it appear that physicians could practice profitably without the incentive of prepayment plans, yet the prepayment system of medical care persists. Despite the extensive development of communications and transportation and the expansion of population in

many of these areas, which have modified their insularity, a psychology of isolation survives. Each mining camp feels that it must have its own doctor; each camp or small group of camps continues a prepayment medical-care plan of its own. Thus, the over-all picture of medical care is that of very numerous, small prepayment schemes of a type originally established to provide medical care when the individual patient had little, if any, opportunity for choice of physicians.[84]

As the Boone Report noted, providing medical care by means of prepayment plans and company doctors undercut the physician's professional autonomy and created opportunities for abuse that both the operators and the union had not been slow to exploit.

Both Management and Labor appear in a few instances to have abused their responsibilities and privileges. This is evidenced by the fact that the physicians were not selected primarily on the basis of professional qualification and the character of facilities and services that were offered, but on the basis of personal friendships, financial tie-ups, social viewpoints, or other nonmedical considerations. Competition among doctors for prepayment contracts may be quite brisk. The quality of professional services that can be offered is a bargaining point, but it is known that doctors have occasionally obtained contracts by their talents for ingratiating themselves with company officials or influencing leaders of the Union.

Several instances were noted where poorly qualified physicians or others not appropriately licensed are receiving the pay-roll deduction for medical care. . . .

Management may exert considerable influence upon the selection of physicians by withholding company-owned office space or living quarters from a doctor whose appointment is not approved by the operator. Management is generally of the opinion that it is wholly within its rights if it refuses to make a pay-roll deduction for transmittal to a physician whose selection it has not approved.[85]

As the Boone Report made clear, the miners had little control over the medical system they supported, a system the operators not infrequently abused for such other purposes as lowering operating costs or increasing their control of the workforce. This system, which was administered by management, was supposed to provide general health care for coal-mining communities and, insofar as the special dangers of the industry were concerned, help miners deal with the injuries and disabilities they suffered as a result of working in the mines. It was not a system designed to discover and mitigate the causes of miners' accidents and diseases. The role of the coal-field physician was to provide treatment, not to interfere with the organization of production by campaigning for preventive measures, and the social circumstances in which he practiced made broadening his range of concern extremely difficult and professionally hazardous. And it is important to note that although John L. Lewis was successful in transfering the cost of the health-care system to the operators and control to the union, he did not call for a reconceptualization of the system's purpose. Thus, until the federal government intervened in 1969, the predominant view within the industry continued to be that as far as occupational health and safety were concerned, the duty of physicians was to cure, not prevent, injury and disease.[86]

The health and welfare program Lewis created had two funds: a welfare and retirement fund financed by a 5-cent-per-ton levy paid by the operators, and a medical and hospital fund financed by pooling the payments being made to the existing medical funds.[87] Founded in 1946, the UMWA Health and Retirement Fund soon established a record of heroic achievement and tragic inadequacy. It "made the coal operators financially responsible for the health and welfare of miners and their dependents, from the cradle to the grave, and started a revolution in health care delivery throughout the coalfields in the South and Midwest."[88] The operators' royalty payments were increased during the early years of the Fund, so that by 1952 they were paying 40 cents per ton. By that date Lewis had also installed himself as chairman of the Fund's three trustees, while his protégé Josephine Roche served as the "neutral" trustee.[89] In the 1950s the Fund built a series of Miners' Memorial Hospitals in the coal fields and launched a massive rehabilitation program for injured miners. But when the market for coal collapsed in the late 1950s, the Fund's financial base began to shrink. By 1962 it was forced to sell the Miners' Hospitals, and by the end of the decade a variety of factors, including the corruption of Lewis's successors, had fatally undermined the Fund. Although utterly transformed by subsequent reorganizations, the Fund will always occupy a place of honor in the history of the American coal industry.

The actual experience of caring for miners and their dependents varied from one community to another and from one year to the next, the controlling factor being the relative affluence and economic security of the mining company involved. Here, as in so many areas of the industry, the corporate structure of the industry was crucial. Small, undercapitalized coal operations that moved in and out of production in response to short-term cycles in the market for coal and hovered on the edge of bankruptcy were hardly in a position to make major investments in improved health facilities for the settlements in which their miners lived. The coal camps associated with such companies therefore generally had the unsanitary and ramshackle appearance commonly and justifiably called to mind by the term "company town." Medical care in such circumstances was equally primitive, its availability depending entirely upon the ability of the miners to continue their payments to the medical plan.

But there were also coal companies that were well capitalized and that built company towns designed to provide their inhabitants with the amenities enjoyed by workers in comparable industries elsewhere. Many of these towns were built by steel companies when they opened mines that were to send their entire output directly to the parent company's mills. These so-called captive mines were thus assured a stable market, administered prices, and protection from direct competition with independent coal suppliers. These companies therefore had both the means and the long-range commitment needed to build attractive and durable coal-field towns, and many of them did so.

Wheelwright, Kentucky, was one such company town.[90] Located in one of eastern Kentucky's tight mountain valleys, Wheelwright was settled in 1916 when its first coal mine was opened, even though the nearest rail line was still 18 miles away. It remained a typical coal camp until 1930, when the Inland Steel Company bought the mineral rights to the coal in the area and set about turning Wheelwright into a model company town. The first order of business, of course, was to rehabilitate the mine itself, which was worked by members of the UMWA, and after that task was well underway, improvements in the town were begun. The valley in which the town was located is only a mile and a half long and when fully settled could accommodate a population of only 3,600. To improve the community, the company built a water filtration plant and piped water into every home, paved the town's one street, tapped a local gas well and made gas available to all houses, installed an automatic telephone system, built a sewage collection system and a sewage disposal plant, arranged to have plumbing installed in every house, assisted with other housing renovations and additions, built a garbage and trash incinerator, loaned money to the county to build the first of four new school buildings, built a town swimming pool, and constructed a community center that included a small public library. To improve the town's medical facilities, the company reequipped the small hospital and recruited a medical staff of three doctors, a technician, and two nurses. House and office calls averaged 150 per day, and several programs for sanitary improvement and innoculation were begun. The justification for such an investment was in no way tainted by welfarism we are told in a report on Wheelwright: "Wheelwright was planned and created, not in the futile hope of gratitude, but out of one sober conviction: That doing everything possible to make a wholesome, attractive community would prove to be thoroughly 'good business.' "

Living in Wheelwright must have been infinitely more pleasant than living in a squalid coal camp, even if from a professional point of view the physicians in Wheelwright had no more autonomy than their colleagues in other company towns. But the number of towns like Wheelwright was small. The large corporations that opened captive mines avoided owning more than about half of the coal-mining capacity they needed. The remainder of the coal they required was purchased on the open market, an arrangement that enabled them to keep their own mines in operation in all but the worst of times. The towns these corporations built were thus islands of prosperity and propriety in a larger sea of insecurity and impoverishment, and they should not be seen as models of the way all company towns could have been, had their owners and inhabitants only cared enough. Indeed, the exceptional nature of such model towns was emphasized by the author of the report on Wheelwright: "It is always a keenly satisfying experience to undertake a project that is unorthodox, that does not have to be done—and see it develop into something sound and worthy. Wheelwright is such a project. There were few, if any precedents for what was done. There was ample precedent for doing nothing—for simply carrying on in the accustomed mining-camp tradition." And, as *The New York Times* labor reporter A. H. Raskin observed in 1947, it was the traditional coal camp that one usually encountered when one traveled in the coal fields:

> There are some towns, I am told, in which the homes are neat, the streets well-tended, the sanitary and recreational facilities up-to-date. The number of such towns is regrettably small. In three weeks of traveling through Pennsylvania and West Virginia, the country's two biggest coal-producing states, the best coal town I saw was on the level of the slum districts one sees from a pullman window on the outskirts of a big city.[91]

Although physicians who cared for miners and their families were hardly in a position to carry on research into the causes of work-related diseases or campaign for measures designed to prevent them, such research and such campaigns were carried on by physicians and others not directly dependent upon those who mine coal. The record of their efforts is noteworthy and laudable, even if on the whole the effect of their exertions on the actual conduct of coal mining was slight. These efforts can be characterized, not unfairly, as Progressive attempts to reform an industry that remained by and large (at least until the 1960s) obdurately unprogressive in its internal structure and therefore immune to persuasion from without. One cannot help applauding the goals of the social reformers involved, but one should avoid overvaluing the significance of their efforts.[92]

Among the specific problems in the coal industry that cried out for reform are several occupational diseases that, in addition to accidents, have made mining an especially hazardous industry.[93] The most important of these afflictions results from the inhalation of coal dust and has been given a variety of names, including miner's asthma and black lung.[94] Unfortunately, accurately diagnosing the various lung diseases associated with mining and establishing the etiology of each is an exceedingly complex problem. As is so often the case, the inability to provide unassailable answers to questions regarding the distinguishing symptoms of the alleged illness, the immediate cause of the condition, and the incidence of affliction has frequently been considered a justification for denying that the problem exists. Long clinical experience with miners persuaded many coal-field physicians years ago that there was a problem, but they were seldom able to construct arguments capable of convincing those physicians who, like most of the miners themselves, were inclined to brush aside the suggestion that the prolonged inhalation of coal dust could cause lung damage. Thus, the author of a 1935 article on "Anthraco Silicosis" published in a Pennsylvania medical journal could blithely report that " 'miners' asthma' is considered an ordinary condition that need cause no worry, and therefore the profession has not troubled itself about the finer pathological and clinical manifestations."[95]

The path that finally brought the medical profession, the coal industry, and the federal government to a direct engagement with the problem of black lung led through the forest of legal compensation rather than from an immediate concern with the prevention of occupational disease. In the late 1920s British medical investigators began the difficult task of distinguishing between silicosis and the pathologies caused by coal dust itself, which they later labeled pneumoconiosis.[96] In the 1930s some disabled British coal miners began receiving worker's compensation benefits for silicosis, even though many physicians believed their symptoms were caused by coal dust rather than silica. In the 1930s and 1940s the British mounted a sustained research effort focused on the diagnosis and prevention of disabling lung diseases among coal miners. The results of these efforts were read with interest in the United States, and as early as 1952 Alabama became the first state to provide compensation for coal workers' pneumoconiosis; yet little was done, and nothing was mandated, concerning prevention.[97] In the early 1950s the UMWA Welfare and Retirement Fund launched a program designed to increase professional understanding of chest diseases among miners, but as in the area of safety, responsibility for actually doing something about the problem, either through prevention or compensation, was assumed to lie with management.

Although workers who contract diseases as a result of the conditions in which they work certainly deserve to be compensated, only in 1969, after nearly seventy years of experience with workmen's compensation laws, was it generally perceived that a legally mandated right to financial compensation for damage is no substitute for legally mandating the prevention of occupational diseases.[98] To establish a claim to compensation, one must satisfy a judge or an administrator acting as a legal officer that the affliction alleged has been accurately diagnosed, that the degree of disability is as claimed, and that the affliction was indeed caused by conditions that prevailed in the place of employment. Companies have an interest in minimizing the number of claims allowed, for they must pay the premiums set by the insurance companies that pay valid claims. In theory this interest should provide an incentive to clean up the workplace so as to prevent occupational diseases, which in coal mining would require reducing dust levels. In practice, however, coal companies have relied on lawyers to contest claims made for compensation and, when this tactic has failed, on the federal government to bail them out when the cost of compensation has become onerous. This response, while harsh from the workers' point of view, is entirely understandable from a business point of view, for few coal companies enjoy the control of markets, the steady level of profit, and the institutional stability that would justify long-range programs aimed at improving working conditions. It is ironic that throughout this century, safety engineers have worked hard to control coal dust levels in mines so as to prevent explosions, which cause business as well as human disasters, whereas it took a federal law explicitly concerned with occupational disease to get them to control the coal dust that has for generations been destroying miners' lungs.

Physicians have played an important if not dominant role in the campaign for occupational disease compensation and prevention in the coal industry. In the 1960s several coal-field physicians were active in the black-lung movement and thereby exposed themselves to the charge of placing political conviction above scientific objectivity.[99] However, because the focus throughout that decade was on compensation rather than prevention, most of the coal-field physicians who got involved in fact put their medical expertise at the service of the lawyers defending compensation cases.[100] Collectively, as represented by state and national medical organizations, physicians were very uneasy about the approach to health problems that was evolving in the coal fields. The American Medical Association strongly opposed the role assigned to physicians by the UMWA Welfare and Retirement Fund, and the medical organizations in those states considering recognizing black lung as a compensable disease remained aloof when they did not join the coal companies in active opposition.[101] After reviewing the history of his nation's efforts to identify, treat, and prevent black lung, a British author concluded, "It must be admitted that medical men by their ill-informed complacency have a heavy load of responsibility to bear for this failure to discover the true state of affairs, a failure which constitutes what is probably the greatest disgrace in the history of British medicine."[102] If this harsh judgment of the part played by organized medicine is appropriate for Great Britain, the nation that pioneered in the diagnosis and prevention of coal workers' pneumoconiosis, how much more severe must the verdict be with regard to the role played by organized medicine in the United States?

Professional Ideals and Institutional Realities

Viewed analytically, professionals can be distinguished from other members of society in terms of the knowledge they command and the purposes that guide their actions.[103] A necessary condition for being a professional is possession of a specialized body of knowledge in the field in which one is an expert. This knowledge need not be scientific or science based, as indeed it is not in the case of the law and the ministry; but in a great many modern professions, including engineering, science itself, and medicine, science—the preeminent form of rationality in modern culture—is central to professional expertise. A second necessary condition for being a professional is a commitment to service that goes beyond the individual interests of the individual practitioner. In science this commitment is expressed as a dedication to discovering truth, while in the more immediately practical professions, the commitment to service takes the form of a commitment to social justice. Professionals claim to be, and generally are considered, privileged members of society in terms of both the authority granted to them and their levels of remuneration. Their privileged status is not seen as inequitable, however, because they are expected to subordinate selfishness and fear to their duty to serve the public good.

It is quite reasonable, given this characterization of professional norms, to expect that when professionals direct their attention to practical problems such as occupational health and safety, they will use their expert knowledge to discover the problems' underlying causes and then, guided by their commitment to the public good, seek to control the problems' occurrence in a way that is most advantageous to all concerned. Professionals, autonomous in their investigations and responsible in their interventions, act through social institutions without being beholden to them. But as has been pointed out in considerable detail, this view of the professional's role hardly describes the way engineers, scientists, and physicians have engaged the health and safety problems of the coal industry during the first seven decades of this century. In actual practice and with very few exceptions, the ways in which they have applied their knowledge and the goals they have served were set by the industry or by the other institutions within which they have worked. And as far as engagement of the problems of health and safety is concerned, they have spent far more time responding to disasters than seeking to remedy the conditions that make underground mining such hazardous work.

Why this great disparity between expectations and practice? Unless the characteristic norms of the professional or the ways in which professionals actually acted in the coal industry have been misdescribed, perhaps the origins of the disparity can be traced back to the industry itself. Indeed, it may be that the very features of the coal industry that made it peripheral within the structure of American industry also created constraints that denied the professionals employed in it the autonomy they needed to fulfill their obligations as professionals. On first encounter this appears to be a likely explanation.

This hypothesis can be examined most easily by asking if the coal industry as an institution has granted special standing to the expert knowledge of the professionals in question or to their supposed commitment to the public good. Obviously, some of the knowledge they had to offer was considered valuable or they would not have found a place in the industry, whereas in fact engineers were hired to organize and supervise production, and physicians were hired to provide medical care for miners and their dependents. But scientific and science-based knowledge had no special authority within the industry; hence, possession of such knowledge in no way legitimized interventions that ranged beyond what management considered appropriate. The same is true of professional commitment to serving the public good. Coal operators struggled to survive in a harsh, competitive environment. If they focused on long-range planning, they were likely to fail in the short run, and if they sought comprehensive solutions to the social problems associated with their industry, they were apt to be eliminated by those who did not. Professional knowledge was legitimated within the industry to the extent it helped them survive; professional concern with service was legitimated insofar as it served the company. To expect a peripheral industry such as coal mining to be more supportive of the wider concerns of its professionals is naive. Coal operators could not afford to even had they been so inclined, and not many of them were.

To really test whether the constraints the coal industry placed on its professionals arose from its being institutionally peripheral, one would have to determine whether engineers, scientists, and physicians in center industries enjoyed greater autonomy. Although this is not the place to pursue this comparison in detail, certain points of contrast are immediately apparent. Whereas peripheral industries lacked the stability, hence the long-range perspective, required to support extensive research and development, many center industries, and most notably those based on scientific knowledge, established industrial research laboratories that gave science a prominence and legitimacy it lacked in other companies. It is certainly not true that all technology-intensive industries were patrons of pure science, but the importance of creating and applying new knowledge was clearly more appreciated in center industries than in peripheral industries. In such circumstances the authority of the expert was likely to carry more weight.

The size, hence the visibility, of center industries also had an effect on their managers' attitudes toward professionals. In industries in which production was in the hands of a small number of large corporations, maintaining a benign public opinion of the corporations was critical. Such companies functioned as quasi-public bodies and had to ensure that their treatment of their employees, their customers, and their neighbors was perceived to conform to contemporary standards. This concern made them at least receptive to the service ethic of the professions and led many center companies to be concerned about worker health and safety, as later they would become concerned about environmental pollution, long before they were obliged to do so by statutory regulations. There were therefore more opportunities to function as a professional within a center industry than in a peripheral industry, even though for most engineers, scientists, and physicians, the differences were not great.

Another way of getting at the problem of the great disparity between professional expectations and professional performance in the coal industry is to turn away from the context defined by the industry and look instead at the professions themselves. Whereas the relationship of the professional to his or her workplace is usually analyzed in individual/institutional terms, clearly the professions are themselves institutions as well. We might then ask what kind of institutions the professions of medicine, science, and engineering were during the first seven decades of this century. More pointedly, and to continue with the mode of analysis we have been using, were these three professions center or peripheral institutions?

Center industries, it will be recalled, organize so as to internalize transactions, a move that shields these transactions from the market by bringing them under administrative control. They have also been characterized as capital, technology, and energy intensive. Although there appears to be no good analogue for energy intensity in the professions, one can ask which professions are education intensive (education being a form of capital) and which are knowledge intensive (technology being a form of knowledge). A center profession, to press the analogy, will have established a high degree of autonomy in coordinating the supply of professionals and the demand for them; it will have effective control over the internal management of its affairs; it will be responsible for validating and establishing the significance of new knowledge in its area of expertise; and it will be largely successful in its attempts to demonstrate that the way in which its members conduct their professional affairs serves the public good. Professions that lack these attributes will be classified as peripheral.

The medical profession in the twentieth century certainly seems to qualify as a center profession. Following the reform of medical education early in the century, entry into the profession was restricted to those who had the educational capital represented by the M.D. degree. The increased emphasis on scientific medicine also raised the level of formal knowledge-intensity associated with being a physician. As advances in medical knowledge brought greater power over disease, the profession of medicine gained ever greater power over its own affairs. Through its oversight of medical schools and their curricula, the profession internalized control over the content of professional training and the rate at which new doctors were produced. Through its control of state certification, it regulated the accrediting of practitioners. Through its leadership in the allocation of research funds provided by private foundations and such federal agencies as the National Institutes of Health, the profession controlled the creation and evaluation of new knowledge. And through its emphasis on the sanctity of the doctor-patient relationship and the advantages of the private health-care system, the medical profession succeeded in convincing the public at large that its members serve the public good.

Whether or not the medical profession has lived up to its image, it certainly has represented the ideal center profession for many decades. Its scientific and service norms have been clearly articulated, and doctors have been widely perceived to be following them in practice. As an institution the medical profession has gained a high degree of autonomy in selected areas of activity, most notably in education, certification, research, and private practice, and it has largely dominated decisionmaking in the institutions in which these activities take place. It should be noted, however, that other forms of transaction that might have been brought under the control of the profession have not been internalized, occupational health being one of the foremost. Perhaps the profession should have been more concerned about such relatively neglected medical problems, but like captains of industry engaged in vertical integration, the captains of the medical profession were building an institution designed to concentrate rather than dissipate their control over the transactions they believed they needed to internalize. As doctors they no doubt wished to rid the world of disease, but as leaders of a highly institutionalized profession they had to avoid coming into conflict with other institutions they could not dominate. That they served themselves and their profession well while also serving the nation is well known. That the carefully nutured institutional autonomy of their profession nevertheless remained vulnerable to the kinds of criticism that have long been directed at center industries has also in recent years become increasingly evident.[104]

Science, like medicine, has managed to transform itself into a center profession. As with medicine, entry into the profession requires a doctorate, and science is by definition knowledge intensive. Because the knowledge scientists produce is used almost exclusively by other scientists, control over the rate at which practitioners are produced has not been a major problem for leaders of the scientific profession—those who fail to stay active in research do not pose a threat to the profession because they no longer compete for the funds that sustain it. It has been vitally important, however, that the content of science curricula and the certification of those entering the profession remain under professional control, and this has been largely achieved. Scientists have also established effective control over the production and evaluation of new knowledge. By orchestrating the influence of such institutions as the National Science Board, the American Association for the Advancement of Science, and the National Academy of Sciences, the leaders of science direct the flow of research funds that supports their profession. And until the late 1960s, scientists, like physicians, were sustained in their efforts by a widespread belief that what they do as professionals ultimately serves the common good.

Although ever since World War II scientists have shown an extraordinary ability to secure public funds, the institutional heartland of science in America has long been the university. The profession of science is most deeply and thoroughly entrenched in the major research universities where, in conjunction with ongoing research, future scientists are trained. University scientists continue to be inspired by the ideal of pure research, whatever rhetorical gymnastics they may be obliged to engage in to obtain funds, and the contrast with federal mission-oriented research and industrial product-oriented research is starkly drawn. This is not to say that professional scientists are necessarily disdainful of practical matters, but rather that within their hierarchy of values, the unfettered pursuit of knowledge stands supreme. That pursuit is what ennobles science, and it is the goal, professional scientists believe, to which the best people in science should devote their lives. Given this value structure, it is hardly surprising that scientists have not been encouraged by their profession to discover and control the causes of occupational accidents and diseases. Viewed an an institution, the profession of science simply is not concerned with such problems.

Determining whether the profession of engineering should be considered central or peripheral is a more difficult task. The importance of the work done by engineers in modern society is not in question, but the institutional characteristics of their profession may be such that, like the coal industry, it should be classified as structurally peripheral. Engineering is not education intensive in the same way that medicine and science are, for the B.S. degree serves as the entry degree for this profession. And although some forms of engineering are undeniably technology intensive, for many engineers the science and technology they learn in college, as perhaps supplemented by occasional short courses, suffices. As Herbert Hoover insisted in a statement quoted earlier, the "vast preponderance of the commercial over the technical" characterizes the daily work of the engineer.

Indeed, it is the intermingling of the commercial and the technical that has prevented engineering from establishing a professional identity as distinct as those of medicine and science. Whereas scientists not engaged in research are regarded as outside the peer group competent to evaluate research proposals and results, engineers continue to be considered engineers even when functioning entirely as managers. Both the commercial and the technical sides of engineering are well-represented in engineering societies, in the engineering curriculum, in the design of engineering research, and in the public perception of how engineering serves the common good. Engineering employment is also more responsive to short-term economic fluctuations than is the case in science and medicine. In many ways, therefore, engineering looks less like a learned profession, such as science, or a vertically integrated practical profession, such as medicine, and more like a loosely connected set of small businesses. And if this is so, it can with justice be called structurally peripheral.

Engineering also differs from medicine and science in that it has not achieved hegemony within its primary institution, which is the business corporation. The engineer in the corporation encounters more value conflict than a doctor in a hospital or a scientist in a research lab. The professions of medicine and science provide unambiguous guidance as to how a professional ought to act, however inappropriate this guidance or the individual's actions may be in practice, and they control certain key institutions in which those values are treated as preeminent. But the engineer, even if he or she works for a center corporation, is always having to adjudicate between technical considerations, where the methods and findings of science pertain, and commercial considerations, where the values of business are of greatest importance. Because it lacks distinctive values and significant institutions of its own, professional engineering seems incapable of internalizing the transactions of its members and therefore has little of the autonomy of medicine and science. Like coal mining, engineering plays a large and vital part in industrial society, but it does so as a peripheral rather than as a center profession.

This chapter began with an analysis of the coal industry's institutional characteristics and has concluded with an analysis of the institutional characteristics of three professions, many of whose members worked in or for that industry. The chapter has emphasized institutional analysis because clarifying institutional commitments within the industry and within the professions seems to be the best way to respond to the question posed at the outset. That question, once asked, immediately calls for an explanation of a nonevent: Why didn't engineers, scientists, and physicians do more to discover and control the causes of occupational health and safety problems in underground coal mining? They did not do so, it seems, because the institutions they worked with and through neither required them to do so nor would have supported such an undertaking.

There is another reason to concentrate on institutions rather than individuals. Throughout the first seven decades of this century, everyone involved with the coal industry wanted to reduce the health and safety hazards of coal mining, but few worked steadily toward this end. Most hoped that the longed-for improvement would come as a happy consequence of reaching some other goal that they considered more pressing. But such hopes were illusory and served merely to deflect attention away from the problems of health and safety. These problems were not in fact seriously engaged until they were addressed directly and the continued operation of the industry was made conditional on their alleviation. Effective reform occurred when relevant institutional commitments were authoritatively and irrevocably reordered. The lesson one can draw from this is that reforming institutions is the most and perhaps the only effective way to achieve enduring social reform.

Notes

1. Cambridge, Mass.: Harvard University Press, 1977.
2. Ibid., p. 5; see also Louis Galambos, "The Emerging Organizational

Synthesis in Modern American History," *Business History Review* 44 (1970): 279–290.

3. For an excellent recent historical overview of the coal industry, see Curtis Seltzer, *Fire in the Hole—Miners and Managers in the American Coal Industry* (Lexington, Ky.: University of Kentucky Press, 1985).

4. Arthur Donovan, "Carboniferous Capitalism: Excess Productive Capacity and Institutional Backwardness in the U.S. Coal Industry," in Arthur L. Donovan (ed.), *Energy in American History,* a special double issue of *Materials and Society,* 7 (1983): 265–278.

5. Chandler, *The Visible Hand,* pp. 240–241.

6. Ibid., p. 242.

7. The option of nationalization, long advocated by miners both within and outside the United Mine Workers of America, was no longer considered credible after 1920, even though all other industrialized nations with extensive coal industries opted for nationalization as the way to deal with the institutional problems of coal mining in the twentieth century. The dismissal of this option was part of the demise of socialism in America following World War I.

8. Indianapolis, Ind.: Bell Publishing.

9. Ibid., p. 41. For a somewhat more extended discussion of this point, see Donovan, "Carboniferous Capitalism," pp. 270–274.

10. For the most recent and most extensive account of Lewis and his career, see Melvyn Dubofsky and Warren Van Tine, *John L. Lewis* (New York: Quadrangle, 1977).

11. Seltzer, *Fire in the Hole,* p. 61.

12. See C. L. Christenson, *Economic Redevelopment in Bituminous Coal: The Special Case of Technological Advance in United States Coal Mines, 1930–1960* (Cambridge, Mass.: Harvard University Press, 1962).

13. Quoted in Seltzer, *Fire in the Hole,* p. 66.

14. For discussions of the likelihood of such a transformation's being fully achieved, see Mel Horwitch, "Coal: Constrained Abundance," in Robert Stobaugh and Daniel Yergin (eds.), *Energy Future* (New York: Random House, 1979), and Seltzer, *Fire in the Hole,* Ch. 13, "The Future of Coal."

15. Carlton Jackson, *The Dreadful Month* (Bowling Green, Ohio: Bowling Green State University Popular Press, 1982), p. 3.

16. For a brief discussion of the attempt made in 1916 to establish uniform state mining laws, an attempt that failed because the representatives from Ohio and West Virginia refused to participate, see William Graebner, "Great Expectations: The Search for Order in Bituminous Coal, 1890–1917," *Business History Review* 48 (1973): 52.

17. Dubofsky and Van Tine, *Lewis,* pp. 376–377.

18. Seltzer, *Fire in the Hole,* p. 101.

19. Dubofsky and Van Tine, *Lewis,* p. 501.

20. George H. Love, *An Exciting Century in Coal! (1864–1964)* (New York: Newcomen Society in North America, 1955), p. 16.

21. In Thomas K. McCraw (ed.), *Regulation in Perspective* (Cambridge, Mass.: Harvard University Press, 1981); see also Thomas K. McCraw, *Prophets of Regulation* (Cambridge, Mass.: Harvard Uiversity Press, 1984).

22. McCraw, *Regulation in Perspective,* pp. 1–6.

23. Ibid., p. 11.

24. Ibid., p. 17.

25. Ibid., p. 21.

26. Ibid., pp. 18–19.

27. Ibid., p. 22.

28. See James P. Johnson, *The Politics of Soft Coal: The Bituminous Industry from World War I Through the New Deal* (Urbana, Illinois: University of Illinois Press, 1979), pp. 19–31; see also Graebner, "Great Expectations."

29. Johnson, *Politics of Soft Coal,* pp. 34–51.

30. Francis S. Peabody, "Coal Wastage," *Transactions of the American Institute of Mining Engineers* 57 (1917): 499–513.

31. Ibid., p. 501.

32. Ibid., p. 502.

33. See the discussion following Peabody's paper in his "Coal Wastage," pp. 505–513.

34. See Johnson, *Politics of Soft Coal,* ch. 4–8; Ellis W. Hawley, "Secretary Hoover and the Bituminous Coal Problem, 1921–1928," *Business History Review,* 42 (1968): 248–270.

35. See Johnson, *Politics of Soft Coal.*

36. See Donovan, "Carboniferous Capitalism."

37. See C. K. Yearley, Jr., *Enterprise and Anthracite: Economics and Democracy in Schuylkill County, 1820–1874,* The Johns Hopkins Studies in Historical and Political Science, Series 74 (Baltimore: Johns Hopkins University Press, 1961); and Anthony F. C. Wallace, "The Ventilation of Coal Mines," ch. 3 in his *The Social Context of Innovation* (Princeton: Princeton University Press, 1982).

38. Many metropolitan literary leftists of the 1920s and 1930s were fascinated by coal miners, whom they took to be prototypical proletarians and thus potential revolutionaries.

39. Peabody, "Coal Wastage," discussion on p. 513.

40. For figures on U.S. engergy industry concentration ratios from 1955 to 1975, see Richard H. K. Vietor, *Energy Policy in America Since 1945* (Cambridge: Cambridge University Press, 1984), p. 211.

41. Quoted in Robert H. Wiebe, "The Anthracite Strike of 1902: A Record of Confusion," *The Mississippi Valley Historical Review* 48 (1961–1962): 243.

42. Ibid., 241–242.

43. Quoted in McAlister Coleman, *Men and Coal,* reprint (New York: Arno, 1969), p. 70.

44. Wiebe, "Anthracite Strike," p. 242. A similar exchange occurred in

England during the coal strikes of 1926, when Prime Minister Stanley Baldwin asked a group of churchmen who wished to act as mediators how they would like it if he invited the Iron and Steel Federation to take over the revision of the Athanasian Creed; Jane Kramer, "Letter from Europe," *The New Yorker,* 15 April 1985, p. 80.

45. It is ironic that President Wilson, having taken charge of coal marketing in 1917, created such serious shortages that he was forced to call upon the industrialists for relief; see Johnson, *Politics of Soft Coal,* p. 53. For an account of President Carter's mismanagement of the 1977–1978 strike, see Seltzer, *Fire in the Hole,* ch. 10.

46. W. P. Tams, Jr., *The Smokeless Coal Fields of West Virginia, a Brief History* (Morgantown, West Va.: West Virginia University Library, 1963), p. 28.

47. W. J. Schuster, "Safety in the Mechanical Mining of Coal," *Transactions of the American Institute of Mining and Metallurgical Engineers* 199 (1954): 524–526.

48. Keith Dix, *Work Relations in the Coal Industry: The Hand-Loading Era, 1880–1930* (Morgantown, West Va.: West Virginia University Institute for Labor Studies, 1977), p. 42.

49. Ibid., p. 43.

50. Schuster, "Safety," p. 526.

51. John Randolph Haynes, "A Federal Mining Commission," *American Labor Legislation Review* 2 (1912): 148–149.

52. Edwin T. Layton, Jr., *The Revolt of the Engineers* (Cleveland, Ohio: Case Western Reserve University Press, 1971), p. 33.

53. Ibid., p. 95.

54. Ibib., p. 12.

55. Ibid., p. 14.

56. Herbert Hoover, *Principles of Mining* (New York: Hill Publishing, 1909), p. 185.

57. Edwin M. Chance, "Portable Miners' Lamps," *Transactions of the American Institute of Mining Engineers* 57 (1917): 198.

58. It is interesting to note that the sociologist William Ogburn, whose well-known theory of "cultural lag" appeared in 1922, used as his favorite example of this phenomenon the lag between the introduction of industrial machinery and the response of workmen's compensation laws; see Dorothy Ross, "American Social Science and the Idea of Progress," in Thomas L. Haskell (ed.), *The Authority of Experts* (Bloomington, Ind.: Indiana University Press, 1984), pp. 167–168.

59. See E. C. Lee, "Merit Rating of Coal Mines Under Workmen's Compensation Insurance," *Transactions of the American Institute of Mining Engineers* 57 (1917): 550–559. Lee was Chief Inspector of the Department of Inspection and Safety, The Associated Companies. I am grateful to Edwin Layton for bringing this article to my attention.

60. Ibid., pp. 551–552.

61. See E. Maltby Shipp, "Report of the Secretary of the Committee on Safety and Sanitation," *Transactions of the American Institute of Mining Engineers* 57 (1917): 253–308.

62. Ibid., pp. 260–262; Herbert M. Wilson, "Mine Labor and Accidents," *Transactions of the American Institute of Mining Engineers* 59 (1918): 654.

63. West Virginia has a Mining Extension Division in its College of Mines, but it is not funded primarily by federal pass-through funds, as is the Agricultural Extension Service.

64. Testimony before a committee of the U.S. Congress, as summarized in Vietor, *Energy Policy in America*, p. 164.

65. The following account is drawn largely from William Graebner, *Coal-Mining Safety in the Progressive Period: The Political Economy of Reform* (Lexington; Ky.: The University of Kentucky Press, 1976); see also A. Hunter Dupree, *Science in the Federal Government* (Cambridge, Mass.: Harvard University Press, 1957), pp. 280–281.

66. Graebner, *Coal-Mining Safety*, p. 47.

67. Ibid., p. 48.

68. For an illuminating case study of the ways in which the needs of a constituent industry can influence the setting of research priorities in a federal laboratory, see Rodney Carlisle, "Impact of Oil Economics on Research Priorities, 1931–1941," in Arthur L. Donovan (ed.), *Energy in American History,* a special double issue of *Materials and Society,* 7 (1983): 339–346.

69. Stuart D. Brandes, *American Welfare Capitalism, 1880–1940* (Chicago: University of Chicago Press, 1976), pp. 5–6.

70. E. E. Bach, "Social and Religious Organizations as Factors in the Labor Problem," *Transactions of the American Institute of Mining Engineers* 59 (1918): 590–611.

71. George S. McGovern and Leonard F. Guttridge, *The Great Coalfield War* (Boston: Houghton Mifflin, 1972).

72. Brandes, *Welfare Capitalism,* p. 124.

73. Far from being an aberration, King's conflation of science, social control, and championing the progressive triumph of good over evil reflected the dominant view on the purposes and implications of the new social sciences; see Ross, "American Social Science," p. 163.

74. Brandes, *Welfare Capitalism,* p. 132.

75. Vietor, *Energy Policy,* p. 165, n. 6.

76. See George T. Mazuzan and J. Samuel Walker, "Developing Nuclear Power in an Age of Energy Abundance, 1946–1962," and Jack M. Holl, "Eisenhower's Peaceful Atomic Diplomacy: Atoms for Peace and the Western Alliance," both in Arthur L. Donovan (ed.), *Energy in American History,* a special double issue of *Materials and Society,* 7 (1983): 307–319, 365–378.

77. For a brief history of OCR, see Vietor, *Energy Policy,* pp. 163–178.

78. Jacqueline K. Corn, *A History of Coal Mine Health and Safety: Part I*, unpublished manuscript.

79. The classic account of such plans is Pierce Williams, *The Purchase of Medical Care Through Fixed Periodic Payment* (New York: National Bureau of Economic Research, 1932); ch. 5 through 8 deal specifically with the coal industry.

80. Brandes, *Welfare Capitalism*, p. 93.

81. Ibid., p. 101.

82. U.S. Coal Mine Administration, *A Medical Survey of the Bituminous Coal Industry* (Washington, D.C.: GPO, 1947).

83. Ibid., p. 2.

84. Ibid., p. 116.

85. Ibid., pp. 123–124.

86. See Seltzer, *Fire in the Hole*, ch. 7, esp. p. 95. The UMWA Department of Occupational Health, the first of its kind in any American labor union, was not established until 1969; Frank Goldsmith and Lorin E. Kerr, *Occupational Safety and Health* (New York: Human Sciences Press, 1982), p. 185.

87. See the 1946 Krug-Lewis agreement, published as an appendix to U.S. Coal Mine Administration, *Medical Survey*, p. 233.

88. Barbara Berney, "The Rise and Fall of the UMW Fund," *Southern Exposure* 6 (1978): 96. See also Leslie A. Falk, "Group Health Plans in Coal Mining Communities," *Journal of Health and Human Behavior* 4 (1963): 4–13.

89. According to one historian of the Fund, Roche "prohibited her staff from involvement in any political effort to gain improved workers' compensation coverage or occupational disease prevention programs," for like Lewis, she felt the industry should manage its own affairs; quoted in Seltzer, *Fire in the Hole*, p. 95.

90. The following account is taken from Lewis M. Williams, "Transformation of a Coal Mining Town," *Mining Congress Journal* 29 (1943): 37–40.

91. A. H. Raskin, "How Miners Live," *American Mercury* 64 (1947): 421–427.

92. For a summary of these efforts, see Ludwig Teleky, *History of Factory and Mine Hygiene* (New York: Columbia University Press, 1948).

93. See George Rosen, *The History of Miner's Disease* (New York: Schuman's, 1943); Edgar L. Collis, "The Coal Miner: His Health, Diseases, and General Welfare," *The Journal of Industrial Hygiene* 7 (1925): 221–243.

94. See Eugene P. Pendergrass et al., "Historical Perspectives of Coal Workers' Pneumoconiosis in the United States," *Annals of the New York Academy of Science* 200 (1972): 835–854; Daniel M. Fox and Judith F. Stone, "Black Lung: Miners' Militancy and Medical Uncertainty, 1968–1972," *Bulletin of the History of Medicine* 54 (1980): 43–63.

95. Quoted in Seltzer, *Fire in the Hole*, p. 94.

96. For a brief historical survey, see Goldsmith and Kerr, *Occupational Safety and Health*, 2, "The Coal Miners' Demand for Occupational Health."

97. Although the respiratory problems caused by coal dust became much more severe when continuous mining machinery was introduced into the mines from the late 1940s onward, operators were aware of the problem and were nervously anticipating legal regulation considerably earlier. In a 1939 annual review of the coal industry, the chairman of the AIME committee on safety reported as follows: "No noteworthy changes in the mining laws of the various coal states occurred during the year. Occupational disease legislation [presumably concerning eligibility for workmen's compensation] has caused most forward-looking operators to pay increased attention to the dust problem, the practice of allaying dust with water on the cutter bar, sprinkling of loaded trips, etc., and to an increased use of respirators." Gordon MacVean, "Safety in Coal Mining," *Mining and Metallurgy* 20 (1939): 50–51.

98. Goldsmith and Kerr, *Occupational Safety and Health,* pp. 189–194, section titled "Occupational Diseases—Workers' Compensation Doesn't Work."

99. See Seltzer, *Fire in the Hole,* ch. 7.

100. Goldsmith and Kerr, *Occupational Safety and Health,* p. 186.

101. Ibid., p. 187; Richard Carter, *The Doctor Business* (New York: Doubleday, 1958), ch. 9.

102. Quoted in Goldsmith and Kerr, *Occupational Safety and Health,* p. 83.

103. Although the literature on professionalism is vast, the topic continues to repay close study. See Kenneth S. Lynn (ed.), *The Professions in America* (Boston: Beacon Press, 1967); Burton Bledstein, *The Culture of Professionalism* (New York: Norton, 1976); Thomas L. Haskell, *The Authority of Experts* (Bloomington, Ind.: Indiana University Press, 1984). I have developed several of the ideas on engineering presented in this section at greater length in two other publications: "Engineering in an Increasingly Complex Society," in *Engineering in Society* (Washington, D.C.: National Academy Press, 1985), pp. 81–132, and "Thinking about Engineering," *Technology and Culture,* special issue on "Engineering in the Twentieth Century," 27 (1986): 674–679.

104. In the 1970s the U.S. Surpeme Court ruled that professions are not exempt from the Sherman Anti-Trust Act, the Justice Department initiated a series of suits charging several professional societies with anticompetitive practices, and the Federal Trade Commission attacked the American Medical Association for price fixing; see Thomas L. Haskell, "Introduction," in Haskell (ed.), *Authority of Experts,* pp. xv–xvi.

3

Failed Warnings: Asbestos-Related Disease and Industrial Medicine

DAVID OZONOFF

It took the prophet Daniel to decipher the handwriting on the wall at Belshazzar's feast, but no special powers were necessary to see that breathing asbestos dust was a threat to health. From the earliest decades the asbestos trade stood out because of its "easily demonstrated danger to the health of the workers, and because of ascertained cases of injury to bronchial tubes and lungs medically attributed to the employment of the sufferers."[1] That was in 1898. Eight years later the Lady Inspector of Factories in England reported that of all the "dusty trades" for which complaints were received, none surpassed the injuriousness of asbestos processes.[2] Her report expressed the hope that better ventilation might improve the conditions in these workshops.

In the more than eighty years since these first reports, this optimistic thought would be repeated at frequent intervals, even as the bodies of asbestos workers piled up. The first death in England was reported in 1907, and the first case of asbestos-related disease in America appeared in the medical literature in 1917.[3,4] By 1930 a specific chronic disease of the lungs attributed to breathing asbestos was well described in dozens of different medical articles involving hundreds of cases. All aspects of the disease were detailed: its signs and symptoms, its natural history, its clinical course, and the minute pathological changes visible only at autopsy. By 1927 the disease had already received the name asbestosis.[5] In 1931 England issued regulations governing work practices in the asbestos industry and began a compensation scheme specifically for asbestos workers.[6] Throughout these thirty years observers expressed the same pious hope that "in the future," conditions would improve. Instead, they took a dramatic turn for the worse.

In 1935 the first reports began to appear that asbestos workers with asbestosis also seemed to be at unusual risk for cancer of the lung.[7] By 1938 German physicians were calling lung cancer an occupational disease of asbestos workers.[8] In the 1940s an even more virulent cancer, mesothelioma, appeared in workers exposed to asbestos.[9] Worse yet, in the 1960s mesothelioma cases were being seen in those only briefly and casually exposed, such as household companions of asbestos workers or those who lived in the neighborhood of an asbestos facility.[10]

By the end of 1964 there were more than 700 articles in the worldwide medical literature detailing the hazards of asbestos exposure.[11] Yet fewer than half of the state governments of the United States had any regulations governing asbestos exposure in the workplace, and those standards were designed only with asbestosis, not cancer, in mind, using data clearly inadequate to the task of setting a safe level of exposure even for that disease. Workers continued to handle asbestos products that carried no warning labels or hazard indications.

That same year most of the world's asbestos experts convened at the New York Academy of Sciences to review the matter.[12] From then on the "asbestos problem" began to absorb the energy and concern of the general public health community, not just that of specialists in industrial medicine.

Asbestos-related diseases have relatively long latency periods (the time between exposure to the agent and the first clinical manifestation of disease). By 1965, the year that the *Transactions* of the New York Academy's meeting was published, workers had already been exposed to risk for many decades. Even if asbestos exposures had ceased from that year on (and they did not), asbestos-related disease would have continued to appear another forty years or more—the entire length of the latency periods. Thus, cases of asbestos-related diseases, such as mesothelioma, would still be appearing into the next century from workplace and environmental exposures that had occurred before 1965.

At the end of July 1982, UNR Industries of Chicago asked the federal bankruptcy court for protection from its creditors under Chapter 11 of the Bankruptcy Code. In the previous two years the company had spent $26 million defending itself in lawsuits brought against it by workers who had used asbestos-containing pipe-insulation products that the company had not made since 1962. Faced with 17,000 more claims, UNR threw in the towel.[13] A week later the Johns-Manville Corporation, the country's largest manufacturer of asbestos products, omitted its quarterly dividend. By the end of that month (August 1982), it too had filed for protection under Chapter 11. Although still solvent, Manville estimated that it might face another 45,000 lawsuits in the years to come and sought protection on that basis. In the industry overall, some 13,500 suits on behalf of up to 30,000 workers had already been filed against some 260 defendant asbestos companies.

History has caught up with more than workers and manufacturers. The use of friable (easily crumbled) asbestos in public buildings, including schools, has potentially exposed millions of citizens to asbestos fiber. In 1984 the U.S. Environmental Protection Agency (EPA) estimated that as many as 14 million school children and 1.3 million teachers and staff might be exposed in the nation's elementary and secondary schools.[14] Many school districts were removing asbestos at great expense, and a new wave of litigation against the asbestos industry began as school districts sued to recover their costs. Asbestos was also found in municipal water supplies and consumer products. And countless homeowners and renters discovered, to their dismay, that their dwellings contained friable asbestos insulation on pipes and boilers. A thriving new cottage industry of "asbestos removal experts" began to occupy more and more column inches in every city's telephone-directory Yellow Pages.

How is it that we allowed ourselves to get into such a dismal predicament? There was no lack of knowledge of the basic dangers connected with asbestos exposure. The medical literature was abundant, and the details had been thoroughly fleshed out. Yet the nature, scope, and depth of what was known had not been translated into practical measures to protect workers and the general public from the evident hazards. In the years after publication of the New York Academy's *Transactions* in 1965, the issue became a live policy controversy, fought out openly in the traditional adversary process that characterizes this country's regulatory system.[15] But what of the earlier years, when the essential elements were known but the problem of asbestos hazard had not yet entered the public debate?

That story involves the asbestos industry, the medical and public health professions—particularly the emerging specialty of industrial medicine—and how each influenced and was influenced by the social and economic context. During this era federal and state governments played only a minor role in ensuring a safe workplace. What emerges is a tale of occasional deception and deceit by powerful special interests, of tragically lost opportunities to protect the public health, and of a medical specialty captured by its origins as a handmaiden to management.

The Asbestos Industry

Briton Hadden, Henry Luce's eccentric partner in the founding of *Time* magazine in 1923, had peculiar amusements. He cared little for golf or tennis but had a shooting gallery in his living room. He also had a suit made of asbestos. Its sole purpose, apparently, was to confound friends and acquaintances by allowing him to put out cigarettes by grinding them against his knees and elbows.[16] This was, of course, a parlor trick, but not the first one with asbestos. It is said that Charlemagne had a tablecloth of asbestos that he would throw into the fire after dinner and later withdraw, clean and intact. That performance, too, was apparently designed to impress his less sophisticated warrior guests.[17]

Not all uses were so frivolous. Royal bodies to be consumed on the funeral pyre were wrapped in asbestos cloth to keep the ashes of the fuel separate from those of the departed. And so asbestos was sometimes referred to as "The Funeral Dress of Kings," not the least of the ironies that litter the tragic history of the "magic mineral."[18]

The Magic Mineral

Until the mid-nineteenth century, asbestos was more of a curiosity than a useful article of commerce—and an amazing curiosity it was. As late as the 1880s its properties were so singular and its occurrence in nature so unusual that it almost defied classification:

> Asbestos is one of the most marvelous productions of inorganic nature. It is a physical paradox, a mineralogical vegetable, both fibrous and crystalline, elastic and brittle; a floating stone, as capable of being carded, spun, and woven as wool, flax, or silk. Occupying the apparent position of a connecting link between the mineral and vegetable kingdoms, it would appear to possess some of the characteristics of both,

while being altogether different from either. In appearance, it is as light and feathery as thistle or eiderdown, while, in fact, it is as dense and heavy as the rock which carries it. Ostensibly as perishable as grass, it is actually older than any animal or vegetable life on earth. So little, indeed, is it affected by the dissolving influences of time that the action of unnumbered centuries, by which the hardest rocks are worn away, has had no perceptible effect on the asbestos found embedded in them. While some portion of its bulk is composed of the roughest and most gritty materials known, it is really as smooth to the touch as soap or oil. Apparently as combustible as tow, the fiercest heat cannot consume it, and no combination of acids will affect the strength of its fibre, even after days of exposure to their influence. Notwithstanding its extreme delicacy, a single strand of it can be spun to weigh less than an ounce to one hundred yards, and a cloth may be manufactured from its fibers which shall weigh less than eight ounces to the square yard.[19]

Marco Polo had been told that asbestos was a product of the woolly salamander, but it was clear from the fact that it was found in rocks that it was a mineral product.[20] Although its exact mode of formation was unknown, its remarkable physical and chemical properties were obvious. The most outstanding were its ability to withstand high temperatures and the destructive effects of acids and alkalis. It also had a tensile strength almost equal to that of steel while remaining quite flexible.

There are many varieties of asbestos. As the Greek origins of the word asbestos (meaning unquenchable or incombustible) indicate, the most salient characteristic of minerals with this name is their resistance to fire and heat.[21] Although asbestos was known in antiquity, its widespread modern use is intimately connected with industrialization. Every bit as much as coal, asbestos is a product of the demands of power.

The Demands of Power

The preeminent source of power in the nineteenth century was the steam engine. Steam produced in a boiler pushed a piston connected by mechanical linkages to pumps, railroad wheels or, later, electric generators. To accomplish this efficiently, the piston had to be fitted to the cylinder in a steam-tight fashion. This became more and more difficult as temperatures and pressures increased. It was virtually impossible to machine cylinders and pistons to fit together exactly, so various kinds of seals or packings had to be used. Most common in the mid-nineteenth century were leather packings or hemp soaked in grease. One method used leather disks secured to both faces of the piston, while another used hemp packed around the cylinder and secured with a flange on each end.[22]

Unfortunately, leather, hemp, and other organic materials deteriorated rapidly under the extreme conditions in the interior of a steam engine, requiring replacement or refitting at frequent intervals. By the 1860s asbestos was being used as a new sealant or packing in steam engines. The asbestos was first spun, woven, or fashioned into a type of millboard for use as a packing. Asbestos was uniquely suited to this use "owing to its power of resisting moisture, friction, high temperatures, and even flame itself."[23]

Heat loss with a consequent waste of fuel was another major problem. As steam engineering advanced, higher steam pressures were accompanied by higher temperatures. These high temperatures and pressures improved the efficiency of the steam engine, allowing more power to be produced, but they also resulted in greater heat loss. It was calculated, for example, that the heat loss from a bare pipe conveying steam at 125 pounds of pressure on an ordinary mild day would be the equivalent of 1.5 pounds of coal per square foot of pipe per working day. On a hundred square feet of pipe, this amounted to a waste of 150 pounds of coal every ten hours: "At the rate of three hundred working days per year, this means an annual waste of forty-five thousand pounds of coal, or twenty-two and a half tons for each one-hundred square feet of unprotected pipe." And this did not take into account any heat wasted from the boiler or places outside the pipe itself, such as flanges and valves.[24]

Eighty to ninety percent of heat waste could be prevented by proper coverings on the pipe and boiler. As with valve packings, a variety of materials were used to insulate the earliest steam engines. Blankets, carpet, chopped hay, feathers, and mixtures of fired clay, charcoal, and sawdust with hair as a binder were all employed with some initial success. The best insulators were those materials which trapped tiny dead spaces of air. Thus, hairfelt and wool were good insulators, but they eventually failed at high temperatures because their extreme dryness allowed them to catch fire easily, often with disastrous consequences. Asbestos fibers mixed with various materials or made into a corrugated paper or millboard did not suffer this disadvantage.[25]

The function of the asbestos was to lend strength and heat resistance to the material whose real insulating capacity was determined by the air spaces in the corrugations of the asbestos paper or the small bubbles in more plasterlike materials. A notable advance was the development in the 1880s of a material called 85 percent magnesia. Magnesia, or magnesium carbonate, had long been a staple of the US Pharmacopeia. In 1885 Hiram M. Hanmore, a pipe coverer, began to mix magnesia with other pipe-covering materials and actually patented his idea. At the same time one of the leading manufacturers of magnesia for medical purposes discovered, in drying his product, that the fine, white magnesia powder so reduced the heat in the drying room that the pipes had to be cleaned continuously. Experiments were soon underway to find the best way to use magnesia as an insulator. Mixing it with asbestos fiber was a natural development. The asbestos fiber acted as a binder to give strength and cohesion to the magnesia sludge, which could be cast or molded into standard shapes and dried. The optimum mix was 85 percent magnesia and 15 percent finely divided asbestos fiber.[26]

The use of asbestos insulation, and of 85 percent magnesia particularly, spread rapidly, especially in the United States. By 1888 the U.S. Navy used coverings of 85 percent magnesia almost exclusively in its capital ships "because by maximum conservation of heat, these coverings enabled ships to steam farther on a given coal capacity."[27] In the boom period of the 1880s and early 1890s, such products could be sold on the basis not only of their efficiency but also of economy. "In the present time of business competition," advised an advertisement for the products of the Salamander Felting Company, "any practical improvements whereby a radical saving can be made in expenses attracts attention." Radical savings, of course, were made possible by the use of Salamander Cement Felting manufactured by the Asbestos Packing Company of Boston.[28]

The Birth of an Industry Giant

The relative indestructibility, high tensile strength, and fireproof nature of asbestos fiber, which made it useful as binder in insulation, also made it valuable as a constituent of building materials. One of the first people to see the virtues of this material was a young man from West Stockbridge, Massachusetts, by the name of Henry Ward Johns. Moving to Brooklyn in 1858 at the age of twenty-one, Johns began a small business handling roofing materials. He soon became aware of the properties of asbestos. One source says that he read about it in the *Encyclopedia Americana* in 1859; however it came to his attention, he began to experiment by incorporating asbestos fiber into various roofing materials.[29]

Johns was fascinated with the properties of asbestos fiber and developed many products using it. Operating in a small basement research and development lab consisting of a stove, tea kettle, and clothes wringer, he developed and patented a new pipe covering made of successive layers of woolfelt, paper, and hairfelt, lined with asbestos paper and made up in prefabricated sections. Johns's business immediately increased from sales of this new insulation in sectional form, precut to standard sizes, which could be wrapped or wired around pipes. The company also sold roofing material, made with asbestos, which Johns had patented in 1868. By 1880 the H. W. Johns Manufacturing Company had a second factory in Brooklyn, manufacturing paints made with asbestos marketed as a fireproofing product.[30]

In addition to his manufacturing employees, Johns also hired a salesman. Soon other companies were selling the products of the H. W. Johns Company. One was Charles W. Trainer and Company of Boston. It advertised that it sold H. W. Johns's patented asbestos materials, including liquid paints, steam-saving materials, and roofing and fireproofing materials. A special advantage was that they could be "readily applied without the aid of skilled labor."[31] Another vendor of Johns's products was a Milwaukee concern, started in 1886 by Charles B. Manville and his three sons. Although the Manville Covering Company also manufactured various types of pipe and boiler coverings, none included asbestos insulating materials for high temperatures, so the company sold Johns's products in the Midwest.[32]

The economic boom times of the 1880s were good to Johns, and his business expanded rapidly. The change in state incorporation laws of the late 1880s and the Sherman Anti-Trust Act of 1890 inaugurated a period of mergers and horizontal combinations in American business, and Johns followed the lead of many others.[33] In 1891, the H. W. Johns Manufacturing Company consolidated with several other firms, namely the Chalmers-Spence Asbestos Company, the Asbestos Packing Company, C. W. Trainer and Company, and the Shields and Brown Company of Chicago. Johns was appointed president, and R. H. Martin of Chalmers-Spence was appointed vice-president, but the company retained the name of the H. W. Johns Manufacturing Company of New York. This new consolidated company now became the largest asbestos manufacturer and dealer in the world, with factories in New York, Chicago, and Philadelphia, more than quadrupling Johns's former production capacity.[34]

Johns's company was taking on all the characteristics of a big business. The several factories tied up a good deal of capital in fixed costs. Those costs, for inventories, debt servicing, and similar items, required that fairly stable levels of operation be maintained, not only to achieve low cost per unit of output but merely to turn a profit. And this required a steady source of new material.

Mining the Magic Mineral

The ability to manufacture such a wide variety of products depended on a ready supply of appropriate-quality asbestos fiber. As the manufacturing sector of asbestos products advanced, so did the mining sector.[35]

In the 1870s the first deposits were mined commercially in the Italian Alps. The quality of the mineral was extremely good, its long fibers permitting the material to be spun. The best deposits were in a remote and high portion of northern Italy. From the plain where the railroad and highway were situated, it took four to five hours of travel, by mule and then by foot, to reach the mining area. About 800 pounds of asbestos could be brought down the mountain in three hours on toboggans or sledges hauled over the rocks by two workers. The crude asbestos was packed in bags and shipped to England in the form of rough lumps, "from the size of a man's head to about as much as one man can lift."[36] The rock was then crushed and the fibers segregated from unwanted particles and from each other. The longer fibers were separated from their shorter fellows and put through the manufacturing process.

Although spinning asbestos was much like spinning wool or cotton, certain special difficulties were encountered with this Italian fiber. When examined under the microscope, wool and cotton fibers show a notched or knobby appearance that allows them to cling together when twisted. The Italian asbestos fibers, however, were straight and smooth, which meant that the fibers slipped past each other instead of clinging to and twisting about each other. Cotton fibers were mixed in with the asbestos to overcome this difficulty and allow it to be spun. Several adaptations of the traditional carding and condensing machines used in textile manufacture were invented, and the long Italian fibers eventually were successfully incorporated into yarn and woven materials.

In 1880 several European mining and manufacturing companies combined to form the United Asbestos Company, Ltd. Between them these companies had a practical monopoly of the Italian mines, and they dominated trade in asbestos and the manufacture of asbestos products from Italian fiber. Because the Johns Manufacturing Company's early asbestos products did not require long fibers for spinning, using instead shorter and inferior fibers for their reinforcing abilities in insulation and roofing materials, Johns had been able to carry on his work in the 1870s without importing expensive Italian fiber. In 1874, for example, a minor deposit of asbestiform materials was discovered on nearby Staten Island. Johns sent over farmers' wagons to load up with asbestos and bring it back to the factory in Brooklyn.[37] However, a source closer to home soon developed.

As early as the 1860s it was known that there were deposits of a mineral in Canada called chrysotile that exhibited all the characteristics of asbestos; that is, it occurred in fibrous form and was highly fire resistent. In the mid-1870s a large forest fire laid bare the area around Thetford, Coleraine, and the entire range near the Black Lake Mountains in the Province of Quebec. While inspecting the territory, a farmer discovered a wooly rock of such singular appearance that he showed it to some mineral experts who judged it to be asbestos fiber of exceptional quality. Within a few years there were four mines operating in the vicinity of Thetford, Quebec. The Canadian fiber, although not as long as that of the Italian variety, had a slight hook on it that enabled easy spinning. Moreover, it was much more accessible than the remote deposits of the Italian Alps.

Production of Canadian chrysotile soon overtook that of the Italian variety. By 1889 the United Asbestos Company had acknowledged the superiority of the Canadian fiber and had itself obtained mines in Quebec. The rapid exploitation of the Canadian deposits, of course, depended upon the growing recognition of the utility of asbestos for modern industrial use, either as a packing for steam engines, insulation for pipes and boilers, or as a component of building materials such as roofing, shingles, or millboard and papers.

The discovery and development of the chrysotile deposits in Canada immediately stimulated an expansion of asbestos manufacturing, and Johns took advantage of this opportunity. He and his American competitors soon became the major consumers of Canadian asbestos. The ease with which the fiber could be worked and the comparatively cheaper price immediately gave the American companies a competitive advantage over their European counterparts.

The mining of asbestos for the most part was carried on in open quarries or pits. Rock was blasted from the face of the pit, and the asbestos-bearing fragments were separated from their barren counterparts. They were then sent to the "cobbing house" where young boys or old men separated the long fibers from the rock by hand using a pick or hammer.

At first only the best and longest fibers were separated and the remainder thrown away as waste. But as the price per ton of asbestos rose with increasing demand, the lesser quality ore was also used, thus requiring the use of large machines, such as rock breakers, rolls, screens, and blowers, to separate the fiber more deeply embedded in the rock. This process produced fibers of varying lengths and qualities. The best qualty was grade 1, with grades 2 and 3 following it. There was no standard grading system, only a qualitative system that varied from producer to producer. The best and longest fibers, grade 1, were used for the manufacture of textiles and yarns. The shorter grade 2 and 3 fibers were used as fillers and binders in cements, plasters, and millboard.

The quality of the material depended not only on the intrinsic character of the fiber but on how well it was freed from various impurities. In the early uses of asbestos for packing in steam engines, for example, it was found that the piston rods frequently became scored by the packing. At first the abrasion was attributed to the asbestos fiber itself, but it was soon discovered that the cause was small pieces of mineral or metallic impurities carried along with the fiber. Freeing the fiber of this foreign matter solved the problem, but this required the use of special machinery and gave an advantage to companies with substantial capital. The H. W. Johns Manufacturing Company was one of these.

By the early 1890s the Johns Company, now consolidated with many of its former competitors, had obtained its own mine. Other asbestos manufacturing companies, in both the United States and Europe, had followed suit. A process of vertical integration now accompanied the horizontal combinations already underway in the industry.

The cost of asbestos per ton had inched steadily upward during the 1880s. In 1889 first-quality fiber ranged from $80 to $120 per ton, the range of prices reflecting a lack of uniformity in grading. In 1890 there was a sudden jump in prices so that by 1891, first-quality asbestos sold for as much as $250 per ton or more. One consequence was a good deal of speculation in mining land as well as in the crude fiber, and many instances of fraudulent "salting" of territory with asbestos fiber in order to sell the land at premium prices were recorded in Italy and Canada. Additional efforts were made to use the cruder fibers and to extract even more fibers from what had previously been considered waste material. Again, the process brought still more capital equipment and machinery into the mining industry.

The financial rewards could be substantial. Although costs varied depending upon the exact difficulty of working a vein of asbestos, the typical cost of production and preparation for market of a ton of asbestos was about $25. With a price of $125 a ton for grade 1, $75 for grade 2, or even $35 for grade 3, large profits could be made in asbestos mining. This was, of course, a considerable enticement for capital. With the introduction of machinery, the costs of production dropped still further to about $15 dollars a ton, although the old prices, depending upon market conditions, remained the same. Little wonder, then, that a noted mineral expert recommended asbestos mining as an ideal investment:

> When failures occur, they may almost certainly be traced to want of practical advice in the first instance, to incompetency or extravagance in the management, or to overcapitalization; but with due care, economy, and honest and capable management, there are but few things which will pay better or with more regularity and certainty than mining for asbestos.[38]

Collapse and Consolidation

Yet the asbestos business could be risky, too. Much of the increase in prices in the late 1880s had to do with speculation in asbestos, a material whose value was now being recognized. At the same time, American concerns were competing with each other in bidding up the price of the raw material. The boom collapsed suddenly in 1892 as the speculators unloaded their stocks at the same time that Johns and his competitors consolidated and formed a combination. With enough stock on hand, these manufacturers ceased to buy at all. Prices for grade 1 fell by 50 percent, and production plummeted. The overproduction of 1889 to 1891 was correcting itself.

The years after 1893 were even worse. The panic of 1893 resulted in one of the severest depressions the country had ever experienced.

Europe too suffered depression conditions, sharply curtailing any American export. The building industry, which was the main consumer of Johns's products, was especially recession sensitive. The economic downturn that started in 1893 lasted for four long years. During one six-month period, 8,000 businesses failed, but Johns's concern managed to survive. Yet neither Johns nor his business were in good health. In 1898 Johns died of scarring of the lungs, perhaps the result of exposure to the product that he pioneered. His son took over the company but finished the century deeply in debt to the Fourth National Bank.

William Robbins Seigle, a bank employee, paid a visit to Johns to see what could be done about his financial problems. He first engineered the sale of the Johns paint business and then arranged a buyout of the entire Johns Company by the Manville Covering Company of Milwaukee (Seigle stayed with the new Johns-Manville Company and eventually, thirty years later, became chairman of the board.)[39]

With a Canadian source of supply assured, the new consolidated Johns-Manville Company further diversified its product line.[40] Although Johns-Manville was recognizably "big business," it was in many ways similar to other family-oriented, one-man shows. *Fortune* magazine likened Manville to the Ford Motor Company. The new president of the Company, Thomas F. Manville, son of Manville founder Charles B. Manville, was a good salesman and loved selling, adding many items to Johns-Manville's catalogue, including automobile horns, fire extinguishers, spark plugs, and hundreds of other products not related to asbestos. A small town, Manville, New Jersey, grew up around the factory, although it contained little but the factory itself and a big hotel that T. F. Manville built. Manville himself lived there, and guests to the factory were put up in fine style. Unlike his predecessor Johns, who considered research and development essential, T. F. Manville cared little for it and is reputed never to have spent a nickel on laboratories or chemists.

Instead, Manville established an extensive network of sales offices with salaried agents throughout the country. Over fifty such offices were listed in the company's 1927 annual report. While the company integrated forward to the retail level, it continued to develop its backward integration to the sources of supply in Canada. The Canadian Johns-Manville Company, Ltd., quarried from 50,000 tons in bad years to 115,000 tons in good years and was said to account for as high as 40 percent of the total Canadian output.

By the fall of 1925, when he suddenly dropped dead in his hotel, Manville had run up sales of almost $40 million a year and had a catalogue of 2,000 products. The Company suffered in bad years, such as 1907, 1914, and particularly 1921, but did exceedingly well in good years. When the economy made a strong recovery in 1922 following the deep post-war slump of 1921, Johns-Manville roofed so many houses and insulated so many pipes that T. F. Manville could declare an extra cash dividend of $40 a share.

The Competition

Johns-Manville, of course, was not the only asbestos company in the United States, nor even the only one with its own asbestos mines. Keasbey and Mattison of Ambler, Pennsylvania, and Philip Carey Company of Cincinnati were among other companies that had their own mines. Both competed with Manville for manufacturing, roofing, and insulation products. Moreover, a number of Canadian asbestos mines had merged to form the Asbestos Corporation, which equaled or perhaps even exceeded Johns-Manville in the production of raw asbestos. At the same time that these companies competed with Johns-Manville on its own turf, other companies arose to dominate new specialty areas of asbestos products.

One was the manufacture of "friction products," primarily brake bands and clutch facings for automobiles and trucks. Both the brakes and the clutches of automobiles required materials of similar properties, as each involved the engagement and disengagement of rapidly moving parts. Early brakes and clutches used a leather-on-metal or metal-on-metal arrangement. Either type was the source of periodic difficulty because they required frequent adjustment and they changed operating characteristics with use:

> Metal to metal clutches and metal to metal brake shoes wear rapidly until tool marks are effaced and the surfaces smoothly glossed over, and early adjustment of these important parts are likely to prove necessary in a new car which is "finding itself." . . . The leather forming the friction bands of clutches is often stiff and harsh in a new car, causing the engagement of the power to be jerky and violent. With use and proper treatment with a suitable unguent, the leather seems to become more pliable and better adapted to effect a gentle clutch engagement.[41]

In 1907, brake shoes and clutch facings with an asbestos and wire composition were introduced. The long sections in automotive handbooks on the preparation and treatment of the leather began to disappear. The newer automotive handbooks sang the material's praises:

> The introduction of this kind of material has undoubtedly effected a great change in the recent practice of motor car clutches, as it is found that, unlike leather, this material is capable of being heated until it reaches a high temperature: even then, although the metal around it may be almost approaching a red heat, the fabric surface only appears to be blackened without burning up the entire body of the fabric as in the case of leather. . . . A true understanding of the whole question of the friction clutch can only be attained by realizing that it is the surfaces which are all important; and having secured satisfactory surfaces for contact, the problem becomes one of mechanical design, to which attention must now be turned.[42]

One of the companies that entered the field of friction materials using asbestos was the Raybestos Company, which was formed in Connecticut in 1916 with Sumner Simpson as president. It made brake linings, clutch bearings, and some miscellaneous asbestos products. Another was the General Asbestos and Rubber Company of Charleston, South Carolina, which had started in 1895 making asbestos textiles and later branched out into friction products, including brake linings. And still another was the Manhattan Rubber Manufacturing Company, which began in New Jersey in 1893 making transmission and conveyor belts and then went into the asbestos brake lining and packing business with a plant in Passaic, New Jersey. In 1925 Raybestos bought out the General Asbestos and Rubber Company, and in 1929 it bought out the Manhattan Rubber Company, forming the consolidated Raybestos-Manhattan Company the same year. It thus became the country's largest manufacturer of friction products, making twice as many brake linings as Johns-Manville itself.[43]

Just as the spectacular economic recovery of 1922 and its attendant building boom gave a boost to Johns-Manville, so did the marked increase in automobile sales help Raybestos and the other friction product companies. In 1919 Oregon, New Mexico, and Colorado financed their road building by putting a tax on gasoline. By the end of the 1920s every other state had done the same thing, and the money raised was used to match federal road construction subsidies. The 1921 federal Highways Act melded each state's system of roads into a regional network. The mileage of concrete roads in the United States increased from 7,000 to 50,000 miles between 1918 and 1927, and new road construction added another 10,000 miles a year. In 1920, 8.25 million automobiles were registered in this country, but by 1927 that figure had more than doubled.[44] And all those vehicles had brakes and clutches that required asbestos friction products.

Brake linings in particular were a large consumer of asbestos, and the brakes were considered one of the most important safety features of an automobile. Automobile hazards were much on the minds of the public and the car manufacturers in the 1920s. The increase in automobile traffic without adequate experience soon led to a serious safety problem. As early as the 1920s, 25,000 people were killed each year and up to 600,000 injured.[45] A nationwide campaign for greater safety on streets and highways began to have an effect on the purchase of new automobiles. Willim R. Strickland, the assistant chief engineer of the Cadillac Motor Company, called attention to changes in brake design that would increase safety:

> While the personal equation is still the biggest factor in safe driving, many features of car design have a very definite relation to safe operation. The greatest feature is brakes. With the increase in the number of cars in operation and the added fact that the individual car is driven many more miles per year than was the case formerly, resultant highway congestion made an undeniable demand for four-wheel brakes. The ease with which cars equipped with four-wheel brakes pass brake tests made by policy officials in the various cities of the country has been a source of satisfaction not only to the drivers, but to municipal authorities to whom is entrusted the safety of city streets. They have decelerating ability and a consequent factor of safety fifty to seventy-five percent greater than that of cars otherwise equipped. So much has been said about four-wheel brakes that some drivers have considered them as the chief safety feature, regardless of other factors in their design and operation which may effect [sic] control of the car.[46]

The conversion from two-wheel to four-wheel brakes was very rapid in the mid-1920s. In 1924, for example, twenty-two of 135 new car models, or approximately one in six, were made with four-wheel brakes.[47] Just four years later, eighty-one of ninety new car models, or 90 percent, had four-wheel brakes. This increased automobile safety and also greatly increased the business of the Raybestos Company and its competitors.

Johns-Manville and the Industry in 1927

By the late 1920s the building products and insulation sector of the asbestos industry was dominated by the Johns-Manville Company, and the friction products sector was dominated by the Raybestos-Manhattan Company. By that time the Johns-Manville Company had ceased being a family-owned business. When T. F. Manville died in 1925, he was succeeded to the presidency by his younger brother, Hiram Edward Manville. Old T. F. Manville had left his stock in three blocks, one to his son T. F., Jr., one to his daughter, and a third to the Manville employees. Hiram Edward was not eager to carry on as president of the company but was concerned about T. F. (Tommy), Jr., who cared more about blonde showgirls than he did about the company. Tommy had already been through two of his five marriages and had generated a good deal of scandalous publicity. Hiram Edward decided to centralize lest someone buy up the employees' stock and gain control of the company. He bought out the stock of Tommy, Jr., and purchased enough employee shares to become the majority owner. He promptly turned around and sold most of his holdings to the banking house of J. P. Morgan. Hiram Edward Manville then went into semi-retirement as chairman of the executive committee, still retaining a large block of Manville stock.[48] That was in 1927, the same year that W. E. Cooke coined the term asbestosis for an industrial lung disease caused by breathing fibers of the magic mineral.

The Triumph of Medicine and the Fall of Public Health

As the asbestos industry developed, warnings sounded that asbestos could be as harmful as it was useful. Soon after the asbestos industry emerged at the end of the nineteenth century, the British factory inspectors were finding serious health problems. The Annual Report of Her Majesty's Women Inspectors in 1898 specifically mentioned asbestos textile work and described the effects of the dust in vivid detail:

> In the majority of cases the evil is very insidious and the general symptoms produced by dust on the various respiratory organs are to the lay mind so similar to those produced by other causes that it is not always easy to trace the connection. The incessant "sore throat," the irritation

of bronchial passages, the frequent "colds on the chest," and "hoarse voice" and "morning cough" from which girls employed in dusty processes suffer, are all symptoms which to casual observers might easily be accounted for in other ways. . . . The worker falls into ill-health and sinks away out of sight in no sudden or sensational manner.[49]

One such fatal case was described to the British governmental committee reviewing compensation for industrial diseases by Dr. H. Montague Murray, Senior Physician at Charing Cross Hospital and a pioneer in the use of X-rays for medical diagnosis.[50] This case is not the first such death reported in detail, but the first with a post-mortem description of the victim's lungs, described as extremely tough and fibrous, especially in the lower parts. Montague Murray's thirty-three-year-old patient had worked fourteen years in the carding room of an asbestos works, claiming to be the only survivor of the ten people who were working in the room when he went into it; the others had all died around the age of thirty.[51]

The first American cases were also described by a pioneer in X-ray diagnosis, Henry K. Pancoast of the University of Pennsylvania. Pancoast was no stranger to occupational disease. He had seen his predecessor at University Hospital suffer severe radiation burns to his hands, which progressed to cancer. The amputation of a single finger was followed by successive amputations of the hand, forearm, and finally the upper arm at the shoulder joint, all to no avail.[52] In 1915 Pancoast and his colleagues turned their attention to X-ray examinations of the chest and the diagnosis of tuberculosis, examining workers exposed to a variety of dusts, including asbestos.

Initially, the dangers of asbestos dust exposure were not clearly differentiated from other kinds of known hazards such as quartz (free silica) dust. In 1917 in the first American paper to mention asbestos disease, Pancoast reported on his investigation of the X-ray appearance of dust exposure, which lumped together potters, metal grinders, cement workers, coal miners, and marine firemen with asbestos workers: "The effects are the same in general but may vary in degree."[53] In the discussion following the oral presentation of the paper at a medical meeting, a noted occupational medicine specialist rose and announced that the work had great economic importance:

This must be apparent when we realize that in 1915 there were not less than 143,000 deaths from pulmonary tuberculosis in the United States, . . . more than half of those deaths occurred among industrial workers, who constitute only about one-third of the adult population. That fact seems to show a clear relationship between the undue prevalence of tuberculosis in the industrial worker and pneumoconiosis as a fundamental predisposing cause.[54]

The economic effect of tuberculosis and any factor that increased its risk also concerned the insurance industry. In 1918 Frederick Hoffman, chief actuary of the Prudential Life Insurance Company, made a special study for the U.S. Bureau of Labor Statistics of "Mortality from Respiratory Diseases in Dusty Trades (Inorganic Dusts)." In his company's records, three of thirteen deaths among asbestos workers were from pulmonary tuberculosis, and all occurred in workers ranging from twenty-five to forty-four years old; thus, these young workers suffered a proportionate rate of mortality from tuberculosis of 25 percent. Acknowledging a dearth of data on the hygienic aspects of the industry, Hoffman judged it clear that the industry was very dusty and therefore involved "considerable dust hazard." Nor was this obvious only to him: "It may be said, in conclusion, that in the practice of American and Canadian life insurance companies asbestos workers are generally declined on account of the assumed health injurious conditions of the industry."[55]

Hoffman called urgently for "more qualified and extensive investigation of the health aspects of asbestos manufacture," noting as he did so that asbestos dust had already been identified as the primary cause of death in at least one worker (Montague Murray's case). Yet for decades to come, even as the scientific literature on asbestos hazards continued to accumulate, little in the way of effective protection was forthcoming for those exposed to the fiber. Neither the medical profession, nor public health scientists and reformers, nor the fledgling specialties of occupational medicine and industrial hygiene seemed oriented to translating knowledge into action. Why not?

The Organizing of American Medicine

In 1901, the same year that Manville bought out H. W. Johns to form the new Johns-Manville Company, the American Medical Association (AMA) also reorganized itself and laid the foundation for its emergence as the most powerful professional lobby in American political life. Although more than a half-century old in 1900, the AMA still represented only 8,400 physicians out of an estimated total of

100,000. The restructuring that occurred as the new century began can best be understood not in terms of its future success but in terms of the problem that it was meant to solve. That problem, purely and simply, was ruinous economic competition within the over-crowded health care professions.[56]

Throughout the nineteenth century, anyone could become a doctor either by apprenticeship to a practicing physician or by obtaining a diploma from a medical college qualified to issue it. As long as there were few such schools, the situation for most practitioners was not serious. But the process of westward expansion in the nineteenth century quickly led to an enormous expansion of degree-granting institutions. The new territories required a source of local physicians, and the demand could not be supplied by a small number of elite and distant institutions.

The new schools that sprang up to meet this need could also be highly profitable. And the flood of new practitioners they produced resulted in intense competition. In the first fifty years of the nineteenth century, the population of the country increased five times, but the number of "regular" practitioners increased from only a few thousand to over 40,000, and the number of medical school graduates increased more than fifty times. As if competition from these orthodox practitioners were not enough, a "regular" doctor had to compete with a variety of alternative practitioners. Thomsonians, botanics, homeopaths and others seemed to many of the public and their elected representatives to be both morally and therapeutically superior. In fact, the public may have been right. With few effective therapies available, the less invasive techniques of the nonregular practitioners may indeed have been less dangerous.

In 1847, local medical societies organized in an effort to exercise some control over the schools that were producing their competition at such a prodigious rate. They met with representatives of some of the better schools to discuss higher standards for education, hoping that a voluntary restriction in enrollment could be established. Not surprisingly this organization, which called itself the American Medical Association, received no support from either the bulk of schools or the many physicians who depended on the apprenticeship system for income and cheap labor and thus opposed any tactic making a diploma a prerequisite to practice. The AMA, divided internally and lacking a grassroots constituency, limped along, more of a yearly social gathering than an effective professional association.

The original objectives of the Association gave it an implicitly egalitarian nature within the profession. Those objectives were to help all those who suffered from the economic threats of over-production of regular practitioners and the existence of irregular ones. Charles Reed, the AMA president, recognized that the interests of the ordinary physician needed to be the focus of AMA actions. In 1901 he recommended that the Association reorganize itself around the state and local societies, a reflection of the need to unify the profession not at the top but at its most elementary level: "On the success of the county organization depends all above us; it is the foundation of the whole superstructure."[57]

Reed's conception struck a responsive chord in the profession. Reorganization proceeded with spectacular ease. By 1905 the AMA staff reported that only Virginia and Maine were not in essential accord with the AMA's model plan, which called for the state societies to be governed by representatives from the county level, with each state organization selecting delegates to the national level in numbers proportional to their membership. Many of the newly reorganized societies were also experiencing phenomenal growth. The Kentucky Medical Society grew from 400 to 1,600 members in two years and the Michigan society from 500 to 1,800 in the same period, while the Tennessee society tripled in an equally short time after reorganization. The picture at the county level was the same. In 1901, 35,000 physicians belonged to some local society. By 1908 this number had doubled to over 70,000.[58]

Along with this growth at the local level went the growth of the AMA itself. The AMA's total membership grew from 8,400 in 1900 to 83,000 in 1920, the same years during which the asbestos companies grew from their embryonic beginnings in insulation, building products, or friction materials to moderate-sized or big business. As the asbestos industry strove to stabilize itself on the economic front, the professional guild of the hard-pressed medical practitioner did so on the political front. State societies set up legislative committees to survey pending bills in their legislatures and lobbied for the profession's interests. Prime among those interests were licensing laws that stipulated minimum standards and required a level of preparation that put many schools out of business.[59]

By 1920 the AMA had achieved its primary goal, dominance over the process of medical education and licensing in the United States. But the political and economic power accrued in the struggle to regulate competition would have unintended side effects on medicine's sister discipline of public health and the nascent specialty of industrial medicine. The result for public health would be an uncoupling from its origins in social reform; for industrial medicine, the result would be a shift in focus from the individual employee to the interests of the employing firm.

Virtue Renounced: Public Health at the Turn of the Century

Early in the new century Dr. Alice Hamilton of Chicago's Hull House Settlement went to the library in search of information on industrial disease in America. A muckraking newspaper account of an industrial disaster was the occasion for her search, but her interest was more than academic, because at Hull House she was brought into daily contact with laborers and their wives who related to her many examples of occupationally derived disease.[60] By her own testimony she learned little at the library:

> It was all German, or British, or Austrian, Dutch, Swiss, even Italian, or Spanish—everything but American. In those countries industrial medicine was a recognized branch of the medical sciences; in my own country it did not exist. When I talked to my medical friends about the strange silence on this subject in American medical magazines and textbooks, I gained the impression that here was a subject tainted with Socialism or with feminine sentimentality with the poor. The American Medical Association had never had a meeting devoted to this subject, and except for a few surgeons attached to large companies operating steel mills, or railways, or coal mines, there were no medical men in Illinois who specialized in the field of industrial medicine.[61]

In fact, Hamilton's judgment is not quite accurate on the state of the American literature in 1907. A preliminary bibliography on occupational diseases and industrial hygiene prepared by the American Association for Labor Legislation shows more than 280 American entries, ranging alphabetically from Adler's "Report of a Case of Chronic Mercurial Poisoning" in the *American Lancet* of 1890 to Zenner's 1886 article on "Auctioneer's Cramp" in the Cincinnati *Lancet-Clinic*. Asbestos disease would soon make its first American appearance.[62] Yet insofar as industrial medicine focused on the diseases of a particular social class, it represented a dangerous topic out of step with the turn away from social reform that the public health profession was taking.

Public health reformers such as Hamilton were frequently of

upper-class and aristocratic origins, quite unlike the usual medical practitioner, the majority of whom lived economically marginal existences in an overcrowded profession riven by factions and sectarianism. By contrast, the tradition of sanitary reform in the nineteenth century rested on a totally different and firmer foundation, the bedrock of moral authority. Science, for public health reformers, was a means to reveal moral truths, expressed in terms of universal laws of nature and health. With the help of statistical compilations, reformers tried to demonstrate that violation of these laws by individuals or groups led inevitably to disease and disorder. By collecting data on large populations, they sought to reveal the laws of health and on this basis were responsible for initiating the systematic recording of vital events that became an obsession with nineteenth-century health reformers such as Lemuel Shattuck.[63]

Yet the ultimate task of public health was moral preceptorship, requiring the authority of the morally upright individual. For although the laws of health were simple and open to the understanding of all, the preventive measures they required—such as altering the behavior of others by example, stopping a company from fouling the public water supply, or seeing to it that the streets of the city were clean—demanded a degree of probity and disinterestedness thought to be in short supply in late nineteenth-century America. In the last analysis, a public health authority needed to be an expert not in science, but in virtue. And the operational definition of virtue was an individual "above politics," meaning not partisan but class politics. Public health decisions were not to be left to the "people" (whose morals were suspect) or to their elected representatives (who were contaminated by "the special interests") but rather to individuals whose social position, hence character, were presumed to insulate them from the vulgarity of personal ambition. The high-mindedness of the public health profession contrasts with a public perception of the venality of the medical profession and makes it all the more remarkable that the reformers' prestige and influence could be so effectively eroded in the space of two short decades.

One important development in this process was the triumph of the germ theory in the period from 1880 to 1900. In public health, particularly, the effect was immediate and sometimes dramatic. The new science of bacteriology had direct practical application in many areas of sanitation, especially regarding water and sewage purification. It now seemed that the insulation from politics that had once been sought by listening to the private voice of moral purity could henceforth be guaranteed by the public voice of value-free science. All through the early decades of the twentieth-century, in fact, science became the new touchstone whereby a disordered and class-ridden society could be made whole again. Only the scientific method and the scientists who understood and wielded it could be trusted to act in the name of reason and not in the name of self-interest. William Thompson Sedgwick, a leading sanitarian and teacher of public health, expressed these typical Progressive Era sentiments in a 1911 address entitled "Scientists and Technicians in the Public Service": "Scientists and technicians alike— must be employed and paid by the people, to rule over them as well as to guide them, to constitute a kind of official class, a kind of bureaucracy constituted for themselves by the people themselves."[64]

A New Order in Public Health

Public health's embrace of science also contributed to a shift in focus away from the environment and toward the individual. The years from 1905 to 1920 were not only years of crucial importance in the history of public health and medicine, but also years of change and turmoil in American society in general. The Panic of 1907 began a wave of bank and business failures that left in its wake a high level of unemployment that lasted for eight years. Whereas the average unemployment rate from 1900 to 1907 was only 2.9 percent, from 1908 to 1915 it averaged 6.6 percent. Although unemployment never reached 5 percent before 1907, in the eight years of stagnation following the Panic, it dipped below 5 percent only in a single year, reaching to 8 percent in 1914 and 10 percent in 1915.

The recession and the hardship it worked were accompanied by several spectacular and well-publicized episodes of labor violence. The Industrial Workers of the World (IWW) engaged in long and bloody free-speech fights in cities throughout the West and Northwest, and IWW involvement in the huge Lawrence and Patterson strikes of 1912 were international events. The dynamiting by union organizers of the Los Angeles Times building in 1911 and the infamous "Ludlow Massacre," where strikers against John D. Rockefeller, Jr.'s Colorado Fuel and Iron Company and members of their families were savagely killed by company thugs deputized as lawmen by county sheriffs in 1914, were each in their own ways taken as object lessons by those who hoped or feared that the existing social structure could not survive the anarchistic and socialistic elements that seemed to be springing up everywhere.

Perhaps most hopeful (or most ominous, depending on the point of view) was the rapid development of a class-conscious Socialist Party that was working hard to win votes and capture the trade unions. Even though it had not made any great gains between 1904 and 1908, by 1910 the Party was picking up momentum again. In that year, the first socialist congressman was elected, and the mayoralty of Milwaukee went over to the Party. In 1911, seventy-three other municipalities followed suit, and there were some 1,200 lesser Socialist officers elected in 340 towns and cities across the country. In the presidential election of 1912 the Socialist Party candidate Eugene Debs more than doubled his previous vote and received over 6 percent of the total votes cast.[65]

Within this context the dominant themes among those concerned with preserving the existing social order tended to be humanistic and meliorative but also carefully devoid of all class content. Leaders in the public health movement were no exception. Charles V. Chapin, the health commissioner of Providence, Rhode Island, cautioned his fellow health officers to beware of advocating public health projects on purely economic grounds, grounds that emphasized, for example, the huge dollar amounts lost from the premature death of laborers or the lost productivity to employers from lack of physical vigor and absenteeism. With the existing surplus of labor, he noted, it was hard to convince a worker that a decreased death rate would mean anything but more competition for jobs, and the argument that increased health meant increased productivity implied just that much more profit that the worker did not expect to share. As for management's view of these arguments, Chapin observed that unlike the cost of replacing a machine, the replacement cost of a laborer was essentially zero. When a manager is in need of an employee, Chapin noted, "in a short time help will come from Italy, from Syria, from Russia, and without cost to him or to the community in which he lives." The best strategy, Chapin countered, was to place the profession on a higher level by resisting the tendency to measure public health in purely economic terms. "Is it not enough," he asked, "to urge expenditures for the preservation of health because the happiness of mankind will be promoted thereby?"[66]

It was not that business standards, so much a part of Progressive-Era thinking, were shunned in public health. Chapin himself was a leading advocate of sound management in the health field, and he continually exhorted his colleagues to keep the kinds of records that would enable them to spend their budgets in the most efficient way. It was in terms of this stress on record keeping that the main features of the shift from an environmental to an individual-centered (medical) perspective began to appear.

Early in his career Chapin became convinced that the most important sources of infectious diseases were infected people, and that the most important mode of transmitting infection was personal contact. He consistently downgraded the importance of almost all other routes of infection except contact contagion. This was at first an iconoclastic and unpopular position. In an address to the American Public Health Association in 1902, he announced that "with minor exception, municipal cleanliness does little to prevent infection or decrease the death rate. Municipal cleanliness is no panacea. . . . It will make no demonstrable difference in a city's mortality whether its streets are clean or not, whether the garbage is removed promptly or allowed to accumulate, or whether it has a plumbing law."[67] Four years later, he declared that to believe that inanimate objects, called fomites, could cause infection was purely speculative. "In most cases of alleged infection by fomites, the fact is not proven at all," he asserted, adding, "direct exposure to infected persons is the probable source of the infection in most cases of contagious disease."[68] For Chapin, the mechanism of infection was social, not physical.

Chapin's ideas had occasioned debate for more than a decade within public health circles, and it was with the expectation of continued controversy in 1910 that Chapin sent off the manuscript of his textbook, *The Sources and Modes of Infection*.[69] In it he reviewed the world literature on the subject of contagion and reached the conclusion that the great preponderance of infectious disease resulted from contact with sick but undiagnosed cases or healthy carriers, that is, infected people. The great environmental routes, such as water and milk, contributed only a small portion to the total amount of infectious disease. Now, however, the book found an enthusiastic reception, with one admirer even proclaiming that it marked "the real beginning of scientific public health in America." This signalled that a sudden discontinuity in American thinking on public health was taking place. It would soon result in the complete displacement of the science of the safe environment from center stage.

Chapin's argument for the primacy of contact infection was based on evidence that there were many mild, unrecognized cases and healthy human carriers of infectious diseases. By means of these agents, disease could appear without any known contact with a previous case. Although the existence of missed cases and carriers had been known since the 1890s, in 1907 the affair of Typhoid Mary, an Irish cook who had infected an entire series of well-to-do households and was forcibly detained by the New York City Health Department, brought the subject to public attention in dramatic fashion. The image of the dangerous individual whose irresponsibility was the cause of disease seemed to be the perfect medical metaphor for a view that preferred to see labor trouble and social unrest as resulting from demagogic agitators and anarchists. A range of social concerns would now be condensed into the medical image of the individual carrier of disease.

Chapin himself saw the solution to the problem in better education in the principles of hygiene. One of his chief disciples, however, Hibbert W. Hill of the Minnesota State Board of Health, was not so restrained. In a widely read and influential book for the general public called *The New Public Health,* Hill announced the New Order: "The old public health was concerned with environment; the new is concerned with the individual. The old sought the sources of infectious disease in the surroundings of man; the new finds them in man himself."[70] Hill observed that the germs that produced disease were not ubiquitous but resided chiefly in a relatively few people. This reduced the insuperable problem of policing the total environment to the manageable problem of policing a much smaller number of people. Using tuberculosis as an example, Hill reasoned that

> if "general environment" be the great factor in tuberculosis the hundred million people of these United States must have each his or her own individual environment brought up to and kept at some standard level designed to maintain each individual in his or her own alleged "highest state of health." If, however, the infectiveness of the disease be the great factor, only 200,000 people (the actively infective cases) need this supervision in the United States, and they need it not for the improvement of their "general environment" but merely to prevent them from infecting others.[71]

Against this background, the first American reports of asbestos hazard by Pancoast and Prudential's Hoffman take on a new light. The justifiable preoccupation with tuberculosis brought with it a redefinition of the significance of the asbestos hazard. For Pancoast this significance was the possibility that exposure to dust would be mistakenly diagnosed as tuberculosis. For the industrial commentator on his paper and for Prudential's Hoffman, it was the possibility that asbestos workers would be predisposed to (and consequently sources of) this dread disease. Although tuberculosis and dust diseases were understood to be distinct but related diseases, the dominant medical concern was with tuberculosis. And the solution to the problem of tuberculosis placed the individual before the individual's environment.

Many politically conscious sanitarians and reformers were glad to be rid of the environment as a focus. Focusing on the environment risked calling explicit attention to the great disparity in living and working conditions existing in society and also raised questions about the economic value of municipal projects and who benefitted from them. Reformers were much more comfortable operating at the level of the individual while elevating their rhetoric to provide a social vision and humanistic objective that could be shared by all, radicals and reformers alike.

But public health as a profession bought this comfort at a high price. The abandonment of social reform for science and the shift away from the environment to the individual meant that public health practitioners occupied the same political, social, and economic arena as clinical medicine. Placed at a double disadvantage by a self-definition relegating them to the role of custodians for the dangerous and irresponsible and the necessity of working in the social locus of a powerful guild jealous of its professional prerogatives, the social reformers suffered a loss of prestige, and the remnants of their reform instinct withered.

As the needs of industry produced a new type of doctor, the industrial physician, the ideal of social reform could no longer provide a guide for practice. Representatives of an earlier era of public health reform, such as Alice Hamilton, were exceptions. In general, public health reformers did not perceive the environment of the worker as their main interest. Insofar as an asbestos worker's health was of any concern, the focus of attention and intervention was on the individual. But the client-centered norms of the private practitioner were not satisfactory, either. As it turned out, clinical medicine was itself not hospitable to the industrial doctor's role, effectively denying it the model of the traditional doctor-patient relationship. As we will see, industrial medicine turned finally to the firm.

Industrial Medicine and the Industrial Doctor

Industrial lung diseases such as silicosis and asbestosis were well defined in the medical literature by 1930 and were subjects of interest to a small group of medical and clinical specialists. In 1924 Dr. W. E. Cooke described in detail, in the widely read *British Medical Journal*,[72] the clinical signs, symptoms, and autopsy findings of a chronic lung disease in a worker in an English asbestos factory. Three years later Cooke described further details of this case, and he gave the name asbestosis to the unusual fibrosis of the lungs he observed.[73] But Cooke's case as well as others previously reported was complicated by co-existing tuberculosis or pneumonia, making an exact specification of the effects of the asbestos dust less certain. In 1928 H. E. Seiler reported a "pure" case of asbestosis from South Africa in an asbestos textile worker.[74] This report immediately prompted Dr. E. R. A. Merewether, chief inspector of factories in England, to undertake examination of hundreds of asbestos textile workers in that country. His report of that study, issued in 1930, revealed that 26.3 percent of the 363 workers examined had diffuse fibrosis of the lungs attributable to the inhalation of asbestos dust, while another 4 to 5 percent had early signs of the disease.[75]

At about the same time Dr. Anthony J. Lanza, formerly of the U.S. Public Health Service but then with the Metropolitan Life Insurance Company, began to study American asbestos textile workers. He did so at the request of "officials representing the asbestos industry in the United States, who were desirous of ascertaining whether asbestos dust was an occupational hazard in their establishment and if so, what was the nature of this hazard and what should be done to prevent or control it."[76] He was joined in this effort by an industrial hygienist, William Fehnel, whom the Jersey Zinc Company had hired to measure dust levels and who later joined Metropolitan after training at Harvard; and by William J. McConnell, who, like Lanza, had worked in the Public Health Service's Division of Industrial Hygiene. A preliminary report prepared in 1931 showed that of those engaged less than five years in asbestos factory work, 43 percent had X-ray signs of fibrosis; of those with five to ten years' exposure, 50 percent; of those with ten to fifteen years' exposure, 58 percent; and of those with over fifteen years, an astounding 87 percent. There was also an unusual prevalence of enlarged heart, thought by Lanza to be "a compensatory enlargement due to the additional work put upon the heart in efforts to oxygenate blood in fibrosed lungs."[77]

But this preliminary report would not appear in print in a medical journal until 1935. By that time the context within which the dust disease research was done would be radically altered by a wave of civil litigation involving industrial lung disease. The heightened awareness that prompted these damage suits was symbolized by the public outrage over the suffering of the victims of the Gauley Bridge Tunnel disaster.

Gauley Bridge and the New Interest in Industrial Lung Disease

The tunnel at Gauley Bridge in West Virginia was to be a conduit for waters of the New River that would drive the turbines of a hydroelectric power plant after a 129-foot drop.[78] Power from this facility was to operate an electrometallurgical plant of the Union Carbide Corporation. Construction of the tunnel began in 1930 under contract to the firm of Rinehart and Dennis of Charlottesville, Virginia. Coming as it did at the depths of the Great Depression, the project attracted skilled and unskilled miners from far beyond the local area. Many were out-of-work coal miners, and many were black.

Much of the material excavated from the three-and-three-quarter-mile hole being driven through the mountain turned out to be 99 percent pure silicon dioxide, or free silica. This was an added bonus for Union Carbide, which could use it as raw material in smelting ferrosilicon alloy. But for the tunnel workers it was a deadly hazard. Dust diseases of the lung caused by free silica had been known for centuries, and by 1930 there was extensive literature on its pathological, clinical, and industrial hygiene aspects.[79] Inhalation of silica dust causes progressive nodular scarring of the pulmonary tissue, which eventually leads to the slow suffocation of the worker from an impaired ability to ventilate the lungs and exchange gases. A markedly increased risk of tuberculosis is also a prominent complication. Under most conditions silicosis is a disease requiring seven or more years to become manifest, but the conditions at Gauley Bridge were so terrible that within months many tunnel workers became sick with acute silicosis and died—some, literally, "on the job." Within the space of a few years, close to 500 of the tunnel workers fell victim to the disease.

"Wet drilling" the tunnel, a technology known and used for many years, could have prevented the disease. But wet methods are slower than dry methods, and the short, two-year time schedule of the project discouraged their use. Even though West Virginia law required the use of wet methods, later investigations showed that the water was turned on only when the mine inspectors appeared and turned off again upon their departure.

In West Virginia, as in most other states at the time, no compensation was available to the tunnel workers. The worker's compensation system covered only occupational injuries that occurred at a definite time and place, thus excluding any occupational diseases that developed over time. The only other redress was through the common-law negligence suit. Eventually some 500 or more of the 2,500 workers employed in the tunnel did file suit against Rinehart and Dennis.

The Gauley Bridge disaster did not remain a local story. Early in 1934 the young radical playwright Albert Maltz picked up a hitch-hiking miner who related to him the events at Gauley Bridge. Maltz turned it into a short story for the left-wing periodical *New Masses* and shortly thereafter passed it on to an editor of the labor weekly *People's Press.* The story was soon picked up by other labor newspapers. By late 1935 Gauley Bridge had become a *cause célèbre* in the nation's radical press. The progressive congressman Vito Marcantonio of New York held hearings on the affair, which developed into a nationwide scandal. A later historian of industrial medicine was to write that "Gauley Bridge became a symbol of the disease hazards and consequent suffering risked by the industrial worker, just as the apple vendor and bread line came to symbolize his economic plight during the Great Depression."[80]

The law suits instituted in West Virginia as a result of Gauley Bridge were not unique, however. They were in fact part of a national wave of silicosis claims. By 1934 it was estimated that almost $300,000,000 in such claims had been filed against employers.[81] The *Weekly Underwriter,* an insurance industry publication, reported that more than 300 aggregate claims totaled in excess of $12 million. Many of the suits were brought against mines and sand and gravel plants. Some cases had already been tried with resulting heavy damages; $15,000 for a single plaintiff was not unusual. Hundreds of other cases had been settled out of court, with one large insurance company reported to have settled claims amounting to $1,000,000 from group insurance policies that contained disability benefits.

The sudden activity in the legal profession soon stimulated new work in the medical profession. Dr. James W. Ferguson, writing about occupational disease in 1936, noted that

> the importance of the subject is emphasized by the number of commissions lately formed to study the conditions dealing with dust and health and by the number of articles dealing with pneumoconiosis, silicosis, asbestosis, etc., that have appeared recently in medical literature.

It is also interesting to note that in cases concerning dust ills brought before the course of several states, industry has received a verdict of adverse character. All this affects the trend of social thought and, in turn, points out that disease due to the inhalation of dust at one's occupation concerns not only the employee and his dependents, but also the industry and society.[82]

Indeed, the medical journals were filled with articles about silicosis and other dust diseases. The historian Howard Selleck examined a dozen typical issues of *Industrial Medicine,* the official journal of the American Association for Industrial Physicians and Surgeons, and found no less than twenty-five major addresses dealing with medical and legal phases of the industrial lung disease problem between late 1932 and early 1935. Accompanying these major articles were more than seventy reprints, abstracts, and editorials on the same subject.[83]

The Lanza Study

Asbestosis was one of the dust diseases that received increased attention. Anthony Lanza was anxious to publish his industry-sponsored survey, the preliminary results of which were first communicated to Johns-Manville and Raybestos Manhattan in 1931, but by late 1934, issues of compensation loomed large to the sponsors.[84] At the very moment that Lanza sent his galley proofs to Johns-Manville's attorney Vandiver Brown, a New Jersey legislative commission was trying to decide if silicosis should be made a compensable disease under worker's compensation.[85] Brown shared the manuscript with attorney George Hobart, who had earlier negotiated some damage settlements for Johns-Manville and was concerned that the report as proposed might result in the inclusion of asbestosis in the New Jersey legislation as well:

> We have consistently urged that there is a substantial difference between silicosis and asbestosis—both as to the clinical nature of the disease and as to the reasonable probability of its incidence; and you will also recall that in particular we have urged that asbestosis should not at the present time be included in the list of compensable diseases, for the reason that it is only within a comparatively recent time that asbestosis has been recognized by the medical and scientific professions as a disease—in fact, one of our principal defenses in actions against the company on the common law theory of negligence has been that the scientific and medical knowledge have been insufficient until a very

recent period to place upon the owners of plants or factories the burden
or duty of taking special precautions against the possible onset of the
disease in their employees.[86]

It was therefore important, Hobart said, to have a medical report
that drew a distinction between asbestosis and the by then notorious
disease of silicosis. And "by the same token, it would be troublesome
if an official report should appear from which the conclusion might be
drawn that there is little if any difference between the two diseases."[87]

Hobart therefore agreed with a suggestion Brown had already
made in a letter to Lanza—that an important idea contained in the
conclusions of the preliminary 1931 report, but cut from the version
in galleys, be reinstated. Lanza had thought that asbestosis was a
disease clinically milder than silicosis because the severity of symptoms seemed less than might be expected from the appearance of the
X-rays. However, by late 1934 Lanza was aware that other scientists
(including Merewether in England) had found that asbestotics were
dying at a younger age than silicotics and that they seemed to contract
their disease under dust conditions that appeared safe in other industries. The attorney proposed a compromise, that Lanza insert in his
conclusions the following sentence: "Clinically, *from this study,* it
appears to be of a type milder than silicosis"[88] (emphasis added).
Several other changes in a similar vein were proposed and accepted
by Lanza. To him they must have appeared to be changes of marginal
scientific inaccuracy, more errors of omission rather than of outright
falsification. At the same time he could remain on good terms with
interests with which he felt comfortable and which provided him with
some support.

This tendency to give the industry position the benefit of the
doubt was best expressed by a request from Brown to Lanza in reference to the editorial changes of his 1934 galleys:

> I am sure that you understand that no one in our organization is suggest-
> ing that you alter by one jot or tittle any scientific facts or inevitable
> conclusions revealed or justified by your preliminary survey. All we ask
> is that all of the favorable aspects of the survey be included and that
> none of the unfavorable be unintentionally pictured in darker tones than
> the circumstances justify. I feel confident that we can depend on
> you. . . . to give us this "break."[89]

That confidence was well placed for other scientists who, like Lanza,
had developed and practiced their science in a milieu oriented to the

needs and viewpoint of management. Why this easy and comfortable relationship of industrial doctors and hygienists with management? Why not a direct and interested relationship with the workers themselves?

The Industrial Physician

By the 1930s industrial medicine had already had a checkered history. As Alice Hamilton noted about the early years of the century, "for a surgeon or physician to accept a position with a manufacturing company was to earn the contempt of his colleagues as a 'contract doctor.' "[90] This ostracism of the company doctor was a natural consequence of the political struggles of the medical profession to regulate competition during that formative era.

Physicians, especially surgeons, had for some time been employed in the railroad, mining, and logging industries in the late nineteenth and early twentieth centuries. In these geographically isolated and self-contained communities, workers suffered a frightening rate of industrial accidents that by the first decade of the century had become a national scandal and ushered in the workmen's compensation system. Although the principal role for reducing workplace injury went to the engineers, surgeons were still required to treat those who were injured.[91] The doctor usually worked under contract to the company, a form of practice that was anathema to the AMA, which wished to eliminate any interference with an open and free competitive market for its fee-for-service, solo-practitioner constituents.

The main objection to contract practice was that it often went far beyond ministrations at the work site, instead extending to all types of medical care. In 1907 in one state alone, Michigan, a Benton Harbor firm operated a contract plan for 300 employees. At Saginaw there were 750 employees enrolled, and an equal number were enrolled at the American Shipbuilding Company. Even more striking was Michigan Alkali Company's plan with 1,350 enrollees. These contract arrangements represented an enormous market loss to practitioners who were already economically pressed.[92]

The pay the physicians received was often degrading and represented to the organized profession the worst form of price cutting. The Michigan Alkali Company, for example, provided coverage for fifty cents a month, only to be outdone by the Electrical and Mechanical Company, which offered medical and surgical care for only fifteen cents a month. Many other firms charged even less.[93]

Organized medicine anguished over contract practice, much of which concerned industrial populations, but wavered on what to do about it. As the profession grew stronger, calls for sterner measures became more frequent, and at the same time the economic issue began to assume larger-than-life proportions as it was recast as a fundamental question of individual freedom and the sanctity of the doctor-patient relationship. According to this view, the doctor and the patient both were at the mercy of conditions stipulated by the contracting agency, which interposed itself as middleman, purchasing services at wholesale and selling them at retail.[94] While few local societies actually forbade their members to engage in any form of contract practice (as it was too common), they did cast a pall of unsavoriness over it that was to have lasting effects on the industrial medical practitioner.

One pioneer industrial physician of the period was Henry E. Mock of Sears Roebuck. Mock's entry into industrial medicine is especially revealing of the forces at work in this new specialty. In 1908 he was acquainted socially with Sears's company doctor of four years, Jules Gauss. Gauss told Mock that he was about to resign since "the Chicago medical society had refused his membership because they considered his industrial practice unethical."[95] Mock, who was just then beginning a surgical practice in Chicago, was attracted to the post as Gauss's successor for practical reasons: he was just married and in debt. Yet he wished to avoid the problems that Gauss had with the medical society. Mock sought Gauss's advice:

> He pointed out that too many industries were invading the field of general medical practice by having their doctors give home treatment to employees at a reduced rate below that usually charged by the profession.
>
> The pitfall that had ruined Dr. Gauss's ethical standing was the fact that the Sears Mutual Benefit Association used one-dollar house calls on any member of an employee's family, as an inducement to prospective members. Naturally this practice had induced the ire of the general practitioners of Chicago, with the result that Dr. Gauss . . . was classified as unethical. Needless to say, he regained his ethical status, and developed an excellent general practice in Indianapolis.[96]

Mock stopped the practice of cut-rate housecalls, instead charging for a home visit by any Sears doctor at prevailing fees. He also adopted a very "professional" attitude toward his work. He was not just a practitioner but an applied scientist. He viewed the 15,000 Sears employees as a "great human laboratory" whose secret would be revealed by performing complete physical examinations.

In 1916 Mock, together with similary minded men employed by other large industries, formed the American Association of Industrial Physicians and Surgeons (AAIPS). With American entry into World War I imminent, conservation of the nation's labor force and the protection of its productive potential were on the agenda of its largest corporations. When the 125 physicians and surgeons engaged in industrial practice or government service first met in Detroit, their chief task was to define the ambiguous role of the physician employed by industry. Stung by the low regard of the rest of their profession, they genuinely strove to understand their function in the general scheme of things.[97] A similar group, the Conference Board of Physicians in Industry, likened its own role to that of the engineer: "No man can work at a job if he is sick in body or mind," noted Dr. John J. Moorhead, chairman of the Conference Board, "and the physician in industry has a unique opportunity of proving that the medical engineer is an essential element."[98]

One favorite tool was the annual physical exam. As the Conference Board stated, "In time the process of physical re-examination at stated intervals will be recognized as a necessary work of medical engineering, just as essential as the re-inspection of any other kind of machinery to prevent breakdown or shutdown."[99] Shortly thereafter the compulsory physical exam came to be considered "the keystone of medical supervision in industry" and was the primary topic of meetings of the Conference Board and the AAIPS. In the 1920s a survey revealed that 50 percent of firms gave preemployment physicals, and 10 percent required annual physicals of those employed.[100]

The industrial physician was more than a mere inspector, however. He also needed a sound grasp of the special context and objectives of the industrial enterprise. According to a 1922 Conference Board report,

> the physician in industry is one who applies principles of modern medicine and surgery to the industrial worker, sick or well, supplementing the remedial agencies of medicine by the sound application of hygiene, sanitation and accident prevention, adequate and cooperative appreciation of the social, economic and administrative problems and responsibilities of industry in its relation to society.[101]

This nonmedical knowledge, similar to that required of company managers, was absolutely essential, for without it the physician was "individualistic" and "non-cooperative" in the industrial enterprise. Thus, the physicians and surgeons that made up the membership of the AAIPS and the Conference Board identified more strongly with the large corporations for which they worked than did the average "lumps and bumps" contract physician.

Doing Good by Doing Well

The "great struggle between capital and labor" was much on people's minds, but in line with the new approach in public health, the AAIPS and the Conference Board saw their work as unaffected by any disparity of interests between these two great forces. If their work were successful, everyone would be well served:

> To secure the maximum efficiency from the human machine, the industrial surgeon, virtually the human engineer, acts as the agent for stabilizing labor, thereby facilitating production and helping the worker to do a better day's work, prolong the years of his activity and increase his compensation.[102]

Many members of the public sector were also drawn to this position. The first president of the AAIPS was Dr. Joseph Schereschewsky of the U.S. Public Health Service. By 1916 the federal government, having only recently entered the field of industrial medicine, was starting to make its presence felt. In 1907 the Hours of Service Act regulated working conditions nationally for the first time by limiting the services of train employees and telegraph and signal operators. Following a disastrous and well-publicized mine disaster, the Bureau of Mines was formed in 1910, although it largely restricted itself to research on mine rescue procedures.[103] In 1913 the Department of Labor was formed to "foster, promote and develop" the lot of wage workers. (One of its publications of 1918, authored by Frederick Hoffman, has already been mentioned in connection with its discussion of asbestos hazards.) In 1914 the Division of Occupational Health of the Public Health Service was formed, with Schereschewsky as its head.[104] In its early years the Service investigated the granite, pottery, glass, chemical, and brass foundry industries. Another Service doctor active with AAIPS was Anthony Lanza, the specialist in dust diseases and future asbestos researcher.[105]

The influence of the New Public Health was also much in evidence in the orientation of the new elite of industrial medicine. Although the drones of the old contract practice toiled on as traditional doctors, suffering the opprobrium of their colleagues, the new medical manager of the large corporation adopted a different posture that separated him both from his unsavory colleagues and from the clinical practitioner. In preventive medicine the first duty was to the public at large. Medical professionals sometimes opposed measures of public value, wrote C. E. Ford, medical director of the General Chemical Company, because their first duty was to the individual. But the *industrial* physician had the best of both, as he did not have to choose between these different objectives, satisfying both moral imperatives by promoting the mutual benefit of employer and worker.[106]

Despite the rhetoric, the reality centered on the benefits to the corporation, not the worker. The physical exam, the tool *par excellance* of the industrial physician, was praised for its ability to protect employers against "fraudulent" compensation claims, to select employees with lower risks of suffering accidents, and to determine the best type of work for a new employee.[107] The goal of determining who was fit to work gradually became the only goal of the physical exam. This truncated objective allowed an abbreviated physical exam to be accomplished in under ten minutes. As the medical director of AT&T expressed it in 1926, the industrial physical exam was not the practice of medicine, but the application of medicine to the industrial enterprise.[108]

The information generated by the physical exam, such as it was, was not even legally the property of the employee but of his employer. Because the results of tests were rarely followed up, they were in any case of little use to the worker but still of tangible benefit to the corporation, since "false positive" errors were of small consequence to the employer. While the company physician did not have to inform the worker of the results of the examination, he was required by law to inform the employer, who paid for the services of each. As the historian Angela Nugent has trenchantly observed, "The industrial context thus transformed traditionally private medical information into a commodity paid for by business and employed for its needs."[109]

Those corporations which did do more thorough exams were still greatly reluctant to get involved in any way in the employee's medical care. The industrial physician was sensitive to the necessity of not trespassing on the turf of the general practitioner and took pains to assure the organized profession that he was not in competition with it. Indeed, the AAIPS maintained that its members actually created work for their nonindustrial colleagues:

> The industrial doctor, through his program of employee examinations and periodic check-ups, discovers conditions that would otherwise remain unknown to the employees, and he sends them to their family doctors or physicians of their own choice. Thus he expands the demands for outside practitioners' services, helps to develop practice for them that they wouldn't get otherwise.[110]

Yet these outside referrals, when they occurred, did not put the workers in very knowledgeable hands: "Most general practitioners are not primarily interested in industrial medicine. They concentrate most of their attention on problems of internal medicine, acute infectious diseases, obstetrics, metabolic diseases, etc."[111] Thus, any results derived from the "great human laboratory" might benefit science or the corporation but were less likely to be of direct value to the worker.

That science did benefit is evident from the gradual accumulation of knowledge as represented in the scientific literature. Yet, as E. F. Lutz, associate medical director of General Motors Corporation, pointed out, this kind of scientific advance was not high on the agenda of most companies, whose

> top managements are not primarily interested in and do not want to practice medicine. Their primary objective is to manufacture automobiles, washing machines, locomotives, or what have you, and their chief concern is that the article they are manufacturing be of superior quality and that it be produced in an economical manner.[112]

As a result, the status of industrial physicians in the 1920s varied from glorified "finger-wrapper" to out-and-out representative of management. This was reflected in the results of a survey conducted in 1918, which showed that 42 percent of company medical departments reported to company officials whose main object was production, 21 percent to departments handling compensation claims for injuries, 18 percent to administrative officers, and 15 percent to staff departments involved in personnel or labor relations. Only 4 percent possessed "the freedom, responsibility, and authority to which [they were] entitled."[113]

Yet the leaders of the AAIPS and the Conference Board did not despair but continued to strive for a more active role in the corporation, which effectively meant increased managerial responsibility. "Industry is the chief basis for the subsistence of civilized peoples," C. E. Ford asserted. "The maintenance of healthy industries is the state's first duty, because those who are employed in industry are part of the community for which the state is responsible."[114] The ambiguity between an industry that is economically healthy and one with healthy workers was symptomatic of an intrinsically blurred distinction that lay at the heart of early industrial medicine.

These ideas fit nicely into the prevailing techniques of the new breed of corporate managers that gained influence in the years after World War I. The introduction of company welfare programs was only part of an organized effort to foster cooperation and trust between management and labor. In line with traditional Progressive Era thinking, the activities of industrial medicine were thought to be intrinsically unbiased because they were grounded in science. The science referred to was only partially medical in nature, however. "Although fundamentally the science of medicine," wrote Clarence Selby, an AAIPS stalwart, industrial medicine in a corporate setting actually occupied a position "similar to that of employment, safety, and compensation. All are specialties in the science of management."[115] Not only the internal dynamics of industrial medicine but also pressure from organized medicine led in this direction. A 1930 editorial in the *Journal of the American Medical Association* allowed that examining workers for employment fitness, maintaining production efficiency, and providing health and safety education were legitimate tasks for industrial physicians, but the author drew the line at caring for bedridden workers and their families: "Industrial medicine . . . must deal with the worker as a *producing unit* not as a *social* unit." Industrial doctors' failure to heed the proper boundaries of their practice, the editorialist warned, would result in loss of status as specialists and a reversion to their former reputation as "poorly educated, low salaried 'hacks.' "[116]

Thus, by 1930 a distinct specialty of industrialized medicine had emerged, separate from the discredited tradition of contract practice but not part of the mainstream of organized medicine. Strongly influenced by the New Public Health movement, practitioners of industrial medicine saw danger residing more in individual workers than in their environment and adopted as their "preventive" tool the physical examination. This emphasis on fixing the worker rather than the workplace was a product of forces operating within medicine and public health during industrial medicine's formative years, affecting profoundly the way industrial doctors viewed occupational hazards. A modern historian has summed it up nicely:

> Company doctors' elaborate emphasis on occupational hygiene and personal stamina masked a failure to consider environmental hazards. The very tests to which doctors subjected employees expressed a tacit acceptance of industrial hazards, and stipulated physical criteria best suited to resist the stress of different occupations. Company doctors' allegiance to physical examinations in industry committed them to focus attention on the fitness of individuals for work, rather than on the more controversial and more difficult problem, the fitness of the industrial environment for health.[117]

Seeing itself as the natural agent whereby the corporation could do well by doing good (and vice versa), the profession did not explicitly acknowledge that there was any intrinsic contradiction between caring for individual workers and safeguarding the interests of the corporation. This allowed an easy identification with management and produced an unresolved role-conflict that continues to trouble the profession to this day.[118]

The Origins of Industrial Hygiene

Less problematic was the emergence of the industrial hygiene profession, an engineering-oriented discipline that had the task of eliminating hazards by proper design of the workplace and its machinery. The hygienist's goal was a workplace "as free as possible of injurious materials, processes and conditions."[119] The individuals who were attracted to this work usually had an engineering or laboratory background. In the field of prevention of dust diseases, much of the work involved assessing the extent of the hazard by devising and carrying out dust measurements in various industries. One such industry was the manufacture of asbestos products. The growth of the asbestos textile, insulation, and friction products industries and the new litigation-inspired concern with dust diseases in the 1930s attracted the attention of industrial hygienists. The results of their early studies would have lasting effects.

Even more than the doctors, hygienists identified with management, despite the fact that much of their early work was initiated in the public sector. There, the lead was taken by the Public Health Service and the Bureau of Mines. The Service's Division of Industrial Hygiene, headed until 1918 by Dr. Schereschewsky (first president of AAIPS), was subsequently in charge of, among others, Drs. Lanza and William McConnell, both participants in industry-sponsored asbestos research in later years. From 1923 on, the Division carried out a number of extensive dust studies in various trades such as granite, cement, and the cotton textile industries. The work was aided by use of a new dust-measuring instrument, developed jointly by Dr. Leonard Greenburg and George W. Smith of the Public Health Service and the Bureau of Mines, respectively.

The Greenburg-Smith impinger, as it was called, was field tested by a young sanitary engineer named John J. ("Jack") Bloomfield, who is considered by many to be the father of American industrial hygiene.[120] Bloomfield was a Russian immigrant, born Ivan Osepovich Garber, whose father had left Europe in 1905 "because of his health."[121] His brother had preceded him to Haverhill, Massachusetts, and changed his name to Bloomfield. Settling in Dover, New Hampshire, Jack Bloomfield was an excellent high school student and was persuaded by an interested teacher to take a competitive examination for a college scholarship. By this means he received both full tuition and a stipend and graduated in 1920 from the University of New Hampshire as a chemical engineer. (The five who graduated with him were all successful, one later becoming a vice-president of Monsanto and another of Gulf.) Bloomfield also did well, receiving no less than four job offers. One was from the Pittsburgh laboratory of the U.S. Bureau of Mines, whose head had done graduate work at New Hampshire and preferred New Hampshire graduates. Bloomfield decided to go there, and thus began his laboratory work measuring dusts, gases, fumes, and vapors.[122]

On at least one occasion during his three years at the Bureau of Mines, Bloomfield was "loaned" to the American Smelting and Refining Company's plant in Donora, Pennsylvania, to help the company with a lawsuit from farmers who alleged crop damage from sulfur dioxide emitted by an AS&R smelter. Using a portable Bureau of Mines laboratory but paid by AS&R, Bloomfield made sulfur dioxide measurements and testified as an expert for the company at trial. AS&R prevailed, with the judge commenting "that smoke stacks indicated progress." (Recalling the incident more than fifty years later,

Bloomfield laughed at the contrast with the 1970s, "with the EPA running rampage all over the place!"[123]). Thus, the relationship with industry was unusually close and cordial even in the public sector.

In 1923 Dr. Lewis Thompson, who had recently taken charge of the Division of Industrial Hygiene of the Public Health Service, recruited Bloomfield. The Service had no actual laboratories of its own, using instead the facilities of various universities. Bloomfield went to Yale, where he shared an office with Leonard Greenburg and an eminent figure in public health, Charles-Edward Amory Winslow. He stayed at Yale ten years, during which time he used the Greenburg-Smith impinger in study after study of the "dusty trades," coupling his measurements with health studies of workers conceived by Thompson and a Public Health Service statistician, Edgar Sydenstricker (brother of Nobel laureate Pearl Buck). As a result of Bloomfield's work, the Greenburg-Smith impinger became the *de facto* dust measuring instrument in the United States for almost the next fifty years.[124]

Other pioneers in industrial hygiene came to the field from different directions. In 1925 Warren Cook was hired by the Engineering and Inspection Division of the Travelers Insurance Company to look into chemical aspects of worker's compensation and liability insurance. One of the first cases involved the fireworks industry, where exposure to white phosphorous was occurring. White phosphorous was a notorious poison that had been banned years earlier in the match industry. Cook recommended engineering controls on the wrapping machine. Before any of Cook's recommendations could be acted upon, a death from phosphorous poisoning occurred in the fireworks industry, and at the behest of the U.S. Commissioner of Labor, a substitute for the chemical was found.[125] Cook's approach illustrates the typical engineering inclination to solve a problem technologically rather than by asking whether phosphorous needed to be used at all. Cook later was instrumental in developing standards for workplace contaminants, including asbestos.

Theodore Hatch also began work in the mid-1920s. The son of a building contractor, Hatch originally planned to become an architect and studied civil engineering in preparation for this profession. By chance, the chairman of the Civil Engineering Department at Dartmouth had begun his own career in the diamond and gold mines of South Africa and was acutely aware of the effect of this work on the health of miners. He believed that some engineers at least should take into account the effects on the users of engineering constructions. Yet the only engineering specialty that in 1925 recognized the connection between people and their physical environment was sanitary engineering, the product of the great scientific public health reforms of the turn of the century. Hatch left Dartmouth for Harvard for a one-year course of study in sanitary engineering and then took a job with the Sanitary Engineering Division of the Tennessee Health Department. There he worked on improving water supplies, sewage disposal, milk sanitation, malaria control, and rat control, among others of the usual problems of sanitary engineering practice. Hatch might well have remained in Tennessee for the rest of his career had he not received an offer from his old Harvard professor, Philip Drinker, to take part in developing a new field called industrial hygiene. It was to be a joint venture between the Sanitary Engineering Department in the Engineering School and the Department of Ventilation and Illumination at the new Harvard School of Public Health. After just a year in Tennessee, Hatch returned to Harvard where he began a close association with Drinker, his new chief.[126]

The industrial health program at Harvard was one of the earliest in the country. Simultaneously with the formal founding of the School of Public Health in 1918, Frederick C. Shattuck, the retired Jackson Professor of Clinical Medicine at the Harvard Medical School, raised $125,000 from manufacturing firms in New England "to be spent upon the teaching of students and the investigation of problems in industrial health."[127] The principal aim was to train company doctors, and to that end a certificate of public health was issued after completion of a five-month course. Nonmedical students were also admitted, but their role was at first not clearly visualized:

> Students who do not possess a medical degree would seem to have a rather doubtful future in the field of industrial health. If properly qualified they may obtain the Certificate of Public Health at the end of one year's work and will be advised to specialize toward the sociological side of industrial medicine. . . . [However], if it is the purpose of these students to qualify for factory inspectorships, they will be given practical opportunity to learn what such work entails. . . . While we are ready to accept well-qualified students of this type, we are not . . . confident of their future.[128]

The curriculum in 1919 and 1920 reflected the heavy medical emphasis, with only two courses out of sixteen identifiable as industrial hygiene in the engineering sense ("Industrial Sanitation," taught in

Cambridge at Harvard's Engineering School, and "Methods of Air Analysis," taught in Boston at the Harvard-MIT School of Public Health).[129]

By 1919 other schools, among them Cincinnati Medical College, Johns Hopkins's new School of Hygiene and Public Health, and Rush Medical College, had one or more courses in industrial health. But no program was as advanced as Harvard's Division of Industrial Hygiene, financed by Shattuck's Industrial Hygiene Fund from New England's industry. It was headed by Cecil K. Drinker, Philip Drinker's older brother, an applied physiologist with a keen interest in the health effects of industrial environments. Descended from a long line of Quakers going back to the colonial era, Drinker had come to his post by way of Haverford College, the University of Pennsylvania Medical School, and a residency at the newly built and Harvard-affiliated Peter Bent Brigham Hospital in Boston. In 1916 he succeeded Shattuck as Jackson Professor and thus began a lifelong association with Harvard that was eventually to lead to his becoming the second dean of the School of Public Health.[130]

When he assumed control of the semi-autonomous (because of the Shattuck Fund) Division of Industrial Hygiene in 1918, it was principally because it was felt that the "point of view of applied physiology was of course wholly appropriate to the carrying on of teaching and research in the field of industrial hygiene."[131] That "point of view" was still medical, as shown by the governance of the program, which was primarily contributed by the Medical School, not its engineering counterpart:

> Since Industrial Hygiene is regarded as being, in the main, a medical problem, it was felt necessary to ally it very closely with Medical School affairs, and as a consequence the Governing Committee on Industrial Hygiene is entirely a Medical School Committee.[132]

Despite the start given it by Shattuck's collection from New England industrialists, the fledgling program to train company doctors proved a hungry mouth to feed. Shattuck was continually forced to solicit more funds from industry. Monies came from both local textile and steel concerns and national sources such as the Rockefeller Foundation and Carrier Engineering Company. In a 1922 letter to J. P. Morgan the younger, Shattuck describes his efforts to obtain $100,000 from U.S. Steel's Judge Elbert Gary: "It was thought possible that Judge Gary might feel like doing something substantial to offset in part, at least criticism to which he and the Steel Company have been subjected on the ground of inhumanity to their workers."[133]

Expiation of guilt with a public relations bonus was not the only advantage Shattuck offered. Writing to a U.S. Steel official, Shattuck noted that the School of Public Health could also complement the industrial research and development effort that had led many of the new elite of technology-based companies to establish their own experimental laboratories: "The School is supplementary to them, if you like, and in a position to undertake studies which may be highly useful to you but [with] which your established laboratories could hardly deal."[134]

While the search for money went on, the program continued to expand and did so, significantly, in the direction of engineering research. In 1921 and 1922 Philip Drinker, trained as a chemical engineer, joined his brother Cecil and took over teaching of the "Air Analysis" course. The ability to measure and control hazards was a natural accompaniment to the interests of medical men such as Cecil Drinker, and this capability became more important as a new approach to prospective donors emphasized the school's ability to provide a certain amount of free consultation, expressed as a "willingness and eagerness to be of assistance."[135] As Philip Drinker was joined by Hatch and other young engineers, it gradually became clear that the original objectives of becoming a major training ground for industrial physicians was giving way to training engineers whose specialty was designing less dangerous workplaces. The medical men were coming in fewer numbers and staying for shorter periods, while interest from engineers was growing.[136] When the Harvard School of Public Health entered a new phase of development in 1922 with the help of a substantial grant from the Rockefeller Foundation, its offerings in "factory hygiene" had already doubled to four courses, and by 1927 the Schools of Public Health and Engineering were ready to launch a new program in "industrial sanitation" (what we now call industrial hygiene).

The impetus to do so clearly came from industry, which was not interested as much in doctors as in engineers. In a joint statement announcing the program, Professor Gordon Fair of the Engineering School and Philip Drinker of the School of Public Health expressed it clearly:

The increase in the size of industrial establishments, the consistent upward trend in the wage level of skilled workmen, and the rapid development of the policy of group insurance in the United States have created a real demand in industry for sanitary working conditions and the increased physical capacity among wage earners. In the past, the industrial physician has been called upon to investigate and carry through the necessary improvements and, more often than not, he has found himself faced with engineering as well as medical problems—the design or supervision of changes in construction or plant operation, for which his training does not qualify him.

The Harvard Engineering School and the Harvard School of Public Health, through their contact with the industries, have become convinced that there is need for engineers whose special studies have prepared them to cooperate with the industrial physician in problems of plant sanitation and hygiene.[137]

The actual employment of engineers in industry specifically for hygiene purposes was almost nonexistent at the time, although a few examples exist. The Jersey Zinc Company, for example, assigned William Fehnel, one of its chemists, to measure dust levels when the Drinkers were investigating manganese poisoning in its plant in the early 1920s. After a short training course at Harvard, Fehnel returned to the company to continue the monitoring program, but he left soon thereafter to join the staff of the Metropolitan Life Insurance Company, a major industrial underwriter. He later participated in Lanza's asbestos industry studies. Hatch considers him the first person to be deliberately employed by industry to do industrial hygiene work, even though his tenure was short.[138]

In general, however, by the 1930s industrial concerns had yet to discover industrial hygiene as a specialized discipline. The Harvard program was just beginning to produce its first engineering graduates after a beginning that emphasized medical practice, and the U.S. Public Health Service and Bureau of Mines had small but influential groups who were pioneering the techniques of field study. Yet the responsibility for industrial hygiene activities rested with the state and local governments. Although federal health officials conducted research work in the laboratory and in the field, as did a few universities such as Harvard, the application of results rested with the five states and one city (New York) that had official industrial hygiene programs.

The Science and Politics of Asbestos-Related Disease

In 1936 the Social Security Act (SSA) provided for the first time money to states for the development and extension of public health work in all its aspects, and the Public Health Service in cooperation with the Conference of State and Provincial Health Authorities of North America began a program to establish active industrial hygiene work in state and local health departments.[139] The Public Health Service was led to do this out of concern for the many small plants that were not equipped to handle industrial hygiene problems, although there is little evidence that many of the larger industries were making any effort to do so either.[140]

The burden of training new hygienists fell largely on the Service, both because of its long experience in the field and its responsibility to administer the SSA funds set aside for this purpose. In the summer of 1936 it set up a special four-week short course for selected personnel from state health departments.[141] Theirs were jobs that promised little in the way of power or fortune. The main task of these individuals was to educate industry, as state industrial hygiene divisions did not have the authority to enforce their recommendations. Apart from a technical background, therefore, industrial hygienists also needed the "ability to establish contact with plant executives and to enlist the cooperation of executives, foremen, and laborers." This required "initiative; tact; good judgment; and good address." For these qualities doctors trained in industrial hygiene had recommended salaries of $7,500; engineers, $5,800; chemists, $4,000; and nurses, $2,000.[142]

Public Health Service-sponsored training of industrial hygienists had two important consequences for the problem of controlling asbestos hazards. The first was the launching of cooperative field investigations of important hazardous industries in cooperation with the newly formed state units. The short course was only an introduction. The field investigations were "hands-on" exercises. One of the first and most important was an extensive study of asbestos textile plants in North Carolina, headed by Public Health Service doctor Waldemar Dreessen and a team from the Service and the state health department. The second consequence was the establishment of an association of industrial hygienists, the American Conference of Governmental Industrial Hygienists (ACGIH). In the 1940s this voluntary organization took it upon itself to recommend guidelines for levels of hazardous agents in the workplace. As it happened, the ACGIH asbestos recommendation was derived from the results of Dreessen's 1938 study of asbestos textile mills. The ACGIH standard stood as the only national benchmark until the late 1960s.

The Dreessen Study

Dreessen and his federal-state team studied three North Carolina asbestos textile factories at the request of the State Board of Health and the Industrial Commission, the administrators of the state Workmen's Compensation Act. This engineering and medical study had three objectives: medical study of the effects of prolonged inhalation of asbestos dust; identification of the most hazardous processes in the plants and recommendations for protection; and "to find out what concentration of asbestos dust can be tolerated without injury to health."[143] It was the final objective that was to have the most lasting effect.

In all, 541 workers were examined, 242 dust counts were made (using the Greenburg-Smith impinger), and detailed recommendations for dust control were given. Results were issued as an official Bulletin of the Public Health Service and ran for 126 pages. Before the medical examination, an occupational history was taken from each worker. The responses present an interesting picture of the southern asbestos textile worker in the mid-1930s.

Five of six were white Anglo-Saxon men and women (in a ratio of three to one); the remainder were black males. Almost 40 percent (200 out of 541) had worked with other fibers in cotton and wool textile plants. "A large proportion" had worked on farms continuously or intermittently. Of the fourteen occupational groups investigated by the Service, asbestos workers were the youngest, with an average age of just over thirty-two years. Ninety-four percent were under fifty.[144] Only twenty-three had ever worked in a dusty trade prior to their employment in the asbestos textile plants, mostly for very short periods.

The average length of employment was also relatively short, with four of five workers employed less than ten years and more than half employed less than five years. This was partly a reflection of the comparative newness of large-scale asbestos textile operations in the United States. (Only one of the three plants was in operation before 1920). But there were also other reasons for the low average age and short duration of employment. Fifteen months before the study began, approximately 150 workers were replaced by new workers who had little or no previous experience with asbestos.[145]

Medical examinations of the workers were done by two physicians. Each had first toured the factories to familiarize themselves with the various jobs. Then the workers were brought in to a space set aside in the factory for the examination.

> An improvised darkroom was used for fluoroscopy and for processing the X-ray films. In an adjoining room the medical examinations were made by two physicians approximately according to the following schedule: Four persons at 9 A.M.; four at 10:30 A.M.; four at 1 P.M.; four at 2 P.M.; and four at 3 P.M. In other words, about 30 minutes were required per examination. The routine used in the study of pulmonary tuberculosis was followed in the examination of the chest. After the history and physical findings had been recorded, the group of four was fluoroscoped and chest roentgenograms were taken. A few examinations were made in the evening, and other adjustments were made in the schedule so as not to interfere too seriously with the work routine of the employees.[146]

The results were typical for those engaged in dusty trades. Overall, approximately one worker in four showed evidence of the disease and the prevalence of asbestosis rose rapidly with increasing dust exposure. Dust measurements were made with the Greenburg-Smith impinger, which did not differentiate between asbestos fibers and any other fibers found in the air (cotton or cellulose, for example). Dust concentrations were expressed, therefore, in terms of the total dust, asbestos and nonasbestos, and given in terms of the number of million particles per cubic foot of air (mppcf).

Dreessen and his co-workers noted that the prevalence of asbestosis was related not only to the concentration of dust but also to the duration of exposure. They therefore initially proposed to measure exposure by the product of the two, in "millions-of-particle-years." Thus, a worker exposed to 5 mppcf for ten years would have the same exposure as one exposed to 10 mppcf for five years. Using this system, they found that a fifth of workers with an exposure of 50 to 99 million particle-years had asbestosis, and half with over 100 million particle-years had the disease. These exposures were extremely low in comparison to dust levels needed to cause a comparable degree of silicosis.[147]

Of some interest was the result of examining the workers who had been discharged before the study began. Sixty-nine of the 150 were located and showed a prevalence of asbestosis of over 60 percent, more than double the rate of those still on the job.[148] It appeared that as workers sickened they were quickly replaced.

The most important results of the study, however, pertained not to those who had asbestosis but to those who did not:

> From a practical standpoint, one of the most important results of a medical and engineering study such as this is the definition of safe working conditions in the industry under study. Ideally, a threshold concentration of dust should be the highest dust concentration that would not produce pneumoconiosis in originally healthy workmen during their entire working life. The chief difficulty in this study, as in most of the earlier studies of the Public Health Service, is that very few workmen are exposed for a long period of time to low concentrations of asbestos dust. Because of the importance of the problem, it seems to be desirable to use such data as are at hand to define tentative safe working conditions that may serve as standards for the guidance of factory managers and engineers until more complete data are available.[149]

No cases of asbestosis were found at exposures to less than 2.5 mppcf, and only three doubtful cases at exposures to less than 5 mppcf. Of the thirty-nine persons in the lower-exposure category, however, only six had been employed longer than five years. Because asbestosis takes time to develop, the significance of finding no or few cases is doubtful. Nevertheless, Dreessen and his team felt it was important to establish some reference mark, so they tentatively suggested 5 mppcf "as the threshold value for asbestos-dust exposure until better data are available."[150]

There was abundant evidence in Dreessen's own study that 5 mppcf was inadequate as a threshold value. Using particle-years as an index to account for duration as well as intensity of exposure, Dreessen found that 8 percent of unexposed office personnel had cough compared to 14 percent of workers in the 0–25 million particle-year group; 27 percent in the 25–49 million particle-year group; 35 percent in the 50–99 million particle-year group; and 61 percent in the group with over 100 million particle-years. Results were comparable for a variety of other signs and symptoms of asbestosis, including blood-streaked sputum and fixation of the diaphragm (from inelasticity of the lungs).[151] Moreover, a table in the report shows that five of 192 workers exposed to less than 25 million particle-years had early asbestosis. At 5 mppcf, 25 million particle years is an exposure of only five years, hardly a working lifetime. In the 50–99 million particle-year category, fully 75 percent of the workers had asbestosis, indicating a working life of only ten to twenty years at 5 mppcf.

Why, then, did Dreessen ignore the important factor of duration in suggesting 5 mppcf as a tentative threshold value? Neither the Service nor the State Division of Industrial Hygiene had authority to order workplace standards. They could only persuade. After investigating work practices in the engineering portion of their study, they concluded that new dust control technology was capable of reducing dust exposure for the "majority" of workers to less than 5 mppcf. Above that level they found clear-cut instances of asbestosis and therefore at minimum could make the case that dust should be reduced at least to that level. Because exposures in many jobs exceeded 50 mppcf without dust control, reducing levels overall to 5 mppcf would have been a major step forward. At the same time, the explicitly tentative nature of the recommendation anticipated a more thorough investigation using a group with longer work experience at the lower exposures. It would be three decades, however, before the required studies would be done, and the "tentative" standard drastically revised. By that time, tens of thousands of asbestos workers would be exposed to levels of asbestos dust that would kill them.

The Shipbuilding Hazard

A tragic example of an industry where deadly exposure would occur on a massive scale was shipbuilding. Chrysotile asbestos had been used in ships since the late nineteenth century for a variety of purposes. Then, in the wake of World War I, President Harding's Secretary of State, Charles Evans Hughes, proposed a drastic reduction in naval tonnage.[152] This 1921 Washington Treaty among the major powers had an unexpected effect on asbestos workers as the lighter amosite asbestos was substituted for chrysotile, thus allowing heavier armaments for the same capital tonnage.[153] The light amosite asbestos became easily airborne and created an evident hazard for shipyard workers. As the United States moved towards mobilization and rearmament for the impending European conflict of the 1940s, industrial hygienists were called upon to ensure safe conditions in the shipyards.

One prominent member of this new profession was the chairman of the Industrial Hygiene Department at the Harvard School of Public Health. In 1941 Drinker and his staff began giving U.S. Navy medical officers, chemists, and engineers short (120-day) intensive courses in the fundamentals of occupational medicine and industrial hygiene. Thus, when asked by the U.S. Maritime Commission and the Navy to survey health conditions in shipyards, Drinker had already identified personnel that could staff this undertaking. Getting the Navy to assign them to him, however, was another matter. Fortunately, as Drinker recounts, the "old boy network" came to his rescue:

> When I asked for the necessary personnel the Navy said, "No, we need them for combat duty." Then I talked to some of the Navy Medical Corps. They asked, "Do you know anybody in the Navy?" I answered, "Yes, I know Jim Forrestal [then Undersecretary of the Navy] well. We were at school together." And they said, "Well, for God's sake, what's holding you back? Go and see him. Tell him what you want." So I went to see Forrestal, and he was his old self, a darn good fellow. I told him that I wanted eight officers on my staff, two doctors and six engineers, and he said, "Well, that makes sense to me, but I don't like to decide that myself. I'll get Nimitz [Chester Nimitz, Commander-in-Chief of the Pacific Fleet] in." So he rang a bell. Admiral Nimitz came in in all his regalia and Forrestal said, "Chester, this is an old friend of mine, Phil Drinker, from School. Now tell him what you just told me," and I did. Nimitz said, "This makes pretty good sense, Professor, would you please make out a list of the officers you want." I pulled it out of my pocket. They both laughed and I got the men promptly.[154]

Presumably one of the things that Drinker told Forrestal and Nimitz was that there were many hazards connected with building ships, among them asbestos exposures. Many parts of a ship were insulated with asbestos, including the bulkheads, engines, boilers, pipes, and electrical lines. Much of the insulating work was carried out in the cramped and confined quarters below decks. Insulators and other users of asbestos products had been showing up regularly in medical case reports since 1932,[155] and Drinker and his staff easily identified this exposure as a hazard.[156]

An inspection of the shipyard at Bath Iron Works in Maine in 1942 found conditions that presented "a very real asbestos hazard."[157] Two years later, conditions had apparently not improved, and Drinker was forced to send his staff back because of "concern among the pipe covering crews who feared that the amosite [asbestos] was causing some respiratory troubles."[158] Thirty-eight workers, all with at least two years' exposure, were X-rayed, and twelve (32 percent) showed "significant x-ray changes consistent with exposure to a dusty environment."[159] Given these results, Drinker decided to check other yards as well.

Drinker was in a difficult position. For four years he had been in charge of a program for health and safety in shipyards. He had a personal relationship with Forrestal, by then Secretary of the Navy, who had given Drinker the tools he asked for. At Harvard, Drinker had worked closely with management and was sympathetic to and understanding of their point of view. He clearly was not looking forward to uncovering a major health problem in contract shipyards, but as a scientist he had little choice, although he refused to take the results of the Bath Iron Works survey on its own merits: "It was not felt that experience in a single yard was enough to justify any general statements on working conditions in other yards, and certainly was no cause for alarm, but the results warranted check-ups elsewhere."[160] Four more shipyards, all on the East Coast, were selected for further study.

The yards studied were not ideal for the purpose, as the large labor turnover occasioned by wartime mobilization meant that most workers had been at the trade only for a short time. The yards varied in dustiness, but all exceeded 5 mppcf by a wide margin. Overall, only 5 percent of those X-rayed had been exposed ten years or more and only one in six for five years or more. Because asbestosis may take years to develop—a feature of the disease recognized in the 1930s— Drinker should have known that most of the workers examined would be unlikely to show X-ray changes for years to come. Moreover, many men at these yards were not included in the study, for whatever reasons. In the dustiest yard, less than 10 percent were examined, and no asbestosis was found (only three workers out of forty-eight examined had had ten years or more of exposure). The least dusty yard, on the other hand, had 100 percent participation and two cases were found, both among the nine of 168 workers that had had ten years or more of exposure.[161] All told, three cases of asbestosis were found in the 1,074 men examined in the four yards, all among the fifty-one workers who had ten or more years of exposure, for a prevalence in this group of 6 percent.

These data are presented in Drinker's 1946 survey, which appeared in the periodical he edited, *The Journal of Industrial Hygiene and Toxicology*. There is no evidence that anything was falsified or fabricated, but, like Lanza before him, Drinker made an effort to include favorable aspects of the survey and pictured none of the unfavorable aspects in darker tones than circumstances might justify, as Johns-Manville's Brown had put it. Drinker gave the shipyard's management the "break" they needed. The evident dustiness of the pipe-covering operations might have prompted shipyard authorities and manufacturers to undertake immediate remedial measures and continued surveillance of personnel to assess the risk of development of asbestosis. Yet no change in work practices or any further studies of asbestos exposure in U.S. shipyards would be done until the 1960s. By then, the many decades of accrued risk would produce a public health catastrophe for shipyard workers.

The Threshold Limit Value

Drinker's survey revealed that shipyard workers were often exposed to asbestos dust concentrations in excess of Dreessen's recommendation of 5 mppcf. Even Dreessen's tentative standard was based on doubtful evidence, and he had urged that additional studies be undertaken to confirm it. Instead, Dreessen's recommendation was promulgated in 1946 as a standard for asbestos workplace exposures by an official organ of the industrial hygiene community. This standard would remain unchanged for more than two decades.

Until the passage of the Federal Occupational Safety and Health Act in 1970, only the states (and only some among them) had the authority to set standards for workplaces. The principal means for ensuring uniformity among the states was through the activities of voluntary associations of manufacturers, such as the American Standards Association (ASA), or through professional groups. The most important professional group in workplace standard setting was the American Conference of Governmental Industrial Hygienists (ACGIH).

The founding of the ACGIH was a direct result of the official encouragement of industrial hygiene by the Public Health Service using Social Security Administration (SSA) funds. By the end of the second Service short course on industrial hygiene in the summer of 1937, it was decided that the ensuing seminars would be continued by an independent sponsor. Even though the same people were to conduct the seminars, nonofficial status would allow greater flexibility of response to matters that the Service could not handle. The ACGIH's model was the Conference of State Sanitary Engineers, a private group that met yearly with the Public Health Service's Division of Sanitary Engineering to discuss policy and training matters. Indeed, the constitution for the ACGIH was taken directly from that of the Conference.[162] According to this constitution, the purpose of the ACGIH was to promote industrial hygiene in all its aspects and phases; to coordinate industrial hygiene activities . . . by official federal, State, local and territorial industrial hygiene agencies; to encourage the interchange of experience among industrial hygiene personnel in such official organizations; to collect and make accessible to all governmental industrial hygienists such information and data as may be of assistance to them in the proper fulfillment of their duties.

The first meeting was held the following summer in June 1938. By that time the Public Health Service had organized industrial hygiene units in twenty-eight states. These units were represented by forty-three members, one associate, and six guests. The new executive committee met in Jack Bloomfield's home. From the outset the founders realized that their strength did not lie in numbers but in their strategic positions in each state. By coordinating efforts among the states, the ACGIH could have a national effect far beyond its size. To that end the members organized themselves into standing committees. It was at that time that a Committee on Threshold Limits began to function.[163]

Formally established in 1941, the committee was chaired by William G. Fredrick of Detroit's Bureau of Industrial Hygiene and included, among others, Philip Drinker, Leonard Greenburg, and Manfred Bowditch of the Massachusetts Division of Occupational Hygiene. Fredrick charged his fellow members with the task of establishing working limits with a view to issuing their recommendations in a list, to be revised annually to conform to new information:

I feel that a committee like ours, representing nearly all the government enforcing agencies could, with justification, establish arbitrary limits which appear reasonable, for different classes of material which as yet have been inadequately or not at all investigated from the standpoint of the industrial toxicologist. The fact that some folks will disagree with such values should do much to stimulate the needed research and investigation.[164]

Fredrick hastened to add that their work was not meant to disregard or belittle the work of such standardizing groups as the ASA, but only to recognize that such groups worked too slowly to suit the needs of the practicing industrial hygienist in government service: "All of us doing field work know that if samples are taken for any contaminant in a plant, we must produce a limit, right or wrong, for the consideration of the management. Otherwise, they feel quite rightly that we are wasting our time and theirs taking samples in the first place."[165]

Fredrick's fellow committee member, Manfred Bowditch, added that health standards were not the same as the kind of mechanical standards that prompted the establishment of the ASA:

> We are dealing here with standards which cannot be arrived at in the same way that we would arrive at the number of threads per inch that should be used on a machine screw of a given size in order to enable everybody to use screws interchangeably. We are dealing with conditions in factories, as to which those of us who are entrusted with the preventive functions have got to use our very best judgment.[166]

Bowditch was particularly sensitive, having already had some unsettling experiences in Massachusetts. In 1937 the state established a set of maximum allowable concentrations for some forty different industrial chemicals. These standards were not regulations but were kept as informal guides to allow revision from time to time without the need for going to the legislature. One proposed revision was to lower the carbon tetrachloride standards from 100 parts per million (ppm) to 40 ppm. The technical advisory committee endorsed the proposal unanimously, but Bowditch was deluged with letters from the manufacturers.

> That was followed by a visit from a gentleman from New York who presented me with two business cards, one indicating that he was an official of an advertising agency, and the other that he was an official of an agency devoted to technical research. Of course, it was in his latter capacity that he came to see me.[167]

Not only did this visitor disagree with the new proposal, but the ASA chose this moment to reaffirm the old standard of 100 ppm, apparently at the urging of the insurance representatives on the committee. Bowditch was cynical about their reasons:

> While I may be mistaken, it seems to me that it is quite obvious why they should object to such a lowering. . . . It would seem to me that if the standard were lowered from 100, we will say to 40, it would enable industrial workers who had been shown to be exposed to concentrations above 40 but below 100 to make claims and secure compensation which

they would otherwise not be able to secure. Perhaps it is not as simple as that, but that is my interpretation.[168]

The ASA subsequently grudgingly acknowledged that exposures less than 100 ppm could produce nausea in some individuals and suggested that every effort should be made to work toward lower exposures. In response, a colleague of Bowditch wryly commented that a worker might be justified in thinking he was being poisoned if he lost his lunch twice a week.[169]

Although there is no direct evidence that similar forces were at work in the setting of the 1946 asbestos standard by the ACGIH, the results were just as unsatisfactory for workers. Using the "tentative" figure of 5 mppcf of total dust suggested by Dreessen, the asbestos threshold limit (TLV) would stand until 1968, despite abundant evidence that it was unsatisfactory. The very shortcomings in the basis of the standard noted by Dreessen in his report and evident in its results were also noted by others, even as the ACGIH was issuing its asbestos TLV.

The IHF and the Hemeon Report

The most direct comment on the 5 mppcf standard came from a private research institute hired by members of the Asbestos Textile Institute to inquire into the nature and magnitude of the asbestosis problem. The investigation was done by Dr. W. C. L. Hemeon of the Industrial Hygiene Foundation of America, a laboratory connected to the Mellon Institute of the University of Pittsburgh.

The Institute was founded in 1913 by Canadian-born chemist Robert Kennedy Duncan, using an endowment from the Mellon family's banking, mining, and petroleum fortune. He had previously set up the Industrial Health Fellowship system at the University of Kansas. Duncan had been inspired by the close cooperation between European manufacturers and universities, and he wanted to establish a system whereby the chemical industry could support and define university research. By this means industry could have the services of experts, and the university could keep abreast of industrial needs. Discoveries and patents resulting from supported research work would belong to the sponsor. The faculty member could publish the work as long as it did not, "in the opinion of the company, injure its interests."[170]

Duncan was invited to continue his work at a new Mellon Institute for Industrial Research, to be affiliated with the University of Pittsburgh. By 1921 it became entirely self-supported by industrial contribution. Other institutes imitated Duncan's creation, but Mellon remained one of the most successful and visible.

In 1935 the Institute spawned an offspring, originally christened the Air Hygiene Foundation, and later (in 1941), called the Industrial Hygiene Foundation (IHF). The stimulus for the IFH's establishment was the "silicosis problem" that developed in the wake of the Gauley Bridge disaster. According to Harvard's Theodore Hatch, who worked with the IHF as a consultant and later as full-time staff member, the Foundation was formed at industry request to deal with issues beyond its technical competence. By pooling their resources and knowledge, companies hoped to acquire sufficient technical expertise to respond adequately to the litigation crisis.[171]

The asbestos industry was quick to get onboard. In 1935 Johns-Manville attorney Vandiver Brown wrote to the editor of the industry trade magazine, *Asbestos,* reporting on a meeting of the IFH. After recounting the remarks of the IHF's chairman of the Medical Committee, who was none other than Dr. Anthony Lanza, and also that of the Chairman of the Preventive Engineering Committee, Professor Philip Drinker, Brown noted the importance and value of the new Foundation:

> Although the [IHF] is approaching various problems relating to air hygiene from an unbiased viewpoint, it is nevertheless the creature of industry and is the one institution upon which employers can rely completely for a sympathetic appreciation of their viewpoint. Its aim is to take an honest effort to appraise the evil, to advance scientific knowledge of many of its doubtful aspects and to suggest remedies, both preventative and curative. As such, it deserves and should receive the unqualified support of all members of industries faced with a dust disease hazard.[172]

Johns-Manville and its colleagues in the Asbestos Textile Institute (ATI) took advantage of the IHF's expertise in 1947. Hemeon's resulting unpublished report on hazards in the asbestos textile industry was meant to facilitate the exchange of information between member companies on successful methods of dust control and otherwise to promote a general improvement in that field."

In the report Hemeon expressed little confidence in the 5-mppcf threshold limit value:

The information available *does not* permit complete assurance that five million is thoroughly safe nor has information been developed permitting a better estimate of safe dustiness. It is nevertheless of the greatest importance either that such assurances be sought or a new yardstick of accomplishment be found for accurately measuring any remaining hazard in the dust zone below five million for the elimination of future asbestosis depends on the degree of control effected now.[173]

Ironically, Vandiver Brown would soon repeat publicly Hemeon's assessment of the quality of the evidence upon which the TLV was based, but with a reverse twist. In a speech entitled "Management's Viewpoint" to a symposium on dust diseases, Brown addressed the newly established New Jersey workplace standard of 5 mppcf, based on the ACGIH threshold limit value:

So far as I have ever been able to ascertain, no one can state with certainty what is the maximum allowable limit for asbestos dust. I am certain no study has been made specifically directed toward ascertaining this figure and I question there exists sufficient data correlating the disease to the degree of exposure to warrant any determination that will even approximate accuracy.[174]

Although as far as Hemeon was concerned the TLV was too high, Brown used his reasoning to turn the argument around to question whether there should be a TLV at all.

The only way to settle the question would be to do the kind of further study that Dreessen had recommended and which Hemeon now urged on the ATI. Hemeon suggested using the records of the factories of ATI members in North Carolina, where state law required annual X-rays of textile workers. In addition, "a general x-ray and medical survey of workers in one or two plants with a long history of high order of dust control would be of great value."[175] The studies were never done.

The ATI's reluctance to follow up on Hemeon's recommendations may have stemmed from another part of his report. Using whatever scanty company records existed, Hemeon found, among other things, that a Raybestos-Manhattan factory that had average total dust values of only 2 mppcf also had an asbestosis rate among its workers of 20 percent. This was not the kind of information that warmed the hearts of ATI members.

Without industry cooperation, any precise information shedding quantitative light on the TLV would be very difficult to obtain. This was true not only for asbestos but for any chemical agent covered by a TLV. Members of the ACGIH Committee regularly lamented the lack of help given by industry to their work:

> No one seriously questions that factual data derived from human experience are by far the most reliable basis for TLVs. The only significant source of such data is industry. Unfortunately, data of this kind are rarely available to ACGIH—either because industry has not taken advantage of its unique opportunity to develop them or because they remain hidden in industry's files for any one of several reasons.[176]

The Cancer Problem

Clinicians were the first to suggest an association between asbestosis and lung cancer in the 1930s. From all evidence, cancer was not as frequent a complication then, partially because of poor diagnosis but more probably because of the competing risk of asbestosis, which carried its victims away before the cancer had a chance to develop. As dust levels decreased, more workers lived to develop lung cancer.

W. B. Wood and S. R. Gloyne, in a review of one hundred deaths among asbestos workers in 1938, found two cases out of fifty-three with carcinoma of the lung.[177] Little was made of this by the authors, but lung cancer was sufficiently infrequent at the time that the following year K. M. Lynch and W. A. Smith from Charleston, South Carolina, and Gloyne from England published case reports of lung cancer in asbestos workers (a total of three cases).[178] Gloyne noted that in his cases, tumors were found in the area of the lungs where fibrosis from asbestos dust was most advanced.

The following year (1936), three more papers appeared: one by D. S. Egbert and A. J. Geiger, one by Gloyne, and one by E. L. Middleton.[179] Egbert and Geiger's case was from New Haven, Connecticut. They stated that "the irritating effects of the inhaled asbestos particles may in this case have been a significant factor in the development of the primary lung cancer [and] seem sufficiently plausible to be worthy of consideration." Gloyne's case was an oat-cell carcinoma in a packer in an asbestos factory. Middleton reported on fifty-four cases of asbestosis reported to the factory department in England and found three lung cancers (6 percent) among them.

Two years later, in 1938, three more articles appeared, this time from Germany, and an editorial was written in the *British Medical Journal* that reviewed the situation. The first German paper on cancer in an asbestos worker was by F. Hornig.[180] This case, with the two American cases (by Lynch and Smith, and Egbert and Geiger), two British cases (by Gloyne) and one more German case, was summarized and reported on by M. Nordmann.[181] In his paper Nordmann concludes that cancer was an occupational disease of asbestos workers. A third paper, in German by F. Koelsch, records twelve cases of lung cancer coexisting with asbestosis.[182] Koelsch concluded that "among those groups most exposed to carcinoma of the lungs we must cite those working in asbestos dust." An editorial that same year in the *British Medical Journal* reviewed the general question of the relationship between lung cancer and dust diseases and urgently called for further study.[183]

Between 1938 and 1942, six more articles appeared that mentioned a suspected relationship between asbestos exposure and cancer of the lung. In Wilhelm Hueper's landmark textbook, *Occupational Tumors and Allied Diseases* (1942), seven pages were devoted to asbestosis. In this text the evidence was reviewed, and Hueper concluded that "there is an incidence of lung cancer in asbestosis of the lung which is definitely excessive."[185]

The clinical reports did not go unnoticed by the asbestos industry. Soon industry-supported work with animals was also suggesting a cancer connection. The experiments were done at the Saranac Laboratories by Dr. Leroy Upson Gardner. The Saranac Laboratory was founded by Dr. Edward Livingston Trudeau, a pioneer of the antituberculosis movement of the 1890s and early twentieth century. Gardner's career began auspiciously after his graduation from Yale in 1914, when he studied pathology in Boston under F. B. Mallory. After a brief stint as an instructor at Harvard, he returned to Yale as assistant professor and in 1917 entered the Army Medical Service, where he was immediately diagnosed as having tuberculosis. Sent to the Trudeau Sanitorium at Saranac Lake, by 1918 he was sufficiently recovered to begin work as a fellow at the sanitorium laboratory; by 1919 he was its pathologist. Until 1918 the laboratory had worked only on tuberculosis, but at that time it came to Gardner's attention that there was a high tuberculosis mortality rate among granite cutters in Barre, Vermont, while the marble cutters at nearby Proctor seemed to have fewer cases of the disease than expected. Gardner began to pursue a research program to find out the reason for the difference, and before long a significant proportion of the Saranac staff was engaged in investigating the relationship of mineral dusts to tuberculosis.[186]

Yet the outlook for continued activity at Saranac was gloomy in the 1920s because of the loss of support from private philanthropies. Gardner took advantage of the new line of research and began to establish new alliances with industry. By the early 1930s Gardner, the laboratory's director since 1927, was head of one of the few groups with experience and information on dust diseases and found himself in demand. According to the official history of the laboratory, the legal situation made "pneumoconiosis" a most unpleasant by-word with business executives:

> By correspondence and by personal interview Dr. Gardner was being consulted by representatives of state industrial compensation boards, of insurance companies, and of industries such as mining, quarrying, sand-blasting, foundries, and manufacturers and users of artificial abrasives. They were given all information available but invitations to Dr. Gardner to appear in court as an expert witness were refused. Adoption of this policy seemed the only way to preserve the reputation of the Saranac Laboratory as a source of impartial scientific knowledge.[187]

Scientific information generated by the Saranac staff was not so freely or universally available as this authorized version suggests, however. In 1936 almost a dozen companies involved in asbestos brake-lining manufacture were supporting animal experiments on the effects of asbestos dust. In a letter to Gardner, Johns-Manville counsel Vandiver Brown set out the conditions for support:

> It is our further understanding that the results obtained will be considered the property of those who are advancing the required funds, who will determine whether, to what extent and in what manner they shall be made public. In the event it is deemed desirable they shall be made public, the manuscript of your study will be submitted to us for approval prior to publication.[188]

All communications and finances were handled by Johns-Manville and Raybestos-Manhattan, which in turn distributed information and collected contributions from the other participants on a *pro rata* basis.

Gardner readily agreed to the conditions and began his experiments late in 1937.[189] He apparently did not take the confidentiality requirement as seriously as his sponsors, however. In May 1939, Johns-Manville's Brown wrote to Raybestos-Manhattan's Simpson that the Saranac annual report for 1938 had made mention of the laboratory's work on asbestosis. Included were reprints of papers and

addresses by Saranac staff, among them an article by Gardner on the
"Etiology of Pneumoconiosis" from the November 1938 issue of the
Journal of the American Medical Association:

> In this article your attention is directed to a reference to Asbestosis on
> pages 12, 13 and particularly at the top of page 14. The information
> covered by these references has presumably been derived from the ex-
> periments which Dr. Gardner is conducting for, and with funds pro-
> vided by, the group members of the Asbestos Textile Industry. The
> Progress Reports which we have received to date would seem to indicate
> as much. This raises a question upon which I would like to have your
> thoughts, namely whether Dr. Gardner's use of this material is proper in
> view of [the previous agreement].[190]

Simpson was quick to reply:

> I do not believe it is proper for Dr. Gardner to use any of the material
> regarding asbestosis without our consent, or without submitting the
> report to you for approval, and I am a little surprised that Dr. Gardner
> has done so. He is certainly not living up to his agreement of November
> 1936. The reports may be so favorable to us that they would cause no
> trouble, but they might be just the opposite, which could be very embar-
> rassing.[191]

Just how these concerns were communicated to Dr. Gardner is
not known, but by 1943 he was looking for alternative means of
support for a new series of experiments he was planning—on the
cancer-causing potential of asbestos. Already nineteen cases of lung
cancer in asbestos workers had been reported in the medical literature, and many German and English workers took the asbestos-
cancer connection seriously. Gardner himself was skeptical, but in his
animal studies he "was startled to discover that a small group of 11
white mice that had been inhaling asbestos dust from 15 to 24 months
showed an excessive incidence (81.8%) of pulmonary cancer."[192] He
therefore approached the chair of the National Advisory Cancer
Council for federal funds to study the carcinogenicity of asbestos,
noting as he did so that he had received almost $30,000 over seven
years from the asbestos industry for other work, and "I cannot ask
them for further contributions."[193] Gardner was turned down by the
government so he could neither do his projected study nor release his
results without Johns-Manville's permission. Shortly before his sudden, unexpected death in 1946, he was reported by a visiting col-

league to be "very much distressed because he said Johns-Manville wouldn't allow him to publish his findings."[194]

Like Lanza, Gardner believed he could remain true to his science while giving his industry sponsors the benefit of the doubt ("the question of carcinogenic action by asbestos is by no means settled. . . . Until that is done I shall maintain the same [skeptical] attitude and say nothing about our observation [in mice]"). Though distressed, he ultimately played within the rules determined by the industry.

One who did not play by the rules was Wilhelm Hueper, the author of the 1942 textbook on occupational cancer. A pathologist who had once worked for DuPont's Haskell Laboratories, Hueper worked at the National Cancer Institute from the 1940s. By all accounts he could be abrasive and stubborn. But he was nothing if not straightforward. In 1943 he published an article on environmental and occupational cancer in the Bulletin of the American Society for Cancer Control (now the American Cancer Society). In it he suggested that industry was not seriously interested in finding cancer hazards in its workplaces:

> Industrial concerns are in general not particularly anxious to have the occurrence of occupational cancers among their employees or of environmental cancers among the consumers of their products made a matter of public records. Such publicity might reflect unfavorabl[y] upon their business activities, and oblige them to undertake extensive and expensive technical and sanitary measures in their production methods and in the types of products manufactured. There is, moreover, the distinct possibility of becoming involved in compensation suits with extravagant financial claims by the injured parties. It is, therefore, not an uncommon practice that some pressure is exerted by the parties financially interested in such matters to keep information on the occurrence of industrial cancer well under cover.[195]

Throughout the 1940s medical reports continued to appear showing a relation between asbestosis and lung cancer. They included all types of workers, not only those working in manufacturing but also those using asbestos products, such as pipe coverers. The Annual Report for 1947 of the chief inspector of factories in Great Britain was published in 1949. The Report's author was E. R. A. Merewether, who had published the first large-scale study of asbestos textile workers in 1930. Merewether looked at 235 deaths between 1924 and 1946 in which the cause of death was asbestosis or in which asbestosis was proved to be present. Cancer of the lung or pleura was found in 13.2 percent. By contrast, in a similar series of deaths from silicosis, the cancer rate was only 1.32 percent. Shortly after publication of this report, an editorial in the *Journal of the American Medical Association* accepted the causal relationship of asbestosis and cancer of the lung.[196] The same year an article on cancer and the environment appeared in *Scientific American;* it listed asbestos as a carcinogen known to be present in the human environment and indicated that the lung was the target organ. Hueper was cited as the authority.[197]

The ATI was perturbed at these published reports, and its members discussed them at their meeting in 1949 in which the *Scientific American* article was specifically mentioned.[198] In the 1950s Hueper continued to mention asbestos as a carcinogen in his writings, giving rise to further dissension at the ATI. In 1956 the ATI's board of governors heard a recommendation by Dr. Kenneth W. Smith, Johns-Manville's Medical Director, that the ATI embark on "a program of investigation and publicity to counteract the unfavorable publicity presently directed to the asbestos industries as a result of the work of Dr. Hueper."[199] In his report to the board from the ATI's Air Hygiene Committee, Smith had indicated that he had "no evidence that there is *not* a relationship between asbestosis and cancer."[200]

Both the Saranac Laboratories and the Industrial Hygiene Foundation had already proposed to undertake studies on the carcinogenicity of asbestosis. Dr. Gerrit Schepers of Saranac wanted to examine tissue specimens from deceased industry employees. The ATI rejected the idea, however:

> The program was considered ill-advised at this time due to its implication that a relationship existed between asbestosis and carcinogenic development, a condition which, to date, has not been established although it has been given rather widespread publicity in the press.[201]

The Industrial Hygiene Foundation also proposed an epidemiologic study of asbestos textile workers. The foundation had undertaken a study of miners for the Quebec Asbestos Mining Association (QAMA), which was just underway in 1957 when the ATI was considering the IHF plan. The ATI also rejected the IHF proposal:

> 1. It was decided that as the QAMA has a similar program, we should not enter into a program of our own as the results of the QAMA

investigation will be made available to us upon the conclusion of that investigation.

2. There is a feeling among certain members that such an investigation would stir up a hornet's nest and put the whole industry under suspicion.

3. We do not believe there is enough evidence of cancer or asbestosis in this industry to warrant a survey.[202]

The QAMA-sponsored IHF research studied 6,000 miners employed in 1950 who had at least five years' exposure. Cancer of the lung was considered to have been reasonably proved in nine and to be strongly suggested in three more. The nine proved cases were not in excess of the rates for the Province of Quebec, but inclusion of the three suspected cases raised the rate to borderline significance. In his report to the IHF, the author, Dr. Daniel Braun, included an analysis of cancer among asbestosis cases as well. Here there was a definite excess, with 12.5 percent of asbestosis victims also showing signs of lung cancer. "The results," Braun wrote, "suggest that a miner who develops the disease asbestosis does have a greater likelihood of developing cancer of the lung."[203]

When this study was submitted for publication, the section on asbestosis and lung cancer was deleted. Writing to the general counsel of QAMA, Johns-Manville's Smith took note of the missing section:

> We have noted the deletion of all references to the association of asbestosis and lung cancer in this condensation. While we believe that this information is of great scientific value, we can understand the desire of QAMA to emphasize the exposure of the asbestos miner and not the cases of asbestosis. . . . It must be recognized, however, that this report will be subjected to criticism when published because all other authors today correlate lung cancer and cases of asbestosis.[204]

Hueper was one of the first to jump on the critical bandwagon. He dismissed the apparently negative findings of the report as "statistical acrobatics which tend to obscure incriminating evidence on hand by use of a highly biased population group as a 'normal' standard."[205] Hueper was referring to the inclusion of the urban areas of Quebec City and Montreal, with their high lung cancer rates, in the comparison with the rural districts, whose rates were less than a third those of the cities. Using the data provided in the published paper, Hueper

wrote that the conclusions were "patently incorrect and grossly misleading and results in obscuring the existence of a markedly elevated
lung cancer rate for members of this working group."[206]

Hueper suffered continual harassment for the content and forth-
rightness of his views. In an extraordinary memo to Dr. John Heller,
the director of the National Cancer Institute in 1959, Hueper presented a long list of incidents that he asserted described the "dark"
and "somewhat shady" history of his Environmental Cancer Section:

> For quite some time I have gained the impression that many of the
> growing difficulties with which I have been confronted in conducting
> efficiently and effectively the investigation of environmental cancer haz-
> ards since the establishment of the Environmental Cancer Section in
> 1948 are reflections of some extra-governmental influences which are
> more concerned with the practical economic implications of the results
> of such activities of the Section than with the proper protection of the
> health of the American public against environmental cancer hazards, for
> which such parties have been responsible.[207]

Hueper went on to set out the particulars, giving detailed accounts of
restriction by superiors of his meeting, speaking, and lecture engagements; censorship, rewriting, and delay in approval of his scientific
papers and books; curtailment and interference with his participation
in congressional hearings and international organizations; and lack of
support for the epidemiologic and experimental research work of the
Environmental Cancer Section. Hueper also responded to a charge
made by his superior that he had published confidential information.
It had always been his practice, he wrote, neither to solicit nor to
accept any information on occupational cancer hazards on a confidential basis: "I have adopted this policy because I consider it undesirable to acquire knowledge of conditions which may amount for all
practical purposes to a crime about which I would be forced to remain
silent if such information has been given to me on a confidential
basis."[208]

Hueper protested the repeated demands of his superior at the
National Cancer Institute to restrict his interpretations of environmental and experimental evidence to data that had already been published, and not to consider any unpublished data that he might have
in his possession from other sources. Such a restriction would have
forced him at times to indulge in straight lying, were he aware that
interpretations based on published data only were misleading:

I would . . . consider it scientifically dishonest, if I would accept as correct, as suggested to me, the recently published allegation of [the QAMA/IHF study] concerning the frequency of asbestosis cancer of the lung among Canadian asbestos workers because I know that the total number of such cases is much higher than . . . cited by these authors who worked under the sponsorship of the American asbestos industry. . . .

My friends at the Ministry of Labor, Quebec, which has handled cases of asbestosis cancer, moreover, have assured me that [the authors of the IHF study] have not contacted them for information in asbestosis cancer. Under these circumstances I feel that I am not only under no obligation, but in fact also I would commit a scientific offense if I would honor the statement of [the IHF Report] as anything more than specially manufactured scientific merchandise of shoddy quality.[209]

Two years later, in a memo to the National Cancer Institute's associate director for field studies, Hueper explained his refusal to organize three symposia on occupational cancer to which representatives of interested industries would be invited. Two previous symposia, Hueper said, were not followed by any meaningful action by industry or public health authorities. At both meetings the industry representatives "boldly refused to divulge definite figures and facts related to occupational cancer hazards" to the other participants (representatives of public agencies, departments of industrial hygiene, and universities). Not only had industry continued "this spirit of noncooperation and public irresponsibility," he said, it had even attempted to repudiate the existence of cancer hazards so as to escape liability and obligations to its workers. Industry had tried to accomplish this "by having investigators of their choice prepare and publish epidemiologic information based on . . . defective and biased data." Hueper cited as a specific example the QAMA/IHF study.[210]

Three years later Hueper would speak at an international meeting on the "Biological Effects of Asbestos," held under the auspices of the New York Academy of Sciences in October 1964. For the first time, scientists from all over the world assembled to compare notes and present their findings. Hueper was no longer a voice in the wilderness.

Conclusion

The full effect of the failed warnings of the 1930s and 1940s is now being felt with tragic force. One estimate suggests that almost 9,000 cancer deaths per year can be attributed to past asbestos exposure; the toll is expected to rise to almost 10,000 by the early 1990s, tapering off from there to 3,000 in the year 2025. This toll, from cancer alone, averages out to almost one asbestos-related death per hour for the next twenty years.[211] The culpability of the asbestos industry in its failure to provide timely warning to the users of its products entangled reputable scientists in a web of deceit and manipulation that was only partly engineered by clever corporate manipulators. Much of it was a consequence of the social forces that produced the industrial health specialist in the first half of the twentieth century.

The scientists and engineers who had responsibility for control of workplace hazards were industrial medical specialists and industrial hygienists. Many clinical reports of individual cases or series of cases appeared in the medical literature in the more than sixty years from the first reports that asbestos dust could harm workers to the international conference in 1964, but the medical practitioners who wrote these articles were usually not able to see the entire picture. Nor were they usually able to do anything about it, even if they had wished to do so. Only the industrial medical specialists and industrial hygienists were both in a position to interpret what they saw *and* in possession of lines of communication to the industry. These professionals, however, did little or nothing in the face of ample warning.

The development of industrial medicine was constrained and directed by the professions of public health and clinical medicine from which it emerged in the first decades of the century. When public health lost its connection to the reform instinct, industrial medicine also became separated from a tradition of challenge and advocacy. Along with this separation came a new focus on the individual rather than the workplace as the point of application of public health practice. At the same time the power of organized medicine prevented this focus on the worker from evolving into a client-centered, care-giving relationship. Instead, industrial doctors defined their role as management consultants whose advice benefitted both labor and management. Independent scientists and consultants held to the same conception, not just doctors employed by industry. The community of professionals was relatively small and organized in its own association (the AAIPS, separate from the AMA). Among its members were many from the public sector, like Dr. Lanza, who later moved to industry.

The link between management and industrial hygiene was even

stronger. Originally conceived as a branch of industrial medicine where engineering knowledge was required, industrial hygiene soon evolved into a branch of engineering where medicine was left to the doctors. For industrial hygiene, too, the basic compatibility of the interests of the firm and the interests of the worker was assumed.

While clinical investigators were revealing the links between asbestos exposure and disease, the precise data that would permit medical and engineering control could come only from scientists in the public sector and industry. Such control required detailed exposure information and systematic examination of large groups of workers. This was beyond the scope of the individual practitioner, who could report only on those isolated cases which came to his attention. But even governmental agencies such as the Public Health Service required the cooperation of industry to gain access to the plants; and private scientists working with or for industry were reluctant to "rock the boat," repeatedly giving their sponsors the benefit of the doubt. This attitude was partly motivated by the dependence on industry for support (in the case of Gardner) but was also reinforced by training and inclination (in the case of Lanza, Drinker, and Hemeon). As a result, the research agenda and control over the publication of results were strongly influenced if not determined by industry.

Through the period before 1964, private enterprise successfully retained control over conditions in the workplace. Even the compensation system was designed to insulate employers from tort liability, offering workers little if anything in return. Despite the overt manipulation of data and interference with the work of insistent Jeremiahs such as Hueper, it is not clear what a scientist could have done without the cooperation of industry. Hueper did sound a warning, but without result. There was no federal authority to regulate the workplace, and even staunch reformers such as Alice Hamilton depended completely on persuasion and rational argument rather than government coercion. The concern of industry was primarily over compensation costs, not fear that it would be required to institute costly preventive measures.

It was not a lack of moral fiber on the part of scientists and engineers but a lack of social controls that allowed private interests to meet their own needs at the expense of the health of workers, consumers, and the general public. The task before us is to fashion a set of social controls that is effective, equitable, and without the kind of unintended adverse consequences that often result when a complex system is changed. We can only hope that we are now evolving such a system and that the process will be speedy.

Notes

1. *Annual Report of the Chief Inspector of Factories for the Year 1898* pt. II, *Reports,* (London: HMSO, 1898), pp. 1/1–1/2.

2. *Annual Report of the Chief Inspector of Factories for the Year 1906* (London: HMSO, 1907), pp. 219–220.

3. M. Murray, "Reports of Departmental Committee on Compensation for Industrial Diseases. Minutes of Evidence" (London: HMSO, 1907), cd 3946:127–28.

4. H. K. Pancoast, T. G. Miller, and H. R. M. Landis, "A Roentenologic Study of the Effects of Dust Inhalation Upon the Lungs," *Transactions of the Association of American Physicians* 32 (1917): 97–108.

5. W. E. Cooke, "Pulmonary asbestosis," *British Medical Journal* 2 (1927): 1024–1025.

6. *Statutory Rules & Orders,* 341, 344, 1440 (London: HMSO, 1931). Made by the Secretary of State under Section 79 of the Factory and Workshop Act, 1901 (1 Edw. 7.c.22).

7. K. M. Lynch, and W. A. Smith, "Pulmonary Asbestosis. III: Carcinoma of Lung in Asbesto-Silicosis," *American Journal of Cancer* 24 (1935): 56–64.

8. M. Nordman. "Der Berufskrebs der Asbestarbeiter," *Zeitschrift für Krebsforschung* 47 (1938): 288–302.

9. "Case Records of the Massachusetts General Hospital. Case 33111," *New England Journal of Medicine* 236 (1947): 407–412; H. W. Wedler, "Uber den Lungenkrebs bei Asbestose," *Deutsche Medizinische Wochenschrift* 191 (1943): 189–209.

10. J. C. Wagner, C. A. Sleggs, and P. Marchand. "Diffuse Pleural Mesothelioma and Asbestos Exposure in the North Western Cape Province," in A. J. Orenstin (ed.), *Proceedings of the Pneumoconiosis Conference Held at the University of Witwatersrand, Johannesburg* (Boston: Little, Brown, 1960); M. L. Newhouse, and H. Thompson, "Epidemiology of Mesotheliomal Tumors in the London Area," *Annals of the New York Academy of Science* 132 (1965): 674–679.

11. Bibliography compiled by author; available on request.

12. I. J. Selikoff, and J. Churg (eds.), "Biological Effects of Asbestos," *Annals of the New York Academy of Science* 132 (1965).

13. T. Lewin, "Asbestos Now Company Peril," *New York Times,* 10 August 1982, p. D2.

14. U.S. Environmental Protection Agency, Asbestos in Buildings: Na-

tional Survey of Asbestos-Containing Friable Materials, Washington D.C., Office of Toxic Substances, EPA S60/5-84-006 (1984).

15. Selikoff and Churg, "Biological Effects."

16. G. Perrett, *America in the Twenties: A History* (New York: Simon & Schuster, 1982), p. 263.

17. R. H. Jones, *Asbestos and Asbestic: The Properties, Occurrence and Use* (London: Crosby, Lockwood, 1897).

18. Ibid.

19. Ibid., pp. 1–2.

20. Ibid.

21. Originally any fibrous material that had this characteristic was termed asbestos, but today we use it more narrowly to cover fibrous minerals of the serpentine or amphibole groups.

22. W. J. M. Rankine, *A Manual of the Steam Engine and other Prime Movers* (London: Charles Griffin, 1870).

23. G. G. Andre (ed.), *Spon's Encyclopedia of the Industrial Arts, Manufactures and Commercial Products* (New York: E. and F. N. Spon, 1879), p. 340.

24. " '85% Magnesia' and Its Interesting Story," *The Asbestos Worker* 8 (December 1926): 5 (original copyright, the Magnesia Association of America, 1917).

25. "Development of the Air Cell Idea," 7 *The Asbestos Worker* 8 (1928): 12.

26. *The Asbestos Worker,* cited n. 24.

27. " '85% Magnesia' and Its Interesting Story," 6 *The Asbestos Worker* 1 (1927). continued from the December issue, cited n. 24 (original copyright, the Magnesia Association of America, 1917).

28. Advertisement, The Asbestos Packing Company, brochure, 1890.

29. W. R. Goodwin, *The Johns-Manville Story* (New York: Newcome Society, 1972), address delivered at the National Meeting of the Newcome Society in North America, New York, 16 December 1971.

30. Ibid.

31. Advertisement in *Dockham's American Report and Directory of the Textile Manufacture and Dry Goods Trade* (Boston: C. A. Dockham & Co., 1886).

32. Goodwin, *Johns-Manville Story.*

33. See, for example, G. Porter, *The Rise of Big Business, 1860–1910* (Arlington Heights, Ill.: Harlen Davidson, 1973).

34. Jones, *Asbestos and Asbestic.*

35. The description of early asbestos mining is largely taken from Jones, *Asbestos and Asbestic.*

36. Ibid., pp. 94–95.

37. Goodwin, *Johns-Manville Story.*

38. Jones, *Asbestos and Asbestic,* p. 203.

39. "Management by Morgan," 9 *Fortune* 3 (1934): 82–89, 128–46.

40. The description of Johns-Manville after 1900 is largely from the source in *Fortune,* cited n. 39.

41. A. L. Clough (ed.), *The Operation, Care and Repair of Automobiles,* from the files of The Horseless Age (New York: The Horseless Age, 1907), p. 246.

42. W. H. Berry (ed.), *Modern Motor Car Practice* (London: Henry Froude and Hodder and Stoughton, 1921).

43. *Moody's Analyses of Investments* (New York: Moody's Investors' Services, 1925, 1928, 1930).

44. Perrett, *America in the Twenties.*

45. Ibid.

46. "Demand for Safety in Cars Increasing," 76 *Automotive Topics* 12 (January 1925): 1190.

47. Data taken from *Automobile Topics* 74 (June 1924): 563–565, and *Automobile Topics* 88 (January 1928): 864–865.

48. Jones, *Asbestos and Asbestic.*

49. Annual Report, cited n. 1.

50. M. Greenberg, "The Montague Murray Case," *American Journal of Industrial Medicine* 3 (1982): 351–356.

51. Murray, cited n. 3.

52. L. A. Leopold, *Radiology at the University of Pennsylvania, 1890–1975* (Philadelphia: University of Pennsylvania Press, 1981), p. 14.

53. Pancoast et al., cited n. 4.

54. George Kober, transcribed discussion following Pancoast et al., cited n. 4, p. 106.

55. F. Hoffman, "Mortality from Respiratory Diseases in Dusty Trades (Inorganic Dusts)," *Bulletin of the U.S. Bureau of Labor Statistics* 231 (Washington, D.C.: U.S. 1918 GPO), pp. 176–180.

56. W. Rothstein, *American Physicians in the Nineteenth Century* (Baltimore: Johns Hopkins Press, 1972).

57. Editorial, *Journal of the American Medical Association* 36 (1901): 1450, quoted in Rothstein, *American Physicians,* p. 319.

58. J. G. Burrows, *AMA: Voice of American Medicine* (Baltimore: Johns Hopkins Press, 1963), pp. 42–44.

59. Ibid., *passim,* ch. 2.

60. A. Hamilton, *Exploring The Dangerous Trades* (Boston: Little, Brown, 1943), p. 115; B. Sicherman, *Alice Hamilton: A Life in Letters* (Cambridge, Mass.: Harvard University Press, 1984), p. 153.

61. Hamilton, *Exploring,* p. 115.

62. American Association for Labor Legislation, "Industrial Diseases," 2 *American Labor Legislation Review* 2, pub. 17 (1912).

63. B. Rosenkrantz, *Public Health and the State: Changing Views in Massachusetts* (Cambridge, Mass.: Harvard University Press, 1972).

64. Sedgwick, quoted in Rosenkrantz, *Public Health.*

65. J. Weinstein, *The Corporate Ideal in the Liberal State, 1900–1918* (Boston: Beacon Press, 1968), ch. 5 *passim.*

66. C. V. Chapin, *Selected Papers* (New York: Commonwealth Fund, 1934), p. 213.

67. Ibid.

68. Ibid.

69. C. V. Chapin, *Sources and Modes of Infection* (New York: J. Wiley, 1910).

70. H. H. Hill, *The New Public Health* (New York: Macmillan, 1916), preface.

71. Ibid., p. 8.

72. W. Cooke, "Fibrosis of the Lungs Due to Inhalation of Asbestos Dust," *British Medical Journal* 2 (1924): 147.

73. W. Cooke, "Pulmonary Asbestosis," *British Medical Journal* 2 (1927): 1024–1025.

74. H. E. Seiler, "A Case of Pneumoconiosis. Results of the Inhalation of Asbestos Dust," *British Medical Journal* 2 (1928):952.

75. E. R. A. Merewether, and C. V. Price. *Report on Effects of Asbestos Dust on the Lungs and Dust Suppression in the Asbestos Industry* (London: HMSO, 1930).

76. A. J. Lanza, W. J. McConnell, and J. W. Fehnel, "Effects of the Inhalation of Asbestos Dust on the Lungs of Asbestos Workers," *U. S. Public Health Reports* 50 (1935): 1–12.

77. Ibid.

78. The most thorough treatment of the Hawk's Nest tragedy is Deborah Rosen's "Industrial Disease in the Great Depression: The Silicosis Tragedy at Gauley Bridge, West Virginia," senior thesis, Department of History, Princeton University, 1977. I am indebted to Ms. Rosen for allowing me to use her work in preparation for this paper. See also M. Rowh, "The Hawk's Nest Tragedy: Fifty Years Later," 7 *Goldenseal* 1 (January–March 1981): 31–41.

79. G. G. Davis, E. M. Salmonsen, and J. L. Earlywine *Pneumonoconioses (Silicosis): Bibliography and Laws* (Chicago: Industrial Medicine, 1934).

80. H. Selleck, and A. Whittaker, *Occupational Health in America* (Detroit: Wayne State University Press, 1962), p. 223.

81. Ibid., p. 233.

82. Ibid.

83. Ibid.

84. A. Lanza, W. McConnell, and W. Fehnel, *Effects of the Inhalation of Asbestos Upon the Lungs of Asbestos Workers,* manuscript for Industrial Health Services, Policy Holder Service Bureau, Metropolitan Life Insurance Company, New York, 1931.

85. B. Castleman, *Asbestos: Medical and Legal Aspects* (New York: Harcourt Brace, 1984), p. 123.

86. Letter, George Hobart to Vandiver Brown, 15 December 1934.

87. Ibid.

88. Castleman, *Asbestos,* pp. 124–125.

89. Letter, Vandiver Brown to Anthony Lanza, 21 December 1934; quoted in P. Brodeur, "Annals of Law: The Asbestos Industry on Trial," pt. I: "Discovery," *The New Yorker,* 17 June 1985.

90. Hamilton, *Exploring,* pp. 3–4.

91. D. Walsh, "Medicine as Management," Ph.D. thesis, Boston University, 1983, p. 77.

92. J. Burrows, *Organized Medicine in the Progressive Era* (Baltimore: Johns Hopkins Press, 1977), p. 170.

93. Ibid.

94. Ibid., 127.

95. Selleck and Whittaker, *Occupational Helath,* p. 60.

96. Ibid., p. 61.

97. Ibid., pp. 76–77.

98. National Industrial Conference Board, *The Physician in Industry,* special report no. 22 (New York: NICB, 1922), p. 3.

99. Ibid., p. 2.

100. A. Nugent, "Fit for Work: The Introduction of Physical Examinations in Industry," *Bulletin of the History of Medicine* 57 (1983): 578–595.

101. NICB, cited n. 98, p. 2.

102. Ibid., p. 11.

103. A. Donovan, Chapter 2 of this book.

104. Selleck and Whittaker, *Occupational Health,* p. 49.

105. Ibid., *passim;* R. Williams, *The United States Public Health Service, 1798–1950* (Washington, D.C.: Commissioned Officers Association of the U.S. Public Health Service, 1951), pp. 279–286.

106. NICB, cited n. 80, p. 14.

107. Nugent, cited n. 100, p. 585.

108. Ibid., p. 590.

109. Ibid.

110. Selleck and Whittaker, *Occupational Health,* pp. 118–119.

111. Ibid., p. 119.

112. E. F. Lutz, associate medical director, General Motors Corporation, writing in 1953; quoted in Selleck and Whittaker, *Occupational Health,* p. 119.

113. Ibid.

114. NICB, cited n. 98, p. 13.

115. Walsh, cited n. 91, p. 91.

116. Emphasis added; quoted in Nugent, cited n. 100, p. 594.

117. Ibid., p. 595.

118. Cf. Walsh, cited n. 91, *passim*.

119. Selleck and Whittaker, *Occupational Health*, p. 115.

120. Williams, *Public Health Service,* cited n. 105, p. 281.

121. H. Doyle, "Interview with John J. Bloomfield," in C. D. Yaffe (ed.), *Some Pioneers of Industrial Hygiene, Annals of the American Confer-ence of Governmental Industrial Hygienists,* vol. 7 (Cincinnati: ACGIH, 1984), p. 15.

122. Ibid., p. 16.

123. Ibid., p. 17.

124. Ibid.

125. Harris, R., "Interview with Warren A. Cook," in Yaffe (ed.), *Some Pioneers,* p. 49.

126. C. Yaffe, "Interview with Theodore F. Hatch," in Yaffe (ed.), *Some Pioneers,* pp. 87–88.

127. J. Curran, *Founders: Harvard School of Public Health,* (New York: Josiah Macy Foundation, 1970), pt. I, *passim*.

128. G. C. Shattuck, *Industrial Medicine at Harvard,* May 1954 manu-script in the Rare Book Room, Holmes Hall, Countway Medical Library, Harvard Medical School, Boston, p. 27.

129. Ibid.

130. Curran, *Founders,* pp. 192–196.

131. Shattuck, *Industrial Medicine,* pp. 196.

132. Letter from School of Public Health Dean David Edsall to Wade Wright, n.d., quoted in Shattuck, *Industrial Medicine,* p. 17.

133. Quoted in Shattuck, *Industrial Medicine,* p. 194.

134. Letter, Shattuck to G. K. Leet, 1922, quoted in Shattuck, *Indus-trial Medicine,* p. 192.

135. Ibid., p. 49.

136. Ibid., p. 60.

137. Ibid., p. 53.

138. Yaffe (ed.), *Some Pioneers,* p. 94.

139. J. J. Bloomfield, "What the ACGIH Has Done for Industrial Hygiene," *Journal of the American Industrial Hygiene Association* 19 (1958): 338–344; reprinted in M. E. La Nier (ed.), "Threshold Limit Values—Discussion and Thirty-Five Year Index with Recommendations," *Annals of the American Conference of Industrial Hygiene* 9 (1984): 3–10, p. 3.

140. A. M. Baetjer, "The Early Days of Industrial Hygiene—Their Con-tribution to Current Problems," *Transactions of the 42nd Annual Meeting of ACGIH* (1981), pp. 10–17; reprinted in Yaffe (ed.), *Some Pioneers,* pp. 15–20.

141. Bloomfield, cited n. 139, pp. 3–4.

142. Baetjer, cited n. 140, p. 19.

143. W. C. Dreessen et al., "A Study of Asbestosis in the Asbestos

Textile Industry," *U. S. Public Health Bulletin No. 241* (Washington, D.C.: 1938), U.S. GPO, p. 2.

144. Ibid., p. 47.

145. Ibid., pp. 47–48.

146. Ibid.

147. Ibid., p. 89.

148. Ibid., p. 93.

149. Ibid., p. 91.

150. Ibid.

151. Ibid., p. 52ff.

152. Perrett, *America in the Twenties,* p. 129.

153. W. Fleischer, F. Viles, R. Gade, and P. Drinker, "A Health Survey of Pipe Covering Operations in Constructing Naval Vessels," *Journal of Industrial Hygiene and Toxicity* 28 (1946): 9–16.

154. Interview of P. Drinker by J. Curran, 19 May 1964, quoted in Curran, *Founders,* p. 168.

155. Cf. Table 2 in Castleman, *Asbestos,* pp. 268–269.

156. P. Drinker, "Minimum Requirements for Safety and Industrial Health in Contract Shipyards," U.S. Navy, U.S. Maritime Commission (Washington, D.C.: U. S. GPO, 1943).

157. Report of Industrial Health Survey, 24 September 1942. Noted in W. C. Dreesen, and W. Fleischer, *Report on Investigation of Asbestosis from Amosite Pipe Covering at Bath Iron Works,* 19 December 1944 (U.S. Navy), U. S. Maritime Commission, War Shipping Administration, Safety and Industrial Health Program, 1944).

158. Ibid., p. 1.

159. Ibid.

160. Tables 4 and 5 in Fleischer et al., "A Health Survey," p. 15.

161. Ibid.

162. Bloomfield, cited n. 139, pp. 4–5.

163. Bloomfield, cited n. 139, p. 5.

164. W. G. Fredrick, "The Birth of the ACGIH Threshold Limit Values Committee and Its Influence on the Development of Industrial Hygiene," *Transactions of the 30th Annual Meeting of ACGIH* 12–14 May 1968, St. Louis, Mo., pp. 40–43; reprinted in La Nier (ed.), *Annals,* pp. 11–13.

165. Ibid.

166. M. Bowditch, "In Setting Threshold Limits," *Transactions of the 7th Annual Meeting of the National Conference of Government Industrial Hygienists,* 9 May 1944, St. Louis, Mo., pp. 29–32; reprinted in LaNier (ed.), *Annals,* pp. 51–52.

167. Ibid.

168. Ibid.

169. Ibid.

170. Quoted in D. Noble, *America By Design* (New York: Knopf, 1977), p. 123.

171. T. F. Hatch, correspondence in Yaffee (ed.), *Some Pioneers,* p. 91.

172. Letter, Vandiver Brown to C. J. Stover, 4 December 1936.

173. Emphasis in the original, W. C. L. Hemeon, *Report of Preliminary Dust Investigation for the Asbestos Textile Institute,* (Pittsburgh, Pa.: Industrial Hygiene Foundation, 1947), pp. 1, 22.

174. V. Brown, "The Management Viewpoint—Discussion," in A. J. Vorwald (ed.), *Pnumoconiosis: Beryllium, Bauxite Fumes: Compensation,* Saranac Symposium No. 6, (New York: Hoeber, 1950), pp. 567–572.

175. Hemeon, *Report,* p. 20.

176. Committee on Industrial Hygiene and Clinical Toxicology of the Industrial Medical Association [AAIPS], in La Nier (ed.), *Annals,* p. 141.

177. W. B. Wood, and S. R. Gloyne, "Pulmonary Asbestosis: A Review of One Thousand Cases," *Lancet* 2 (1934): 1383–1385.

178. K. M. Lynch and W. A. Smith, "Pulmonary Asbestosis, III: Carcinoma of Lung in Asbesto-Silicosis," *American Journal of Cancer* 24 (1935): 56–64; S. R. Gloyne, "Two Cases of Squamous Carcinoma of the Lung," *Tubercle.* 17 (1935):5–10.

179. D. S. Egbert and A. J. Geiger, "Pulmonary Asbestosis and Carcinoma—Report of a Case with Necropsy Findings," *American Review of Tuberculosis* 34 (1936): 143–150; S. R. Gloyne, "A Case of Oat Cell Carcinoma of the Lung Occurring in Asbestosis," *Tubercle* 18 (1936): 100–101; E. L. Middleton, "Industrial Pulmonary Disease Due to the Inhalation of Dust with Special Reference to Silicosis," *Lancet* 2 (1936): 59–64.

180. F. Hornig, "Klinische Betrachtungen Zur Frage des Berufskrebses der Asbestarbeiter," *Z. Krebsforsch* 47 (1938): 281–287.

181. M. Nordmann, "Der Berufskrebs der Asbestarbeiter," *Zeitschrift für Krebsforschung* 47 (1938): 288–302.

182. F. Koelsch, "Lungenkrebs und Beruf," *Acta Un. Int. Cancr.* 3 (1938):243–251.

183. Editorial, "Silicosis and Pulmonary Carcinoma," *British Medical Journal* 2 (1938): 411–412.

184. E. W. Baader, "Asbestose," *Deutsche Medizinische Wochenschrift* 65 (1939): 407–408; K. W. Lynch and W. A. Smith, "Pulmonary Asbestosis: V.: A Report of Bronchial Carcinoma and Epithelial Metaplasia," *American Journal of Cancer* 36 (1939): 567–573; M. O. Klotz, "The Association of Silicosis and Carcinoma of the Lung," *American Journal of Cancer* 35 (1939): 38–49; J. W. Bridge, *Annual Report of the Chief Inspector of Factories for the Year 1938* (London: HMSO, 1939), pp. 61–67; R. Desmeules et al., "Amiantose et Cancers Pulmonaires," *Laval Medicine* 6 (1941): 97–108; H. B. Holleb and A. Angrist, "Bronchogenic Carcinoma in Association with Pulmonary Asbestosis," *American Journal of Pathology* 18 (1942): 123–135.

185. W. C. Hueper, *Occupational Tumors and Allied Diseases* (Springfield, Mass.: Charles C. Thomas, 1942), pp. 399–405.

186. L. R. Blinn, *History of the Saranac Laboratory,* unpublished manuscript, 1959.

187. Ibid., p. 12.

188. Letter, Vandiver Brown to L. U. Gardner, 20 November 1936.

189. Letter, L. V. Gardner to Vandiver Brown, 23 November 1936.

190. Letter, V. Brown to S. Simpson, 3 May 1939.

191. Letter, S. Simpson to V. Brown, 4 May 1939.

192. Letter, L. Gardner to L. Hektoen, 15 March 1943; quoted in Castleman, *Asbestos,* p. 45.

193. Ibid.

194. As reported by Dr. Harriet Hardy, quoted in Castleman, *Asbestos,* p. 49.

195. W. C. Hueper, "Cancer in Its Relation to Occupation and Environment," *Bulletin of the American Society for Control of Cancer* 25 (1943): 63–69.

196. *Annual Report of the Chief Inspector of Factories for the Year 1947* (London: HMSO, 1949), pp. 78–81; editorial, "Asbestos and Cancer of the Lung," *Journal of the American Medical Association* 140 (1949): 1219–1220.

197. G. Conklin, "Cancer and Environment," *Scientific American* 180 (1949): 11–15.

198. ATI minutes, 7 April 1949, noted in Castleman, *Asbestosis,* p. 54.

199. ATI Minutes, 7 March 1956, quoted in Castleman, *Asbestosis,* p. 81.

200. Ibid., emphasis in original.

201. ATI minutes, 9 June, 1955, quoted in Castleman, *Asbestosis,* p. 82.

202. ATI minutes, 7 March, 1957, quoted in Castleman, *Asbestosis,* p. 83.

203. D. C. Braun, *An Epidemiological Study of Lung Cancer in Asbestos Miners* (Quebec, Canada, 1957).

204. Letter, K. W. Smith to I. Sabourin, 30 December, 1957, quoted in Castleman, *Asbestosis,* p. 86.

205. W. C. Hueper, "Environmental and Occupational Cancer and Hazards," *Clinical Pharmacology Therapeutics* 3 (1962): 776–813.

206. Ibid.

207. Memo, W. C. Hueper to John Heller, 8 June 1959. The Hueper memos were printed in the *Drug Reporter* ("Blue Sheets"), a drug industry newsletter, on 11 January, 1961.

208. Ibid.

209. Ibid.

210. Hueper to Michael Shimkin, 9 May 1961, in *Drug Reporter,* 11 January 1961.

211. Cited in Castleman, *Asbestos,* p. 529.

II

REGULATION, RISK,
AND
UNCERTAINTY

4

Scientists, Engineers, and the Burdens of Occupational Exposure: The Case of the Lead Standard

RONALD BAYER

The toxic effects of lead exposure have long been known, so much so that by the late nineteenth century the consequences of working with lead had become the focus of attention of writers such as Charles Dickens, Thomas Hardy, and George Bernard Shaw.[1] Despite the recognition that lead could maim workers, efforts to control exposure remained rudimentary. For Dr. Alice Hamilton, writing in the early twentieth century, "lead intoxication" was the most prevalent of occupational diseases. Its medical implications were to be found not only in workers but in their children as well. Because lead could be passed on through exposed women to their children, Hamilton termed it a "race poison" affecting not only one generation but two.[2] About a half-century later, the Centers for Disease Control (CDC) reported on an epidemiological study of workers exposed to lead at a scrap smelter.[3] Of the thirty-seven employees who had been followed, thirty displayed signs of toxicity. Nine had at some point been hospitalized with lead-related disorders. Commenting on this evidence, Morton Corn, a former director of the Occupational Safety and Health Administration (OSHA), referred to the "grim" details of "this alarming story."[4]

This discovery on the part of the CDC reveals that although the most extreme examples of lead poisoning had by and large been eliminated from the American industrial landscape by the early 1970s, the toxic consequences of lead exposure remained a critical problem. For those concerned with occupational health and safety, the issue of lead poisoning had a contemporary importance that was amplified by its historical significance. With the creation of a federal presence in matters affecting the health of workers through the enactment of legislation establishing the National Institute of Occupational Safety and Health (NIOSH) and the Occupational Safety and Health Administration (OSHA) in 1970, it was inevitable that efforts would be made to use Washington's new regulatory authority to protect workers exposed to lead. In the bitter, almost decade-long struggle that surrounded efforts to promulgate a national lead standard, it became clear that the ideal of safety and health regulation based upon scientific findings free of the taint of political and social interests was a chimera. At every stage of the process, from the presentation of the science of lead exposure by NIOSH to the promulgation of the final lead standard by OSHA, the centrality of politics was evident. That this was so was not an aberration but an inevitable consequence of the fact that the processes of risk assessment and standard setting entailed not only the technical issue of whether given exposures posed a potential hazard for workers but nontechnical questions of who would bear the burdens of risk. And such questions are inherently political because whatever their empirical bases, they require a confrontation over matters of equity and distributive justice.

Background to the OSHA Lead Standard

Prior to the enactment of the OSHA lead standard, the exposure of workers to lead in the workplace was guided by a series of both public and quasi-public safety standards that were more often exceeded than adhered to. In the 1930s and 1940s the prevailing standard was 150 micrograms of lead per cubic meter of air (150 $\mu g/m^3$ air). This standard, established in response to the implications of a U.S. Public Health Service survey of the health of battery workers in 1928, was far below the once accepted 500 $\mu g/m^3$ air. The standard of 150 $\mu g/m^3$ air was raised to 200 in 1957 on the advice of the American Council of Government Industrial Hygienists. Although the prevailing standard was shifted downward to 150 $\mu g/m^3$ some years later, it again rose when OSHA adopted its first standard for lead exposure in 1971 and incorporated the recommendation of the American National Standards Institute of a 200 $\mu g/m^3$ level.[5]

Despite this constantly shifting standard, the practice of American industry remained such that large numbers of workers continued to be exposed to levels of lead in excess of prevailing "scientifically" grounded recommendations. Thus in 1977, prior to the adoption of the OSHA lead standard, more than 61 percent of workers in the primary and secondary lead smelting industries were exposed to more than 200 µg/m³ air. This was true for more than 20 percent of those who worked in storage battery plants.[6]

It was in 1973, and against this background, that NIOSH issued its first report on the risk posed to workers by lead exposure. In its Criteria Document,[7] the Institute sought to provide those concerned with the future course of regulation with data that reflected the prevailing scientific consensus. NIOSH thus presented, without any attempt at critical analysis, a broad body of research findings, much of which was derived from studies conducted under industry sponsorship. This research, and the NIOSH conclusions upon which it was grounded, incorporated traditional clinical notions of how the pathological was to be defined. By so narrowly drawing the boundaries of its concern, NIOSH placed a significant array of physiological changes in lead workers beyond the range of regulatory concern.

On the basis of this clinical standard, the Criteria Document asserted that workers whose blood lead levels remained at or below 80 micrograms of lead per 100 grams of blood (80 µg/100 g) would be unharmed by their exposure. Although the margin of safety provided by such a blood level could not be established, NIOSH had determined that there would be "few if any cases" of lead poisoning below blood levels of 90 µg/100 g.[8]

To maintain a blood level of 80 µg, NIOSH proposed that no worker be exposed to an air-lead level of more than 150 µ/m³.[9] Thus, rejecting the 1971 OSHA standard as insufficiently protective, NIOSH would have required a return to an air-lead level that had long prevailed as a standard of safe exposure. Returning to such a standard would, however, have required a modification of prevailing industrial practice, which, as noted, often resulted in lead exposures of more than 200 µg/m³ air.

The reaction to the NIOSH findings by representatives of industry and labor prefigured the more bitter confrontation that was to occur when OSHA sought to promulgate a standard of lead safety for workers. At a 1974 conference convened by the Lead Industries Association (LIA) to discuss the NIOSH report, industry representatives and scientific allies found much to recommend in the Institute's efforts. The 80-µg blood level had long been put forth as providing an adequate margin of safety by George Kehoe, the preeminent figure in lead toxicity research, who was viewed by industry as sympathetic to its interests. Concern was voiced, however, over the proposed reduction of air-lead levels. Not only was the scientific basis for the more stringent standard lacking, but the very basis for suggesting that air-lead exposures could provide an appropriate index of occupational hazard was brought into question.[10]

The most critical note during the LIA conference was struck by Sheldon Samuels of the AFL-CIO's Industrial Union Department. He charged NIOSH with participating in a "vile numbers game."[11] The scientific community, by assenting to the Institute's determinations and by providing the empirical foundations for its conclusions, was "engaged in a massive, destructive game of deception greater than this society, perhaps, has ever encountered."[12] Samuels argued that scientists who asserted that the proposed NIOSH recommendations provided a margin of safety for lead workers were making "authoritarian social decisions and labeling them scientific."[13] Not only were essentially social determinations thus being masked, but hidden assumptions about how the burden of risk ought to be borne were being incorporated into the NIOSH calculations. Samuels put forth what was for that moment in the public debate on lead toxicity and the protection of workers a radical proposition. He argued that blood lead levels had to be reduced to 40 µg/100 g—half the standard adopted by those who focused on traditional definitions of the pathological consequences associated with lead exposure. Furthermore, to achieve the required blood lead levels, Samuels demanded that air-lead exposure be reduced to 50 µg/m³ air—25 percent of the prevailing OSHA standard and one-third of the standard being proposed by NIOSH.[14] Those who heard these proposals understood that Samuels was calling for a massive expenditure in resources and thoroughgoing changes in the production process in order to ensure the health of workers.

In discussing the clash between labor and industry's representatives, Irving Tabershaw, editor of the *Journal of Occupational Medicine,* within which the proceedings of the LIA conference were reproduced, expressed his hostility toward those who would radically challenge the professional and social consensus then dominant in the lead industry. "Most revealing perhaps is the emotional attitude of labor towards the scientists and professionals practicing industrial hygiene and occupational medicine," Tabershaw wrote. "The accusation of industry's malfeasance is so broad, nonspecific and unsubstantiated that it defies an answer, but it is illustrative of the climate in which occupational health standards are being developed."[15]

It was within this politically charged climate, a climate characterized by the emergence of strong environmentalist and women's movements and increased sensitivity to risks in the workplace, that social and scientific perceptions of the risks of lead exposure began to change. Changes in the practice of industrial toxicology fueled and were fueled by increasing concern about the ever more subtle effects of lead exposure. As a consequence, no sooner had NIOSH issued its first Criteria Document on lead than the process of reevaluation began. Two years later, in August 1975, NIOSH issued a revised set of recommendations.[16] No longer was a blood lead level of 80 µg/100 g considered safe for workers; the level was now reduced to 60 µg/100 g.[17] Although it was unable to determine the appropriate air-lead level that would produce such a margin of safety for workers, NIOSH did note that it ought to be below the initially proposed 150 µg/m³ of air.[18] There seemed, however, no justification for forcing it down as low as 50 µg, as had been proposed by Sheldon Samuels.

The August 1975 NIOSH recommendations served as a basis for OSHA's preliminary 1975 proposals for a lead standard.[19] Issued as part of a flurry of regulatory initiatives designed to mute the growing dissatisfaction with OSHA's lackluster and sluggish performance, the 1975 proposal was to be characterized by representatives from industry and labor as well as professionals within government as inadequate in its formulation of the scientific and policy issues at stake. Despite these limitations, OSHA's preliminary proposal was noteworthy in a number of respects. It broke with the tradition of lead toxicology that had been dominated by George Kehoe, and indeed with much prevailing professional opinion, by asserting that clinically significant changes might well occur at blood lead levels below 80 µg/100 g.[20] In adopting this position OSHA rejected the conventional toxicological focus on gross manifestations of lead pathology and sought to underscore the relevance of far more subtle occurrences. In the words of the proposal, "lead may produce changes in biochemical and physiological parameters which occur at blood levels lower than those usually associated with overt clinical effects. The point at which subclinical changes become sufficiently serious to represent a threat to health is not clearly defined."[21]

Faced with such uncertainty, OSHA adopted a conservative posture. An appropriate margin of safety for lead workers required that attention be given to "subclinical" changes. The burden of uncertainty was to be shifted from exposed workers to those who would be forced to make the necessary modifications in the production process. Thus, rather than focusing on encephalopathy and "wrist drop," the conventional signs of advanced lead toxicity, the OSHA standard targeted neurological changes that involved the slowing of nerve conduction.[22] Rather than emphasizing gross anemia, a traditional indication of lead poisoning, the OSHA standard expressed concern about hemesynthesis and its effect on blood production.[23] Instead of a standard designed to prevent renal failure, OSHA's proposal was directed at avoiding reduced renal function.[24] Finally, rather than the "race poison" so central to Alice Hamilton's concerns and to those fearful of the potential effects of lead on women in the workplace, OSHA addressed its attention to an entire spectrum of reproductive hazards, including failures of conception and reduced fertility.[25]

The medical and technical shift represented by OSHA's attention to changes in biochemical and physiological parameters had important moral and political implications. So, too, did the preliminary standard's commitment to protecting the most vulnerable groups within the working population. Rather than designing protections for those workers who were especially robust, OSHA believed that the margin of safety being proposed had to be such that all workers could endure work with lead. The effect on those with sickle-cell trait and on women of reproductive age was a matter of special concern: "It is appropriate to consider these sizable groups in setting a standard which applies to all workers."[26]

Having established 60 µg as the body burden that would provide an adequate margin of safety for workers, OSHA next had to address the question of an air-lead standard that would produce that effect. Like NIOSH, OSHA acknowledged that the correlations between air lead levels and blood lead levels were not definitive. The available data simply did not permit a specification of a precise air lead level at which workers exposed to lead would have a mean blood level of 40 µg/100 g and a maximum blood level of 60 µg/100 g. NIOSH had indicated that something below 150 µg but above 50 µg would be necessary. In setting a standard within that range, OSHA adopted a compromise posture that owed as much to a social determination of tolerable risk as to empirically based conclusions: "In the circumstances we believe it is appropriate to propose a PEL [permissible exposure limit] that falls in the middle range: 100."[27]

In setting forth this preliminary lead standard, OSHA called for public comment on five broad areas touched upon in its effort. First, should subclinical effects be considered in the setting of an appropriate standard of safety? Second, does the air lead level of 100 μg/m³ provide an appropriate margin of safety? Third, should biological monitoring supplement ambient air monitoring? Fourth, are there especially susceptible groups, and how should they be considered in the setting of standards? And finally, what is the technical feasibility of the proposed standard?

Hearings on the OSHA Standard: Science, Politics, and the Clash of Interests

It was not until March 1977, eighteen months after the publication of the preliminary OSHA standard, that hearings were held to elicit public reaction. This setting provided an occasion for representatives of industry, labor, government, and the scientific community to put forth responses that were at once empirical, political, and moral. Most striking in the drama that unfolded during the course of the hearings and reproduced in the thousands of pages of testimony was how few surprise turns were encountered. With a predictability that was almost stunning, matters of scientific judgment as well as differing policy perspectives conformed to economic interests. The clash of social interests was reflected not only in responses to the proposed regulatory interventions but also in characterizations of the risks posed to workers from lead exposure. Social interests determined judgments not only of whether the cost of regulation was justified but also of whether the changes required in the production process were at all feasible. Usually called upon because their assessments met the political requirements of antagonistic constituencies, the scientists and engineers who testified before OSHA were enmeshed in a process that was radically partisan.

The long-standing professional and political tension between OSHA and NIOSH was reflected in the lukewarm support given by the latter to the former's recommendations. Although not opposed to the suggestion that the maximum blood lead level should be set at 60 μg/100 g with a mean of 40 μg/100 g, NIOSH could not itself support the position of those whom OSHA would call upon as its expert witnesses, who maintained that the proposed blood level standard be reduced below that which was proposed in the preliminary proposal. NIOSH held that "to go below 60 would place considerable emphasis upon a limited number of observations which have not been confirmed by multiple investigators. To do this would place the recommendations of a blood level in the workplace on less than firm ground."[28]

But for the lead industry and the scientists who testified on its behalf, both OSHA and NIOSH had already gone beyond the realm of empirically based regulation. Four issues were central to the industry's attack. First, it questioned the grounds upon which OSHA had determined the level of risk associated with elevated blood levels. Second, it doubted the appropriateness of setting a standard based upon assumptions of a relation between air lead levels and blood lead levels. Third, it rejected OSHA's determination that the 100 µg/m³ air lead level was necessary to provide an appropriate margin of safety for workers. And fourth, it believed that the standard proposed by OSHA was neither technologically nor economically feasible.

Citing what they termed the "seminal" work of Kehoe, representatives of the lead industry testifying before OSHA asserted "there is no persuasive evidence that even the slightest *clinical* lead intoxication occurs below 80 µg/100 g."[29] A physician testifying on behalf of industry asserted that his "experience over 25 years suggests that in reports of lead intoxication [at blood lead levels below 80], the diagnosis is wrong or the method of establishing blood lead levels is inaccurate or the estimation was delayed for some time after the occurrence of the symptoms."[30]

Most significant in the lead industry's attack on the OSHA standard was the testimony of British expert Michael Williams, a medical advisor to two battery plants since 1962. In his testimony he claimed to have conducted 50,000 routine medical examinations of workers exposed to lead. He stated that "except for 2–3 cases of anemia where blood lead levels exceeded 80 µg/100 g of blood, I have not seen one single case of lead poisoning in these lead workers nor has there been one day's sickness absence due to lead known to me."[31] Williams went on to dismiss the significance of the "subclinical" changes deemed so important by OSHA:

> Nerve conduction velocity is of course of no importance in the short run unless it results in some material deficit or diminution of function. . . . The hemesynthesis argument can, I think, be totally discounted. It is surely reasonable to interpret these changes as one of many thousands of homeostatic mechanisms of the body whereby the effect of an alter-

ation in the external environment is fully compensated by a biological response.[32]

Unlike the proposed standard, which suggested the importance of considering subclinical responses, the industry thus sought to preserve the standard of traditional clinical diagnosis: "We feel that a measure of health is the absence of illness; and we feel that you can correlate the absence of illness with blood lead levels below 80 μg/100 g."[33]

The industry's rejection of OSHA's proposal was not grounded solely on a philosophical difference over the appropriate focus of health regulations, however. At almost every juncture the scientific evidence used to make the case for a reduction in blood and air lead levels was subjected to methodological challenge by the lead industry. The studies upon which OSHA depended, charged the industry, had been conducted in a sloppy fashion. The data upon which it relied were inaccurate and could not provide the basis for stringent controls.[34]

The industry also rejected OSHA's assertion that a meaningful relation could be found between ambient air levels and blood lead levels. Williams claimed that his own study, upon which OSHA had relied in its argument, had been misinterpreted and could not be so used.[35] Kenneth Nelson of ASARCO, a former president of the Industrial Hygiene Association and a founder of the Academy of Industrial Hygiene, emphasized the inadequacy of the scientific basis for postulating a relation between air lead levels and blood lead levels: "I do not think that one can do any predicting at all of individual blood lead levels in connection with any air concentrations of lead as we presently measure them."[36] The conclusion of the 1968 International Conference on Lead, that the relationship of air and blood lead levels was insufficiently precise to warrant the establishment of an air standard, was seized upon by industry to make the argument that such a standard could have no rational justification.

As a consequence, industry's representatives asserted that biological monitoring of individual workers rather than environmental monitoring was the only reasonable approach to the control of lead toxicity.[38] But if such a standard were to be established, the appropriate level would be 200 μg rather than the 100 μg proposed by OSHA.[39] This point was made by Dr. Jerome Cole, Director of Environmental Health for the Lead Industries Association. Acknowledging that "few, if any" major segments of the lead industry were in compliance with the existing OSHA standard of 200 µg, he stated: "This is significant because it means that we simply do not know what health improvements, if any, would be achieved if the industry complied consistently with the present air lead requirements."[40] Faced with indeterminate data and the certain costs associated with the reduction of exposure levels, the industry argued for regulatory restraint: "To require the lead industry to spend millions of dollars for engineering controls which are likely to have no significant impact on employees' health is obviously wrong."[41]

Finally, the lead industry questioned OSHA's assumption regarding the feasibility of the proposed standard. The industry relied on Knowlton Caplan, a prominent industrial engineer, to make its case. The cost estimates of the economic consulting firm hired by OSHA and the results of OSHA's own economic and technological analysis were challenged.[42] Caplan said, "I believe that there are portions of the secondary and primary lead smelting industry that will not be able to achieve the goal of 100 µg/m³ of lead per cubic meter of air."[43] He even doubted the capacity of segments of the industry to achieve the 200 µg level established by OSHA in 1971.[44] According to Caplan, many firms would be forced out of business by the OSHA standard, and the lead industry would suffer, as would the economy as a whole.[45] The picture of an unreasonable government attempt at control thus emerged. Michael Williams captured the spirit of the industry's opposition when he concluded his testimony by stating: "It is wrong to demand action in advance of facts, for that is the way not of reason, but of hysteria."[46]

If NIOSH seemed unwilling to press beyond the blood lead level of 60 µg/m³ and if industry believed that such a standard was "medically unnecessary," scientifically groundless, and practically impossible, OSHA itself had begun to doubt the adequacy of its own proposed standard. In the period between the publication of OSHA's initial standard and the public hearings, Eula Bingham, closely identified with labor's concern for a safe workplace, had assumed directorship of OSHA. Committed to the adoption of rigorous standards that would protect all workers, including fertile women who had been faced with exclusionary hiring practices, Bingham found the initial OSHA proposals weak.

That OSHA had become disenchanted with its own proposal was clear from the testimony of the experts it brought forth on its own behalf. In almost every instance calls were made by OSHA's expert witnesses for standards significantly more restrictive than those proposed in 1975. OSHA's primary witness on the effects of blood lead levels on the nervous system, Finnish researcher Anna Seppalainen, concluded that there were significant effects on the peripheral nervous system when blood lead levels exceeded 50 micrograms per 100 milliliters (50 µg/100 ml) of blood.[47] Richard Wideen, testifying on renal function, asserted that blood lead levels above 40 µg posed a risk to the capacity of kidney function.[48] Vilma Hunt, citing the data on lead's effect on children, asserted: "If there is any good that can come from calamity, we now know that the biological response to lead of a heterogeneous population of children is increasingly manifest as pathological changes when the blood lead levels rise to 30 µg/ 100 ml. Until we can show that all workers are different from all children in their response to lead exposure, we are obliged to use those tragic data for the protection of all."[49]

Involved here was not simply an empirical redefinition of the toxic effects of lead, but a transformation of the very concept of acceptable risk, a reduction in the tolerance for biological changes with *potentially* important consequences for health. Commenting on this shifting perspective, Dr. R. L. Zielhuis noted: "To take into account factors which are not detectable by normal clinical methods and which are not known to give rise to any long-term clinical effects, represents a change in philosophy as to what is or is not acceptable."[50]

This shift in philosophical perspective was clearly reflected in the testimony of Sergio Pionelli, director of the Pediatric Hematology Unit at New York University. Starting from the fact that the alteration in hemesynthesis produces no subjective evidence of impairment of health unless it reaches extreme depression in severe lead intoxication, he concluded:

> I do not believe that it is any longer possible to restrict the concept of health to the individual's subjective lack of feeling of adverse effects. This is because we know that individuals may get adjusted to suboptimal health and believe they are well. . . . We have moved from restrictive medicine to a functional preventive medicine. It is the responsibility of preventive medicine to detect those alterations which may precede frank symptomatology and to prevent their occurrence.[51]

Although there was some divergence of opinion about the appropriate level of ambient lead exposure—not surprising, given the uncertainty about the way in which lead directly affects the body burden— most of those who testified on behalf of OSHA saw the proposed standard of 100 µg/m³ air as unacceptable.[52]

Central to OSHA's position on the protection of workers exposed to lead was the determination that engineering controls had to provide the first line of defense for those at risk. Although it acknowledged that the use of protective equipment and administrative efforts might be necessary to supplement the control of ambient air lead levels, they were viewed as inherently less effective and socially less desirable.[53] As a result, OSHA, in this instance as in other cases affecting the potential threat to exposed workers, stressed the importance of redesigning the workplace to protect the health of workers. In some cases such efforts would entail retrofitting; in others, the building of new plants. Finally, OSHA believed it had an obligation to force the development of new technologies when necessary. But was such a strategy feasible?

OSHA's primary engineering witness, Dr. Melvin First of Harvard University, put forward an exceptionally optimistic picture on the prospects for reducing lead exposure through engineering controls: "Every operation that can be mechanized and automated is capable of being enclosed by tight physical barriers and placed under slight negative pressure to prevent outleakage of dust or fume-ladened air."[54] The prospect of major financial outlays would, he believed, provide the industry with an incentive to design improved and less costly control methods.

The clash that occurred between First and Caplan (the latter speaking on behalf of industry) during the hearings is revealing. Caplan's attention to the details of the lead industry production process was designed to indicate that First grasped neither the technical nor the economic dimensions of the problems posed for an industry being challenged by government regulation. To First's assertions that industry could technically achieve the standards of protection being proposed by OSHA, Caplan responded: "Yes, but you were leaving cost out of here."[55] First acknowledged the importance of economic considerations in all engineering efforts but asserted that Caplan had overestimated the costs that would be generated by OSHA's regulations.[56]

If OSHA was pressed by its own witnesses to enact a stricter standard, labor's representatives too expressed their dissatisfactions with the early proposal. Leonard Woodcock of the United Auto Workers thus asserted: "I must say that if high body burdens of lead cause anemia and low levels of lead disrupt the production of blood, then we want protection from low levels. . . . If it is known that high levels of lead cause kidney failure and low levels cause kidney damage, then we want protection from low levels."[57] Like Lloyd McBride of the United Steelworkers,[58] Woodcock demanded lower exposure levels to lead and indeed argued that no more than 40 μm would be tolerable.[58] For Dr. Sol Epstein, testifying on behalf of the AFL/CIO, the OSHA standard failed to meet the requisite criterion of providing a margin of safety adequate to protect all workers.

For those pressing OSHA to adopt very restrictive standards for air lead and blood lead levels, the burdens of uncertainty were not to be borne by workers but by the lead industry. Ambiguity regarding scientific data was to be acknowledged but not used as an excuse for inaction. Sidney Wolf, testifying on behalf of the Public Citizen's Health Research Group, thus stated: "The Health Research Group does not claim that all of the suspected effects . . . will necessarily be proven by future research . . . [but] if a doubt exists as to the danger of long-term exposure to lead, that doubt must be resolved in favor of the workers."[60] Leonard Woodcock stressed the disjunction between what he saw as the level of protection afforded to the public under conditions of uncertainty and that provided to workers. "Our members," he stated, "are troubled when it is explained to them that a food additive or pesticide must be proven to be safe as it is used, whereas an industrial chemical must be proven harmful before it can be regulated."[61]

Emblematic of how differently uncertainty might be viewed and used in the regulation of toxic substances is the response evoked by one important study that detailed the morbidity and mortality of workers exposed to lead. For the lead industry, the Cooper-Gaffey study, which it had sponsored, proved that current levels of exposure to lead and the pathological consequences of lead toxicity as conventionally appreciated posed no risk to workers.[62] For Sidney Wolf, that same study suggested the need for regulation and reform. "Though not statistically significant, the standard mortality ratios for major cardiovascular and renal disease were increased," he noted.[63]

Most important to labor and recognized by OSHA at the outset of its hearings was the necessity of a provision for medical removal protection with wage rate retention for those whose blood lead levels rose above the maximum permissible levels. Only a provision that would guarantee, at whatever cost, the earning capacity of workers whose health required that they be removed from exposure to lead would be effective and equitable. Without rate retention, workers would refuse to participate in medical surveillance programs so crucial to the standard, and workers with elevated blood lead levels would be forced to bear the economic burdens of toxicity.[64] As one speaker put it, "a worker with excessive blood lead levels should not have to suffer the additional indignity of being unable to support a family."[65]

Labor's representatives were mindful that an adequate standard of protection—one that would include medical removal protection with rate retention—would create added social costs in the production of lead. But from their perspective, it was wrong to ask workers to bear the burden of disease so that the cost of lead products could be kept down: "We just cannot expect a group of employees to be put on a sacrificial table because we happen to need lead and because it is a vital metal and we cannot do without it."[66]

The Final Lead Standard

When at last OSHA issued its final standard in November 1978,[67] the result was a set of regulations far stricter than those initially prepared and indeed stricter than many advocates of reform had anticipated. The acceptable limits for blood lead levels were reduced from 60 μg to 40 μg/100 g;[68] the permissible air lead level was reduced from 100 μg to 50 μg/m³ of air.[69] Medical removal protection with rate retention was mandated.[70]

On the basis of a model of the interaction of blood lead levels and air exposure developed by the Center for Policy Alternatives at the Massachusetts Institute of Technology, OSHA believed that it had resolved the issue of scientific uncertainty that had plagued the hearings on the proposed lead standard.[71] That formulation provided a mathematical basis for asserting that the protection of workers required not only that the prevailing 200-μg standard be reduced but also that the initially proposed 100-μg standard be reduced by half. But even that very strict standard represented a compromise between the demands posed by the goal of worker health and the economic and technological feasibility of modifying the production process. OSHA's model indicated that at a 50-μg lead level, 29.3 percent of exposed workers would have blood lead levels above the 40 μg/100 g established as providing the necessary margin of safety.[72]

Despite its commitment to engineering controls, OSHA recognized that to achieve the mandated reduction in blood lead levels, it would be necessary, for an interim period, to rely upon protective equipment for workers and a variety of administrative devices to limit the exposure of workers to airborne lead. Massive investments over an extended period would be necessary to effect the necessary reduction in air lead levels. Extended periods would be necessary for the redesign of the production process. For the primary lead industry, ten years was provided to achieve the engineering controls necessary to achieve the mandated air lead levels.[73] For the secondary lead smelter and lead battery industry, five years was provided.[74] Even the implementation schedule for the medical removal protection was to reflect the limits imposed by the complex tasks involved in the modification of lead production.[75]

Rejecting the counsel of those who argued that the lead industry could not so radically transform itself, OSHA asserted that its commitment to the health of workers required it to act as an agent of technological change. Thus, in the primary lead smelting industry, OSHA believed that the health of workers ultimately would make it necessary to replace pyrotechnology by hydrotechnology,[76] although there was very limited evidence to suggest the feasibility of such a transformation.

From a societal perspective the demands that were to be placed on the lead industry, and ultimately on the consumers of its products, could be defended on both moral and economic grounds. The failure to impose stringent controls would create private burdens for those least able to bear them, workers and their families. The most elemental principles of equity could thus be called upon to defend the argument that those burdens would have to be redistributed by increasing the social costs of lead production. Furthermore, a failure to control the toxicity associated with exposure to lead, and even the risks of such toxicity, would generate medical and social costs that would not be reflected in the costs of lead production. The OSHA standard could thus be justified as entailing the internalization of the negative externalities associated with work in the lead industry.

From the point of view of the industry, however, and especially of those firms which might be forced to close because of their inability to meet the costs associated with the implementation of the OSHA standard, the new regulations appeared not only unfair but irrational. The inherent tension between the private and the public is thus underscored here in an especially acute fashion. It is not surprising, therefore, that engineers speaking on behalf of the industry generally and for particular firms specifically would find the final OSHA lead standard unacceptable and infeasible. Nor is it surprising that the Lead Industry Association would seek to thwart the OSHA decision by

appealing to the courts, where the Association would charge the
agency with a failure to meet the administrative requirement that
standards be based upon a rational consideration of scientific evidence and the feasibility of implementation.

When the District of Columbia Court of Appeals handed down its
decision on August 15, 1980,[77] it upheld the OSHA lead standard with
some minor exceptions involving the adequacy of some of the feasibility studies upon which decisions were made for marginal elements of
the industry. The court acknowledged the difficulty in reviewing such
standards that require the application of a "substantial evidence test"
to regulations that it viewed as essentially legislative. Agencies were
compelled, the Court held, to make "inferences from complex scientific and factual data," and "such determinations necessarily involved
highly speculative projections of technological development in areas
wholly lacking in scientific and economic certainty."[78] Faced with such
uncertainty, it was for OSHA and not the court to weigh the potential
burdens associated with alternative policy options.

Despite the legal delays and despite the variances that have been
granted in recent years for political and technological reasons, there
is already clear indication that the lead standard has begun to affect
the body burden of workers. A report prepared for the Office of
Technology Assessment on the effect of the standard[79] reached four
broad conclusions:

1. The blood levels of workers had declined in primary and secondary smelters and in battery plants. Thus, the number of workers
   with blood lead levels over 40 μg/100 g had been reduced by about
   one-third. Blood levels over 80 μg/100 g, which had been found in
   earlier studies in 16 percent of workers in the secondary smelting
   industry, 6 percent of workers in battery plants, and 2 percent in
   primary smelters, were practically unobserved in workers in the
   post-standard period. Finally, dramatic changes in the proportion
   of workers found to have blood lead levels in the 60–80 μg/100 g
   range had also been observed.[80]
2. Although air lead levels in plants had come down, a 50 μg/m³ level
   had not been reached in either secondary or primary smelters or in
   battery plants. Indeed, in primary and secondary smelters, compliance with the 200-μg level had not yet been achieved.[81]
3. Interestingly, the reduced body burden of lead that had been
   found in workers was not solely a consequence of OSHA's efforts.
   Between 30 and 50 percent of the observed reduction in blood

lead levels could be attributed to the effect of regulations adopted by the U.S. Environmental Protection Agency.[82]

4. The costs of medical removal protection, by forcing an internalization of the costs associated with elevated blood lead levels, had been a driving force for change, creating an economic incentive for the reduction in air lead levels.[83]

How far change will progress in the current political and economic climate is unknown. Efforts by industry representatives to force a reopening of the issue of the health effects of lead exposure have been resisted by the professional staff of OSHA, although it has come to believe that the feasibility of developing engineering controls to attain a 50-μg level is increasingly remote, especially given the financial structure of the lead industry.

Conclusion

In its evaluation of the efforts of both the Environmental Protection Agency and OSHA to regulate exposure to lead, the National Research Council has underscored the extent to which regulatory agencies faced with politically contested alternatives have at times sought to justify their actions by relying on the protective mantle of value-free science.[84] Although OSHA explicitly acknowledged that it could not await the resolution of the full range of scientific controversies surrounding the health effects of lead before issuing its standard, it did seek to ground its much-disputed air lead exposure limit on a mathematical model. For the National Research Council, however, "the data base that supported [both the EPA and OSHA] models was small, and neither the exact form of the mathematical function nor the slope of the resulting curve [could] be determined with great accuracy."[85]

That OSHA had sought to provide a scientifically objective basis for its policy determinations should come as no surprise. Like other regulatory bodies it must, either because of demands placed upon it or because of the ideological commitments of the scientists upon whom it relies, adopt a posture in which the tasks of hazard evaluation and risk assessment are viewed as above politics and the influence of social values. The controversy surrounding the regulation of lead demonstrates, however, that even the putatively technical tasks of hazard evaluation and risk assessment inevitably involve judgments that are social and moral. As a consequence, these tasks, as much as the more explicitly political ones of risk management and regulation, must be judged within a broad ethical framework that has as its centerpiece the issue of distributive justice. Thus, the widely read report of the National Research Council Committee on the Institutional Means for the Assessment of Risks to Public Health, *Risk Assessment in the Federal Government: Managing the Process,*[86] which seeks to draw a sharp distinction between the value-free task of risk assessment and the value-laden undertaking of policymaking, must be viewed as flawed and as an oversimplification.

Because scientists, engineers, and other professionals are called upon to make determinations on the basis of data of highly variable quality, with often ambiguous implications for policy and regulation, their interpretations inevitably will be affected by social and political interests.[87] In the struggle that took place over the adoption of the lead standard, scientists confronted each other as partisans. For some, this was an unseemly encounter. However, if the perspective presented here is correct, then such conflicts must be viewed as unavoidable. Indeed, efforts to eliminate them can only result in a process of obfuscation, one in which social values and interests will be masked.

Notes

1. V. Hunt, *Work and the Health of Women* (Boca Raton, Fla.: CRC Press, 1979), p. 201.

2. Ibid., p. 202.

3. R. J. Levine et al., "Occupational Lead Poisoning, Animal Deaths and Environmental Contamination at a Scrap Smelter," *American Journal of Public Health* 66 (1976): 548–552.

4. M. Corn, "Lead Poisoning in Industry, 1976," *American Journal of Public Health* 66 (1976): 531–532.

5. U.S. Department of Labor, Occupational Safety and Health Administration, "Lead: Occupational Exposure; Proposed Standard" (hereafter OSHA 1975), *Federal Register*, 3 October 1975, p. 45934.

6. D. R. Hattis et al., "Airborne Lead: A Clearcut Case of Differential Protection," *Environment* 24 (1982): 14–42.

7. National Institute of Occupational Safety and Health, *Criteria for a Recommended Standard. Occupational Exposure to Inorganic Lead* (Washington, D.C.: U.S. GPD, DHEW(NIOSH) No. 73-11010, 1972).

8. Ibid., V-4.

9. Ibid., V-5.

10. "Standards for Occupational Lead Exposure," *Journal of Occupational Medicine* 17 (February 1975): 95.

11. Ibid., p. 80.

12. Ibid., p. 81.

13. Ibid.

14. Ibid.

15. Ibid., p. 75.

16. OSHA 1975, p. 45934.

17. National Institute of Occupational Safety and Health, *Criteria for a Recommended Standard. Occupational Exposure to Inorganic Lead, Revised Criteria-1978* (hereafter NIOSH 1978), (Washington, D.C.: U.S. GPO, DHEW (NIOSH) No. 78-158, 1978), XII-3.

18. Ibid.

19. OSHA 1975.

20. Ibid., p. 45935.

21. Ibid., pp. 45935–45936.

22. Ibid., p. 45935.

23. Ibid., p. 45936.

24. Ibid., p. 45937.

25. Ibid., p. 45935.

26. Ibid., p. 45936.

27. Ibid., p. 45938.

28. NIOSH 1978, XII–18.

29. Lead Industries Association, "Comments, Objections and a Summary of Evidence by the Lead Industries Association to the Proposed Standard for Exposure to Lead," 16 January 1976 (hereafter LIA 1976), p. 17.

30. Ibid., p. 19.

31. U.S. Department of Labor, Occupational Safety and Health Administration, Informal Public Hearings on Proposed Standard for Exposure to Lead, *Transcript of Proceedings,* pp. 1886ff. (hereafter *Transcript*).

32. Ibid., p. 1886.

33. Ibid., p. 3094.

34. Ibid., pp. 610, 4183.

35. LIA 1976, p. 47.

36. *Transcript,* p. 4032.

37. *Transcript,* p. 4056.

38. LIA 1976, p. 52.

39. Ibid., p. 76.

40. *Transcript,* p. 3017.

41. LIA 1976, p. 52.

42. *Transcript,* p. 3923.

43. Ibid., p. 3931.

44. Ibid.

45. Ibid., p. 3856.

46. Ibid., pp. 1886ff.

47. Ibid., p. 123.

48. Ibid., p. 1732.

49. Ibid., p. 661.

50. R. L. Zielhuis, "Second International Workshop on Permissible Levels for Occupational Exposure to Inorganic Lead," *International Archives of Occupational and Environmental Health* 39 (1979): 59–72.

51. *Transcript,* p. 464.

52. Ibid., p. 489.

53. OSHA 1975, p. 45940.

54. *Transcript,* p. 2230.

55. Ibid., p. 2350.

56. Ibid., p. 2370.

57. Ibid., p. 5040.

58. Ibid., p. 2959.

59. Ibid., p. 5041.

60. Ibid., p. 4135.

61. Ibid., p. 5041.

62. LIA 1976, p. 44.

63. *Transcript,* p. 4134.

64. Ibid., p. 1035.

65. Ibid., p. 2967.

66. Ibid., p. 2971.

67. U.S. Department of Labor, Occupational Safety and Health Administration, "Occupational Exposure to Lead, Final Standard," *Federal Register,* 14 November 1978, pp. 52952–53014.

68. Ibid., p. 52954.

69. Ibid., p. 52963.

70. Ibid., p. 52973.

71. Ibid., p. 52963.

72. Ibid.

73. Ibid., p. 53008.

74. Ibid.

75. Ibid., p. 52974.

76. Department of Labor, Occupational Safety and Health Administration, "Occupational Exposure to Lead, Attachment to the Preamble for the Final Standard," *Federal Register,* 21 November 1978, p. 54480.

77. *United Steelworkers of America,* AFL-CIO v. *Marshall,* 647 Fed. 2d 189 (1980).

78. Ibid.

79. R. Goble et al., "Implementation of the Occupational Lead Exposure Standard" (November 1983), mimeo, 3:10–3:15.

80. Ibid., 3:10–3:15.

81. Ibid., 3:3–3:9.

82. Ibid., 1.3.

83. Ibid., 3:28–3:48.

84. National Research Council, Committee on Lead in the Human Environment, *Lead in the Human Environment* (Washington, D.C.: National Academy of Sciences, 1980), p. 231.

85. Ibid., p. 213.

86. National Research Council, Committee on the Institutional Means for the Assessment of Risks to Public Health, *Risk Assessment in the Federal Government: Managing the Process* (Washington, D.C.: National Academy Press, 1983).

87. R. Crandall and L. Lave (eds.), *The Scientific Basis of Health and Safety Regulation* (Washington, D.C.: The Brookings Institution, 1981), pp. 14–16.

5

Moral Dimensions of Occupational Health: The Case of the 1969 Coal Mine Health and Safety Act

CURTIS SELTZER

The Federal Coal Mine Health and Safety Act of 1969 (PL 91-173) established precedent-setting protections for American coal miners. The act set forth strict safety standards designed primarily to reduce underground explosions, which had claimed about 7,500 lives since the early 1900s. The Department of the Interior—and later the Department of Labor—was to enforce these standards and subsequent regulations through periodic inspections, civil penalties, closure orders, and injunctions. Although several coal-safety measures had been enacted in the twentieth century, the 1969 act was the first to impose meaningful safety standards and require federal enforcement. For that alone the act stands out in the history of workplace legislation. But its more far-reaching breakthroughs came in the area of occupational health. The purpose of the 1969 act was

> to provide, to the greatest extent possible, that the working conditions in each underground coal mine are sufficiently free of respirable dust concentrations in the mine atmosphere to permit each miner the opportunity to work underground during the period of his entire adult working life without incurring any disability from pneumonconiosis or any other occupation-related disease during or at the end of such period.[1]

This language is notable for its forthright, and perhaps naive, call for a risk-free work environment. Although Congress stated that no miner should incur "any" disability from "any" occupational disease, the legislation did not establish a risk-free dust standard. Congress established a compensation program for coal miners who were disabled by coal workers' pneumoconiosis (CWP), which the act recognized as a work-related respiratory disease.[2] The legislation also created a cumbersome procedure for sampling the mine atmosphere for respirable coal dust.

All this was new ground for federal legislators and administrators. Earlier coal legislation had said nothing about occupational health. A federally imposed standard for respirable coal mine dust had never been considered before 1969; indeed, Congress and the executive branch had never even shown much curiosity about dust sampling before then. Although a few precedents existed for compensating victims of workplace negligence, Congress had never before enacted a compensation program of such scope and significance. The year-long debate over this legislation provides a framework for thinking about the moral issues that scientists, engineers, and doctors face in the field of occupational health.

Choosing Sides: Science and Medicine in the Coal Fields

Coal mining is an industry whose history suggests that it has often forced those it touched to choose sides, to choose between those who manage and those who work in the mines.[3] The line of division is deep, and few bridges were constructed over it that would allow health and safety professionals to stand comfortably on both sides.[4]

The division was expressed in coal-field health care through the company-doctor system, by which mine operators provided medical services of their choosing to their employees, who were compelled as a condition of employment to finance the arrangement.[5] It is fair to assume that most doctors who signed on with a company accepted management's perspective on employee health matters. Such doctors chose to provide health care within a system bounded by the requirement that the employer—the coal operator—produce coal at a profit. Doctors' income depended more on the company's ability to stay in business and less on the ability of their patients to pay. In coal's competitive market, costs related to preventing workplace injuries and disease, public sanitation, and individual medical treatment could substantially reduce the rate of return. Even the most well-intentioned doctor would have had trouble maintaining independence in circumstances in which professional interests were so awkwardly juxtaposed with those of personal finances.

Deciding to become a company doctor was the key moral choice. The company's interest framed the perspective of the health provider and structured his practice. This career choice fit the doctor into an established corporate ethical framework for resolving most, if not all, professional questions about industrial safety, occupational disease, and public health. The company's financial interests were superimposed on the practice of medicine and became the matrix within which these decisions were made. Where a company doctor felt professional and ethical conflict, he faced a choice of either finding new work or swallowing his objections. Some doctors undoubtedly left, but most seemed to have made peace with the arrangement and developed ways of avoiding issues that caused discomfort.

The history of worker and community health in the American coal-mining industry through World War II shows two curves running conjunctively. One is the abysmal record of community and occupational health in the mining camps;[6] the other is the stunning professional silence of the physicians who worked there.[7] No evidence of company doctors acting collectively as health advocates on behalf of their patients and communities has yet been uncovered, nor have cases been found of doctors resigning to protest poor workplace conditions or inadequate support—although some probably did. Company doctors either left after a few years or adapted to the system by choosing not to see problems whose existence would otherwise cause them professional or moral conflict. A federal survey of health conditions in the coal fields in 1947, the Boone Report, attributed physician ignorance of workplace hazards to "disinterest":

> With very few exceptions, coal mine physicians are not familiar with the miner's working environment, the physical capacities required to do several types of mining work, and the industrial accident and occupational disease hazards of the particular mines they serve. . . . This observation indicates the general disinterest of management and physicians in the modern concept of industrial medical care.[8]

"Disinterest" is a shallow explanation. Blindness and deafness were doctors' mechanisms for adapting to the ethical conflicts that the company-doctor system generated. Silence was the result.

As early as the 1870s, a professional literature appeared on coal workers' respiratory disease.[9] But with the decline of the miners' self-insurance associations in the late nineteenth century and the rise of the company-doctor system, medical professionals seemed to have lost interest in the lung ailments of the nation's several hundred thousand coal miners. The broad current of medical opinion was that a unique, dust-related disease did not exist in coal miners, and that if one did, it did not do much damage. Of the few professional articles that appeared in American journals from the 1890s to the 1950s, most claimed that the lung symptoms of mine workers were either benign or normal, and often both. Miners' asthma was a common name for these symptoms. A typical proponent of this view is Earl H. Rebhorn, who wrote that " 'miners' asthma' is considered an ordinary condition that need cause no worry and therefore the profession has not troubled itself about its finer pathological and . . . clinical manifestations."[10]

Some doctors attributed these lung symptoms to poor personal hygiene and unsanitary individual life styles.[11] Some said breathing coal dust might actually help miners because it was quite possible that the dust had "the property of hindering the development of tuberculosis, and of arresting its progress."[12] Others opined that miners who claimed disability from miners' asthma were actually malingerers or, alternatively, suffering from a psychological fear of mining.[13]

Even as most private physicians dismissed miners' respiratory symptoms, some portentous evidence surfaced from researchers in the public sector, especially in Europe. The U.S. Public Health Service studied coal miners' health three times between 1914 and 1945. In the 1930s the Service discovered that more than 40 percent of the bituminous miners X-rayed showed excessive fibrous tissue in their lungs (pulmonary fibrosis). Nevertheless, the researchers found little correlation between fibrosis and lung impairment. Further, they believed that silica—particularly among anthracite miners—rather than coal dust produced the fibrosis.[14] When inhaled, "even in large quantities, [pure coal dust] produces little or no fibrosis," the Service study reported.[15] Despite the continued denial of American researchers, British scientists began to identify dust-related disease. In fact, in 1943 Great Britain officially recognized coal workers' pneumoconiosis as a work-related disabling lung disease and introduced a program of workers' compensation.

What explains the failure of American medicine to probe the linkage between mine work and respiratory disease? Why did it take so long for a connection to be made? Were medical practitioners and researchers obtuse? Had they failed as professionals to measure effects and determine cause? Were other factors affecting their behavior?

The majority of coal-field medical practitioners had no interest in discovering—and a powerful interest in not discovering—that business-as-usual methods in the coal industry were routinely damaging thousands of their patients. Researchers and physicians did not feel a need to explore the subject as long as they either denied the existence of symptoms, thought them harmless, or attributed them to ignorance in the victimized population. Occupational medicine tends to look for a single, specific disease. As long as American researchers denied the existence of a distinct coal workers' disease, no research was required. Was the science of medicine and industrial health too undeveloped to have asked the right research questions? Was there too little financial support available for those who might have wanted to study the problem? Was the coal industry so politically powerful, or so weak financially, that public agencies simply chose not to sponsor research that might add cost to the production cycle? Some truth is probably to be found in all these hypotheses.

But it was impossible for a doctor to practice among miners without hearing their coughs, seeing their black spit, and observing their breathlessness. Nor could it be denied that this set of symptoms was common to coal miners. How was this to be explained? Any coal-field medical professional who raised questions about dusty working conditions would soon find himself beyond the periphery of tolerated curiosity. So alternative explanations were advanced—cigarette smoking, poor living conditions, and bad diet—that shifted the blame for injury to the victim himself. And if these hypotheses fell short, a nonwork-related disease—tuberculosis, bronchitis, emphysema—was available. It is perhaps simply our greater scientific knowledge and the advantage of hindsight that makes these practitioners appear so kept.

John L. Lewis, president of the United Mine Workers of America (UMWA) from 1920 to 1960, established the first worker-centered counterforce in coal-field medicine after World War II when he persuaded the unionized sector of the industry to finance what became a UMWA-controlled health and pension plan.[16] The UMWA Welfare and Retirement Fund provided nearly comprehensive medical coverage to UMWA miners for several decades.[17] However, the Fund's administrators quickly realized that improving medical insurance would be wasted without improving health-care delivery. Consequently, the Fund built a chain of ten hospitals and several dozen clinics throughout the coal fields in the 1950s, which were staffed with salaried doctors whose loyalties lay with their employers—the Fund and its patients. The UMWA's alternative health-care system provided a base from which a handful of pro-miner doctors would question conventional medical wisdom about the causes and nature of respiratory disease among coal miners.[18]

It is easier to understand the silence of physicians in the industry's employ than the behavior of many of their UMWA-associated colleagues. Even though a few doctors associated with the UMWA Welfare and Retirement Fund published their observations of lung disease in professional journals, the UMWA and the Fund in the 1950s and most of the 1960s did less than might have been expected to alert their constituents or public policymakers about occupational lung disease.[19] They, too, conformed to the policies of their employer.

The UMWA, which exercised effective control over the Fund, had ended years of turmoil with unionized companies in 1950 when Lewis signed a collective bargaining agreement that became the first act in a two-decade-long industrial partnership. Circumstances forced him to protect the big unionized companies from small, nonunionized producers and from cheap alternative fuels in a demand-constrained market that kept coal prices low. Lewis supported the unionized operators' drive to modernize their mining systems, raise productivity through the substitution of capital for labor, reduce production and labor costs, and drive small coal producers into bankruptcy.[20]

This union-management partnership had several direct and related effects on the occupational health of American coal miners in the 1950s and 1960s. The new continuous-cutting underground mining machines seemed to increase respirable dust over levels generated by the older blast-and-shovel techniques. Neither the UMWA nor the companies thought to reduce dust as coal was cut from the advancing face. Few companies took dust samples. Both measures would have increased production costs, and as long as coal dust was assumed to be benign, neither appeared necessary.

Lewis financed the Fund through a tonnage royalty, which had the effect of coupling the Fund's ability to provide health-care services to the quantity of coal that unionized companies produced. Had Lewis forced these companies to install expensive dust-control devices or modify their mining methods to reduce dust, they would have lost markets to nonunion companies. And an even harder time would have been faced in competing against low-cost oil and natural gas. To Lewis, the benefits the Fund provided to miners were more important than costly dust controls in the workplace. He traded prevention for treatment. The respiratory health of working miners was exchanged for a system that would care for them and their families.

The Fund, whose professional staff believed in the principle of preventive medicine, faced a troubling situation. Some of its doctors were beginning to challenge the conventional medical wisdom about coal dust. In 1951 the Fund asked one of its staff employees, Dr. Lorin Kerr, to become versed in dust disease. Kerr sought to persuade the scientific community that coal workers' pneumoconiosis was a work-related disabling disease caused by inhaling coal dust. To that end he collected research, organized conferences, and wrote several articles in professional journals over the next two decades. But the opinions of physicians such as Kerr profoundly threatened industry economics and the UMWA's partnership with the leading companies. The Fund responded by doing very little about what it was beginning to understand.

Most of the Fund-employed doctors did not take up black lung in their profession or in nonscientific arenas. Why? The answer is discouragingly simple. These doctors were as captive to the Fund's political agenda as most coal-field doctors were to the industry's. In both cases, many health professionals ranked their employer's interest and their own pocketbooks over scientific inquiry and professional responsibility. An additional consideration operated with the Fund's professionals. Many of its staff and doctors shared left-wing political views and had lost jobs in the late 1940s and early 1950s because of their beliefs. The Fund had taken them in, protected them from the hysteria of McCarthyism, and had given them an opportunity to put many of their political/medical principles into practice. One price of this opportunity was putting black lung on the back burner.

The UMWA also had an interest in limiting the Fund's work in coal dust disease, although miners themselves had debated the subject as early as their 1942 convention. The *UMWA Journal* carried only a small story or two about dust-caused disease until the late 1960s. The union did not raise the issue in Congress until that time, and it appears the Fund was content to urge public health agencies to conduct studies. The Fund's administrator, Lewis-confidante Josephine Roche, "prohibited her staff from involvement in any political efforts to gain improved workers' compensation coverage or occupational disease prevention programs."[21] She understood the economics of the union's partnership and knew the Fund could not afford to pay benefits to miners disabled by lung disease. And so the Fund and the

UMWA—the two institutions that should have been strong health advocates on this issue—did much less than they should have. If there was grumbling among the Fund's staff and doctors, it was not made public. Nor did it have much measurable effect until the late 1960s.

Cracks in the wall of denial began to appear in the late 1950s and 1960s. Fund doctors and a few others pressured the Pennsylvania Department of Health to X-ray 16,000 bituminous miners in 1959. The survey found some measure of CWP in from 14 to 34 percent of the sample, varying with age and length of exposure.[22] A few years later the Public Health Service found X-ray evidence of CWP in 9.8 percent of working miners and 18.2 percent of inactive miners.[23] Pennsylvania, Alabama, and Virginia recognized CWP as a work-caused disease for the purpose of compensation.

Despite these advances, this occupational health issue remained largely in the closet of the scientific community until three maverick doctors, some organizers, and a couple of gadflies opened the door in West Virginia in the late 1960s. Drs. I. E. Buff, Donald L. Rasmussen, and Hawey A. (Sonny) Wells practiced in West Virginia: Buff as a Charleston cardiologist, Rasmussen as the chief of the pulmonary section of the Appalachian Regional Hospital in Beckley, and Wells as the one-time chief of pathology at the federal Appalachian Laboratories for Occupational Respiratory Diseases (ALFORD) at Morgantown. Rasmussen and Wells were research scientists who had examined thousands of miners in the course of their work. Buff was a popular hellraiser by temperament who drew a connection between miner lung disease, cor pulmonale (a form of heart failure), and heart attack (which was not accepted as a compensable work-related cause of death). They formed the Committee of Physicians for Miners Health and Safety in 1968 after failing to interest UMWA officials in their research findings,[24] and they took their message directly to miners through a series of sometimes raucous public meetings. Congressmen Ken Hechler, a Democrat from southern West Virginia, supported them, as did Ralph Nader. So, too, did a handful of young community organizers in the federally funded Volunteers in Service to America (VISTA). They called the miners' disease "black lung."

The black lung meetings evoked the response of a revival. Suddenly, hundreds of miners understood why they could no longer walk up a hill in deer season, handle a garden tiller, or do their mining jobs. The message came at a propitious time. The rank-and-file membership of the UMWA was restive after years of subordination to Lewis and his successor, W. A. (Tony) Boyle, both of whom kept miners in the dark about union finances and suppressed democracy to maintain control of the organization.[25]

Black lung became an issue that gave the still forming elements of rank-and-file resistance an axis on which to turn. Boyle responded to grassroots interest in black lung by allowing the Fund's Dr. Kerr to address the union's September 1968 convention. Kerr made a powerful speech, and the UMWA's leadership channeled membership activism into a resolution urging miners to seek compensation at the state level.[26]

Many took this as a serious assignment. A few dozen miners formed the Black Lung Association in January 1969 to press the West Virginia legislature for adequate compensation. This effort drew national media attention when almost every miner in the state stopped work for three weeks in February to force passage of their bill. The black lung strike came just a few months after seventy-eight coal miners died in a Consolidation Coal mine near Farmington, West Virginia, in the northern part of the state. There, Boyle had praised the company for its safety efforts, which had angered many working miners who believed Consolidation had precipitated the explosion by failing to use sufficient ventilation. These events combined to force the issues of coal-mine health and safety onto the congressional agenda.

Black Lung Disease as a National Political Issue

Congress faced black lung amid an atmosphere of political and moral contrition caused by the Farmington disaster and the perception of inequity surrounding mine health and safety. The hearings on the 1969 act are filled with the laments of legislators acknowledging their failure to express concern at an earlier point. They bewailed the dreadful dynamic that allowed them to respond only after seventy-eight preventable deaths had weakened the coal industry's influence on national politics. Congressman Carl Perkins, chairman of the Labor and Education Committee that reported the bill to the House, introduced the subject to the Representatives sitting as a Committee of the Whole on October 27, 1969, saying:

> Like almost all legislation on this subject, the bill before us was triggered by a coal mine disaster—one in which 78 men lost their lives. Every significant advance in federal coal mine safety law has required

that men die—that they die dramatically and in substantial numbers—before the Congress would undertake to afford them a greater measure of protection. The majority of coal miners killed on the job, however, do not lose their lives in dramatic disasters. They die by ones and twos in accidents that do not generate national headlines. And more, many more, are killed not on the job but by the job, victims of the insidious "black lung" disease that results from the daily breathing of coal dust.[27]

The safety legislation that Congress had passed over the years was terribly flawed. Occupational health was never included, and the safety protections were inadequate and inadequately enforced. Congressman John Dent, chairman of the labor subcommittee that developed the 1969 legislation, confessed that

the fault lies not so much in the fact that they (the coal operators) have not obeyed the regulations but that Congress has not passed the kind of regulations that were needed. . . . The ones at fault, in reality, are the members of the Congress of the United States and the members of the various state legislatures, because private enterprise is in business to make money and the miners are in business to get what they can out of the money that is made and between the two they are too busy to write regulations.[28]

Although Congress was willing to confess to negligence, it was industry that had failed to protect its employees and on which the onus of responsibility fell.[29] The Senate subcommittee's report of July 31, 1969, stated that

a fatalistic attitude regarding the inevitability of coal mining hazards appears to have permeated the industry and to have anesthetized it from the shocking reality: men are maimed and killed in mine accidents, or their lives are slowly ground out in the struggle with black lung, because the industry has not been willing to spend the funds necessary to protect the workers from such fates. . . . We know that 100,000 U.S. miners are afflicted with pneumoconiosis. But we also know that in this age of space exploration the incidence of this disease can be completely prevented by implementing existing technology and undertaking the research necessary to reduce the level of respirable dust. The problem lies not in the lack of technical competence, but in the lack of will to invest in health and safety.[30]

Science and Medicine in the Congressional Arena

Scientists were called upon to give expert testimony, and Congress attempted to fashion legislation in a context that was at once moral and political. Pressure to rectify past neglect did not eliminate political opposition. The Nixon administration, for example, proposed a weak bill compared with those of Senator Harrison Williams and Representative Hechler. Other coal-field legislators—John Dent, Carl Perkins, and Jennings Randolph—submitted weak bills. The UMWA, which had had separate health and safety bills introduced, was outflanked by the *ad hoc* group of miner advocates, including Hechler, Representative Phil Burton, and Ralph Nader. (UMWA president Boyle claimed these "Johnny-Come-Latelies" wanted to subvert the union and embarrass its leadership.) The major coal operators worked principally through Senator Randolph. They could not oppose legislation in principle but hoped that certain provisions could be eroded. Furthermore, they were willing to accept a federal dust standard and a taxpayer-financed compensation program. The small coal companies opposed any dust standard but conceded the need for further research and, perhaps, machine-mounted dust collectors.[31]

Testimony from health scientists, doctors, and engineers fell along a continuum of scientific thought that matched the political continuum. Each political/economic interest found an expert willing to support its position. Health scientists clashed with each other through the medium of legislative hearings. Their positions were embraced by congressional allies looking for "expert" advice to justify their political positions. Two issues divided expert and politician alike: the definition of coal miners' lung disease and the stringency of the dust standard that Congress should impose to prevent future lung disease.

The Ethics of Definition

After years of denial and neglect, political events in 1968 and 1969 forced the American medical community to concede that coal miners experienced work-related lung impairment. Basic policy choices would follow from how politicians interpreted what scientists told them about this occupational health problem. What caused the impairment? Was there a single work-related disease or were there several? What diagnostic tests should be used? And how was disability to be determined?

Black lung is a term of description rather than medical diagnosis. It is a clear, understandable vernacular that relates inhaling coal dust to difficulty in breathing. The problem for many experts was that black lung is not a "disease." The victim sees it as a set of work-related symptoms. The scientist observes discrete sets of symptoms, some of which might be related to inhaling coal dust for many years.

The experts who testified before Congress divided into two battle lines. The scientific mainstream tried to limit the issue to a single identifiable disease—coal workers' pneumoconiosis (CWP)—that was unquestionably related to the long-term inhalation of respirable coal dust. The others argued that many complexities and much uncertainty was involved in establishing a single agent as the cause of many symptoms. They focused on a broader concern, preventing and compensating all work-related lung ailments in coal miners. Several of their number insisted that a disease process distinct from CWP, bronchitis and emphysema, was also in evidence.

The weight of scientific testimony favored confining congressional attention to CWP, a disease caused only by respirable coal dust. Dr. William H. Stewart, surgeon general of the Public Health Service, defined CWP within this context:

> Coal miners' pneumoconiosis is a chronic chest disease caused by the accumulation of fine coal particles in the human lung. In its advanced form, it leads to severe and premature death. Coal miners' pneumoconiosis is a distinct clinical entity, resulting from inhalation of coal dust. . . . Medical researchers in both Britain and the United States have repeatedly shown that coal miners suffer from more respiratory impairment and disability than does the general population. These respiratory problems are frequently accentuated by chronic bronchitis and emphysema, the causative factors of which remain to be clarified.[32]

Dr. Stewart, representing the Nixon administration, and other scientists such as Drs. Ian Higgins of the School of Public Health at the University of Michigan and Keith Morgan, chief of the Appalachian Laboratory for Occupational Respiratory Disease, drew a very tight connection between respirable coal dust (defined as particles 5 micra or less in diameter) and CWP, a disease that scars the lower part of the lungs where gas exchange occurs. Dr. Higgins said:

[CWP] . . . causes disability in its advanced stages and also reduces expectation of life. But most of the cases which are found in X-ray surveys are examples of the disease at earlier stages, often of simple pneumoconiosis, which does not cause much disability and does not reduce life expectancy. A certain portion of miners with simple pneumoconiosis go on to develop PMF (progressive massive fibrosis, or "complicated" CWP). Chronic bronchitis and emphysema are more important causes of disability than pneumoconiosis in the great majority of cases. These conditions are not unique to coal workers but occur in any occupation. The most important factor in their causation is cigarette smoking. Miners and ex-miners do, however, seem to have a consistently higher frequency of bronchitis and emphysema than other workers. . . . It is impossible in the individual to say how much his bronchitis and emphysema is due to his work or to his smoking or to other factors in the cause of these diseases. It is not practicable to compensate all persons who have bronchitis and emphysema. It is not desirable to compensate persons who have pneumoconiosis but no disability, because such compensation may lead to disability through the compensated man believing he ought to be breathless and consequently becoming so. . . . It is desirable that disabled men should receive adequate compensation.[33]

This interpretation of scientific knowledge fit with what the leaders of the coal industry were willing to concede. Dr. Paul Gross, a research professor of the pathology of industrial diseases and director of Industrial Hygiene Research in the Department of Occupational Health at the University of Pittsburgh, supported Higgins's position from the perspective of a pathologist:

The testimony I shall give is my own, [but] it also reflects the best judgment of leading scientists and professionals in this country and abroad. . . . Disabling lung disease in a coal miner may or may not be of occupational origin. When it is occupational in origin, it is usually a particular form of coal workers' pneumoconiosis.

Chronic bronchitis and emphysema are lung diseases that are separate and distinct from coal workers' pneumoconiosis. . . . These two conditions are often found coexisting in the same lungs and are spoken of collectively as "chronic obstructive bronchopulmonary disease." [This] disease causes disability and shortens the expectancy of life. . . . It is possible to find miners disabled from chronic obstructive bronchopulmonary disease who have little or no evidence of pneumoconiosis.

When asked by Senator Williams if he had ever found such a miner himself, Dr. Gross replied that he had not. He went on to say that coal dust without a significant silica content, that is less than 1 percent, would be about as harmful as clay, and clay is considered a nuisance dust. . . . A dust like bituminous coal without significant silica content has the ability to be spit up again once it has become deposited. The proof of that statement is the fact that a coal miner who retires to the country will continue to spit up black sputum for years or for the rest of his life, indicating that the coal which has been securely locked in his lungs is gradually being given up.[34]

The view of Dr. Gross and others suggested that Congress need only respond to a relatively uncommon disease and should not be stampeded into throwing money at disability caused by smoking.[35] Coal dust, he said, was basically a nuisance, not a hazard. Bronchitis and emphysema, not pneumoconiosis, were the chief agents of lung disability among coal miners. Cigarettes, not coal dust, caused them. Disabling CWP affected only between 1 and 4 percent of the miners studied.[36] Of the 130,000 active and inactive miners estimated to have some stage of CWP, 50,000 were estimated to be disabled, but only 1,300 to 5,000, Dr. Gross said, were disabled from CWP's most advanced stage, progressive massive fibrosis (PMF). He maintained that 45,000 disabled miners were victims of smoking-related bronchitis and emphysema and therefore should receive no compensation.[37] Dr. Gross never allowed for the possibility that inhaling mine dust could cause lung impairment other than CWP or that coal mine dusts could contribute to bronchitis and emphysema.

Four important conclusions were to be drawn from the testimony of Drs. Morgan, Higgins, Gross, Stewart, and others. First, PMF occurred in a comparatively small number of miners.[38] Second, disability occurred only among those with "complicated" (advanced) CWP, the stage of progressive massive fibrosis. Third, X-ray evidence was the only reliable means for diagnosing CWP. Finally, all other respiratory symptoms and disease in coal miners were not work-related. These conclusions formed a tidy scientific package that fit nicely with the customary models of cause and effect. They justified a small compensation program that would placate liberals and be acceptable to conservatives.

But the black lung-as-CWP thesis left many things unexplained. State-of-the-art science could not dismiss larger coal dust particles as possible illness-causing agents with anything approaching 100-percent confidence. Coal dust as well as cigarette smoking could contribute to upper-respiratory disease such as bronchitis. Furthermore, the Morgan-Higgins-Gross-Stewart school did not explain why the correlation between CWP and disability was so imperfect; some miners with substantial X-ray evidence of CWP were not disabled while others—even nonsmokers—with little CWP evidence displayed substantial disability. Finally, as Dr. Leon Cander, chairman of the Department of Medicine at the University of Texas Medical School, noted, chest X-rays did not measure disability and were not even a foolproof method of diagnosing CWP because of variability in machines and radiological interpretation.[39]

Researchers and practitioners who were sympathetic to the miners pointed out the incompleteness of the black lung-as-CWP model. Dr. Werner Laqueur, director of Laboratories at the Appalachian Regional Hospital in Beckley, West Virginia, suggested that "the disease . . . in the language of the law . . . be referred to as 'Coal Workers' Dust Disease'." His studies, he testified, indicated a 20.5 percent prevalence of complicated pneumoconiosis, and those with simple pneumoconiosis showed "the greatest functional impairment, the largest amount of retained dust in the lung . . . , and the highest incidence of death related primarily to the cardiopulmonary disease."[40] Laqueur went on to say:

> Our observations . . . have been challenged by coal corporations and physicians related with them; and, if not challenged, they are not used by the United States Public Health Service. The reasons are a bit difficult to understand. It would border on the ridiculous to deny that coal miners . . . subject to the dangers of smoking are prone to contract any lung disease afflicting the general population, but it is likewise inconceivable to deny accumulative effect of lung damage due to dust and other factors causing respiratory impairment. . . . Everybody who has ever worked with an open mind in coal field communities knows that the incidence of respiratory ailments is much greater in coal miners than in the general population. . . . There is sufficient evidence from our work . . . on living and dead miners to form a strong opinion in these matters, even if strictly scientific proof has not been delivered.[41]

One of Laqueur's Beckley colleagues, Dr. Donald L. Rasmussen, chief of the Pulmonary Section at the Appalachian Regional Hospital, directly challenged the Morgan-Higgins-Gross-Stewart picture of coal workers' disease. On the basis of an evaluation of 3,000 miners in his laboratory, Rasmussen argued that two-thirds were disabled from a kind of impairment associated with injury to or destruction of the lung's small blood vessels. He believed that dust deposits around the smallest muscular arteries of the lungs caused the injury. Like Laqueur, he challenged the conclusion of industry and mainstream researchers who sought a narrow and restrictive definition of coal miners' disease. The industry's call for more research to justify congressional dust control he asserted, "should be regarded as evidence of a total lack of regard for human life and health."[42]

Congress had to choose between these alternative models of lung disease. The policy implications of the Morgan-Higgins-Gross-Stewart model were modest: a few thousand compensation claims, a lenient dust control standard, a limited federal dollar commitment, and no wholesale condemnation of the private sector. The Laqueur-Rasmussen model's implications were more ominous: many thousands of claims, a strict dust standard, a large federal commitment, and an implicit indictment of the coal industry, the Public Health Service, and many well-known researchers.

What drove each model? Were the differences between them simply the result of a division among impartial scientists who drew equally valid conclusions from available evidence? Or were political goals pushing the science? Did good science require the most cautious reading of the evidence? Were pro-miner scientists such as Rasmussen reaching for scientific conclusions because of their concern for their patients' well-being? Were the industry-oriented doctors and Public Health Service administrators using rigorous science to protect their own careers by shielding corporations from health-related responsibilities? Considering the negligent history of American medicine with respect to mine-worker lung disease, were the Surgeon General and his colleagues simply giving an inch of acknowledgment to preserve a mile of denial?

Thousands of pages of congressional records do little to reveal motives, although some clues appear. Without in-depth interviews, historians cannot say how individual scientists weighted competing values or what they believed the policy implications of their science were. But all must have been aware of the enormous political and economic implications of their "clinical" debate. The division between the disease models even seemed to shape the research. The Service researchers at ALFORD, for example, stopped doing the blood-gas tests which the Beckley group used, after their initial results agreed with Rasmussen's findings.

The most forthright in linking political beliefs and science were Rasmussen, Buff, and Wells, who risked considerable professional and personal reprisal for their nontraditional activism. Each acted to make the public aware of the implications of their collective scientific understanding, and each rejected a narrow definition of a profession-al's role. For them, victims had a right to know, and theirs was the duty to enlighten.

These doctors gave legislators a clear statement about why they had chosen to act. Rasmussen, for example, told the House subcom-mittee on April 15, 1969, that he was present "because of my con-cern primarily for the health of bituminous miners. My concern arises from almost daily contact with miners who suffer from pulmo-nary insufficiency of varying degrees.[43] Dr. Murray Hunter of the Fund-related Fairmont (West Virginia) Clinic spoke plainly about his "bias": "I have a bias. . . . I am not talking about statistical bias. I am talking about an emotional affair." To this, Senator Williams replied, "You are soft on people. I spotted that." Dr. Hunter re-sponded: "Thank you, that is a compliment. I do believe that miners have increased respiratory disability as a result of their occupation with or without X-ray change."[44]

Unlike the physicians who spoke for and represented the "estab-lishment," some such as Dr. Kerr seemed haunted by their personal experience with coal miners:

> I can vividly remember, twenty-one years ago when I came with the UMWA Welfare and Retirement Fund, the constant stream of wheez-ing, breathless coal miners coming to the Area Medical Office in Mor-gantown, West Virginia, seeking relief from the struggle to breathe. I can also remember how overwhelmed I felt. Never in my earlier profes-sional experience had I observed or heard of a single industry with so many men who seemed to be disabled by their jobs. I say "seemed to be disabled by their jobs" because doctors said these men rarely had silico-sis and it was unusual to find a physician who even suspected that coal dust might be dangerous.[45]

Those who argued for a narrow definition of coal miners' lung disease shifted the burden of uncertainty related to diagnosis and compensation to the miners. Those who sought a broad definition placed the burden of uncertainty—the costs of radically reducing dust levels and compensation—on the private sector and the public in general. Their dispute was not, and could not have been, a narrow scientific affair. It was suffused with issues of equity and economics. Historical reflection underscores that the scientific debate existed within and contributed to a framework of political economics, which shaped the science and ultimately determined how science would be applied through public policy.

The Ethics of Prevention

The question of where to set the dust standard linked science with the weighing of potential economic costs against potential social benefits. The politicians asked a simple question: should a respirable dust standard be set at 2 milligrams per cubic meter (2.0 mg/m³), 3.0 mg/ m³, 4.5 mg/m³, or higher? The questioners, as might be expected, wanted a scientific consensus, and it was not forthcoming.

The science behind this question was disputed. No one in the United States had done a dose-response study. No one, in fact, had even systematically sampled dust and collected data prior to 1969. The one small survey done by the U.S. Bureau of Mines in 1968 showed mean dust concentrations of between 2.1 mg/m³ and 8.7 mg/ m³, depending on the particular job.[46] American researchers and legislators were forced to rely on British dose-response correlations derived from a survey of 4,122 coal-face workers over a ten-year period involving twenty mines.[47] The British study, however, was not as methodologically sound as it should have been. The survey did not attempt to sample actual dust exposures for each worker on each work day. No attempt was made to ascertain whether the samples taken were representative of conditions when the samples were not being taken. The survey, instead, relied on a "stratified random sampling procedure."[48] Not only were there methodological problems with this study, but dose response curves derived from the data were not available in published form in 1969. American experts and legislators were therefore forced to infer as best they could what they thought the British data would show.

For much of the year the debate raged over whether the new federal standard should be set at 2.0, 3.0, or 4.5 mg/m³. But in the context of so much uncertainty, the debate over numbers was really a political struggle between legislators responsive to rank-and-file interests and those more sympathetic to industry and the UMWA.

The debate over the dust standard raised the issue of economic costs and benefits within the context of historical neglect. Compared with later legislative debates, the level of cost-benefit analysis found in the 1969 hearings was primitive. The industry never presented firm dollar-cost calculations. The dollar costs, both public and private, of preserving the status quo or of alternative standards were never considered. The cost of a compensation program was never calculated with even approximate precision, since the definitions of disability and disease were so vague.

The small coal companies opposed any dust standard, and the larger ones eventually backed a phased-in 4.5 standard. Pro-industry scientists and engineers had no trouble arguing against a 3.0 standard. James R. Garvey, vice-president of the National Coal Association and president of Bituminous Coal Research, Inc., presented a detailed analysis of dust-sampling methods, from which he concluded that the industry-supported interim standard of 4.5 mg was best. Respirators, he said, could be used to comply with this standard where the operation of any dusty mine was threatened.[49] Garvey argued that any standard Congress decided to pass was "arbitrary," as "we don't know or we don't have . . . medical evidence relating any specific level of dust to a health effect."[50]

Mining engineers and state mining officials generally supported the industry's position. Charles T. Holland, dean of the School of Mines at West Virginia University, testified that

> of all the [dust] standards that have been suggested here in the United States . . . not one is a medical standard. Every one of them are [sic] engineering standards. . . .It is not correct that we have not had standards suggested before this. The Association of Industrial Hygienists have set standards of dustiness and it adds up to. . .about 5 or 5-1/2 milligrams per cubic meter. . . . I haven't anything to quarrel with [about that standard].[51]

D. M. Ryan, an Ohio mining engineer with fifty years of service, testified that if a 3.0-mg standard were "enforced in this country using present mining methods, most of the industry would have to quit."[52] W. Foster Mullins, Virginia's chief mine inspector, wrote to Senator Williams's subcommittee on June 3 to say that the 3.0 standard "has no practical or theoretical background for support."[53] The National Coal Association summed up the private sector's position in an October 21, 1969, letter to Congress by warning that a 3.0 standard would "close many coal mines . . . [and] jeopardize the public welfare by bringing on a nationwide power and steel shortage. . . .Gentlemen, [if the 3.0 standard is enacted] the wolf is here."[54]

Pro-miner advocates, who supported a phased-in 3.0 standard, chose to counter this expert testimony with moral appeals rather than economic analysis. None of the health professionals testifying on the miners' side could do much more than endorse the 3.0 standard in principle. Their position was the less dust, the better, inasmuch as the only study and all the data were elsewhere. Lacking conclusive research findings, pro-miner professionals and legislators drifted into calling for reason and humanity. Representative Hechler told his colleagues on March 19, 1969:

> The . . . serious issue confronted by this Congress is whether or not to accept the administration-recommended dust standard of 4.5 milligrams per cubic meter of air, as against 3.0 milligrams as recommended by all competent medical authorities. I strongly support the lower standard, and cannot understand the philosophy of those who would give up the fight before it starts, on some vague assertion that it is neither "technologically possible" or "economically feasible" to try and [sic] obtain a mine atmosphere of 3.0 milligrams. . . .This committee and the Congress, in conjunction with the coal industry and the miners, face an awesome responsibility which involves an age-old question: Just what is a human being worth?[55]

Although he supported an eventual 3.0 standard, the Surgeon General recommended that Congress impose an initial interim standard of 4.5 mg within six months of enactment because, he argued, the immediate imposition of the stricter standard was not feasible.[56] The 3.0 advocates felt that the administration was likely to keep the interim 4.5 standard indefinitely for reasons of technological feasibility and cost, even though Surgeon General Stewart admitted that the "ideal standard would be zero," because "there is a linear relationship between the amount of dust inhaled. . .and the progression of the pneumoconiosis."[57]

The debate over the numerical dust standard was clouded by the absence of any shared criteria by which to answer Representative Hechler's question about the worth of a human life. Surgeon General Stewart said the recommended 3.0 standard "should represent no more than a reasonable degree of risk to our miners, given our present technology," although he acknowledged that the 4.5 standard "will have a 50-percent more progression [of the disease] than 3.0."[58] "Reasonable risk" was never spelled out in terms of dead and diseased miners. When they became available, the British probability curves suggested that with a 3.0 standard, about 5 percent of those exposed for thirty-five years would show evidence of simple CWP and about 2 percent would have more advanced stages of illness. Thus, the Surgeon General defined "reasonable risk" as exposing the individual miner to a 1-in-50 chance of getting serious CWP over his work life. With a population of 200,000 miners, the "acceptable" cost of the 3.0 standard would have been about 4,000 advanced CWP cases.

Most pro-miner legislators and experts accepted the assumption of worker-borne risk and cost. No one proposed a 0.0 standard or even a 1.0 standard—a "no cost" standard. The Senate's basic working document—S. 2917 introduced by Senator Williams—included an interim 3.0 standard leading to a 2.0 standard at the end of three years. This bill, on which the 1969 act was based, declared its purpose to be to provide a mine atmosphere that would "permit each miner the opportunity to work underground during the period of his entire adult working life without incurring any disability from pneumoconiosis or any other occupation-related disease during or at the end of such period."[59]

Many legislators not directly concerned with coal-field politics endorsed S 2917's falsely optimistic language in principle. In the absence of credible projections of the dollar costs for a taxpayer compensation program and an industry-borne dust control program, the rhetorical commitment to a zero-risk work environment embedded in the legislative language helped to establish a presumption to protect that ultimately justified a *2.0* standard.

Despite his explicit intention, Senator Williams acknowledged when presenting his report that even a 2.0 standard would take some toll on miners' health. It was Senator Gaylord Nelson, a Wisconsin Democrat rather than a health professional, who pointed out on September 29, 1969, that a 2.0 standard would not offer full protection:

> The interim standards of 3.0 milligrams of coal dust per cubic meter of air within 3 years and 2.0 milligrams within 6 years are only interim standards and should only be considered as such. At the interim standard of 2.0 milligrams, thousands of miners would still be expected to contract pneumoconiosis, the black lung disease, before the end of their normal working career. This is unacceptable for any miner and for the Nation. Black lung disease does not have to be an accepted fringe liability for American coal miners. It seems to me that the air any miner breathes should be as pure as is breathed by any other worker or any other citizen.[60]

Like the debate over disease definition, the conflict among scientists over the new dust standard was framed by politics and economics. Given the high degree of uncertainty and disagreement within the scientific community, politicians and interest groups could easily justify different standards. In the end, the outcome turned on the matter of social equity and politics.

Congress finally passed legislation that required a 2.0 mg/m^3 standard three years after enactment following an immediate interim standard of 3.0. The 2.0 standard was stronger than what even pro-miner experts had supported in the hearings. The act's zero-risk language was retained as a way, it appears, of establishing congressional intent. The act provided "black lung" benefits for victims of pneumoconiosis, which was defined as a "chronic dust disease of the lung arising out of employment in an underground coal mine." In an artful synthesis of two opposing scientific opinions, black lung was defined as pneumoconiosis and pneumoconiosis was defined as black lung. Over the coming decade, Congress and the executive branch would redefine these terms several times. Each time the process of redefinition was driven by political considerations more than by new scientific findings.

Despite the confessional tone of the 1969 debate, it is doubtful that the pro-miner forces could have secured a black lung compensation program had not the U.S. Treasury been designated the bearer of almost all its costs, now approaching a 17-year total of $20 billion. No legislator, economist, or health professional proposed that the coal industry pay for both prevention—the dust control program—and rectification—the black lung benefits. Both were politically feasible as long as the federal government subsidized the far more expensive of the two.

Conclusion

Scientific truth is rarely as clear as we would like on occupational health issues. Uncertainty provides the context within which scientists and engineers must make decisions, draw conclusions, and recommend policies. How the burden of uncertainty should be distributed cannot be resolved with a calculus that denies politics, economics, and individual values. When a scientific consensus does not exist, protective policy is delayed and workers are frequently kept at risk. Caution is a virtue in scientific research but not in the policymaking process, when it leads to paralysis. Those who make occupational health policy have an obligation to consider empirical data with care but an equal obligation to respond to those at risk who suffer the practical consequences of delay. Scientists and engineers should recognize that it may be better to protect health amid uncertainty than to do nothing. The cost of giving workers the benefit of the doubt may be high in dollars but more than reasonable compared with the alternative.

The political role of science and scientists was clear in the black lung debate; so was the role of self-interest (whether defined as income, professional standing, or career planning). Such self-interest and political commitment cannot be eliminated from occupational health sciences. Appeals for objectivity are thus naive and can have little weight. As a consequence, it would be a mistake to shield scientists, doctors, and engineers from the kind of ethical scrutiny that most politicians endure. The history of the 1969 Coal Mine Health and Safety Act underscores the importance of compelling scientists, doctors, and engineers to confront the moral context and ethical implications of their work.

Notes

1. Federal Coal Mine Health and Safety Act of 1969 (Public Law 91-173), Title II, Sec. 201(b). The phrase "to the greatest extent possible" can be interpreted in one of two ways as a qualification on a declaration of intent: either to accomplish the objective consistent with technological feasibility and other mitigating considerations, or to accomplish the objective to the maximum extent of which American society is capable. The legislative record indicates that the second of these interpretations is most in keeping with congressional intent.

2. Ibid., Title IV, Sec. 401. Congress defined pneumoconiosis as a "chronic dust disease of the lung arising out of employment in an underground coal mine." Surface miners and surface workers in and around coal miners were included subsequently.

3. Curtis Seltzer, *Fire in the Hole: Miners and Managers in the American Coal Industry* (Lexington, Ky.: The University Press of Kentucky, 1985).

4. The terms "professionals" or "health professionals" have been substituted for the cumbersome phrase "health scientists and engineers" throughout.

5. In the mid-1800s miners in Great Britain and America were establishing self-financed associations to provide themselves with medical care.

Mining companies eventually suppressed these efforts and took over this function in the latter part of the Century. See Leslie A. Falk, "Coal Miners' Prepaid Medical Care in the United States—And Some British Relationships, 1792–1964," 4 *Medical Care* 1 (January–March 1966): 37–42.

      6. The dimensions of community and industrial health in the American mining industry can be pieced together from many sources. Congress investigated labor-management turmoil and living conditions on numerous occasions beginning in the 1880s. The presidentially appointed U.S. Coal Commission found in the early 1920s that of the 713 camps surveyed in the bituminous fields, more than 85 percent of the houses depended on external water sources, one-third had six or more families sharing a single water source, and less than 4 percent contained internal flush toilets. Open privies and typhoid went hand in hand. A Public Health Service survey of sixty-four company towns and fifty-nine independent mining communities at that time reported:

> The fact that manure is a fly-breeding material of first importance is practically unrecognized in the places surveyed. Ordinances or requirements for the systematic and frequent removal of manure are conspicuously absent. . . . Screening against flies may be said to be generally inadequate. . . . Control of disease carriers and communicable disease contacts appears to be an unknown art. (Edward E. Hunt et al., *What the Coal Commission Found* [Baltimore: Williams and Wilkins, 1925], p. 147.)

Conditions had improved by the end of World War II, although a 1947 federal survey of community health—the Boone Report—at 260 mines with 72,000 miners reported that coal counties had substantially higher infant mortality rates than the national average, and almost half of the communities used water that was contaminated by industrial waste or untreated sewage. The survey found that the vast majority of coal-field physicians were in general practice and "have not been made responsible for adequate programs of industrial hygiene and preventive medicine." About 70 percent of the miners surveyed were covered by a company-organized prepayment plan for health care. The doctors in these plans "were not selected primarily on the basis of professional qualifications. . ., but on the basis of personal friendships, financial tie-ups, social viewpoints, or other nonmedical considerations." The report concluded that "the present practices of medicine in the coal fields on a contract basis cannot be supported. They are synonymous with many abuses. They are undesirable and, in numbers of instances, deplorable" (U.S. Department of the Interior, Coal Mines Administration, *A Medical Survey of the Bituminous-Coal Industry* [Washington, D.C.: U.S. GPO, 1947], pp. 59, 92, 123, 164).

      For an excellent discussion of the social foundations of occupational disease among miners, see Barbara Ellen Smith, "Digging Our Own Graves: Coal Miners and the Struggle Over Black Lung Disease," Ph.D. dissertation, Brandeis University, 1981.

7. Smith, "Digging Our Own Graves," p. 44. Smith points out that nineteenth-century doctors in the anthracite coal fields published professional papers on the work-related lung diseases of miners until the company-doctor system became widespread.

8. U.S. Department of the Interior, *Medical Survey,* p. 92. The survey is often referred to as the Boone Report in deference to its author, Admiral Joel T. Boone.

9. Smith, "Digging Our Own Graves," pp. 29ff. Dr. John T. Carpenter in 1869 informed the Schuylkill County Medical Society in the Pennsylvania anthracite region that

> The respiratory apparatus presents us a very large percentage of cases of disease among [coal] miners. Bronchial irritations are continual. . . . A peculiar asthmatic character of cough is generally noticed; emphysema and nervous distress in breathing. These chronic troubles may last a lifetime, without being rapidly fatal, or necessarily so. . . .[A] chronic softening of the lungs may occur, in other words, phthisis [tuberculosis or consumption], which is a frequent disease among these men, and generally an incurable one. (Report of the Schuylkill County Medical Society," *Transactions of the Medical Society of Pennsylvania Fifth Series,* pt. II [June 1869], p. 490, quoted in Smith, "Digging Our Own Graves, p. 29.)

Dr. Henry C. Sheafer reported in 1879:

> Any one who has seen a load of coal shot from a cart, or has watched the thick clouds of dust which sometimes envelop the huge coal-breakers of the anthracite region so completely as almost to hide them from sight, can form an idea of the injurious effect upon the health of constant working in such an atmosphere. The wonder is not that men die of clogged-up lungs, but that they manage to exist so long in an atmosphere which seems to contain at least fifty per cent of solid matter. (Henry C. Sheafer, "Hygiene of Coal-Mines," in Albert H. Buck, *A Treatise on Hygiene and Public Health* [New York: William Wood, 1879], vol. 2, pp. 243–245, quoted in Smith, "Digging Our Own Graves," p. 30.)

Novelists such as Upton Sinclair and Émile Zola saw profound lung disability in the coal miners about whom they wrote. Frederick Engels, in the 1890s, described "the peculiar disease" of coal miners, "black spittle, which arises from the saturation of the whole lung with coal particles, and manifests itself in general debility, headache, oppression of the chest, and thick, black mucous expectoration" (Frederick Engels, *The Conditions of the Working Class in England* [London: Panther Books, 1892; reprint ed., 1969], p. 272).

10. Earl H. Rebhorn, "Anthraco Silicosis," 29 *The Medical Society Reporter* 5 (May 1935): 15.

11. Dr. Emery R. Hayhurst wrote in 1919 that "housing conditions, and hurtful forms of recreation, especially alcoholism, undoubtedly cause the major amount of sickness. The mine itself is not an unhealthful place to

work" (Emery R. Hayhurst, "The Health Hazards and Mortality Statistics of Soft Coal Mining in Illinois and Ohio," 1 *Journal of Industrial Hygiene* 7 [November 1919]: 360, quoted in Smith, "Digging Our Own Graves," p. 53).

12. Andrew Meiklejohn, "History of Lung Diseases of Coal Miners in Great Britain: Part II, 1875–1920," 9 *British Journal of Industrial Medicine* 2 (April 1952): 94.

13. W. Donald Ross et al., "Emotional Aspects of Respiratory Disorders Among Coal Miners," 156 *Journal of the American Medical Asociation* 5 (2 October 1954): pp. 484–487.

14. U.S. Department of the Treasury, Public Health Service, *The Health of Workers in Dusty Trades,* bulletin 208 (Washington, D.C.: U.S. GPO, 1933), pt. III, p. 3, 15, 19, quoted in Smith, "Digging Our Own Graves," p. 58.

15. Ibid., p. 18.

16. For analysis of the UMWA Welfare and Retirement Fund, see Janet E. Ploss, "A History of the Medical Care Program of the UMWA Welfare and Retirement Fund (M.A. thesis, The Johns Hopkins University, 1981); Seltzer, "Health Care by the Ton: Crisis in the Mine Workers' Health and Welfare Programs," *Health/PAC Bulletin* 79 (November–December 1977); and Warren F. Draper, "The Quest of the UMWA Welfare and Retirement Fund for the Best Medical Care Obtainable for Its Beneficiaries," paper presented to the annual meeting of the American Association for the Surgery of Trauma, Hot Springs, Va., 1 November, 1957.

17. One of the first programs the Fund undertook was to arrange rehabilitation and remedial services for an estimated 50,000 union miners, many of whom were homebound or bedridden from their work injuries. The Fund's services included inpatient and outpatient hospital care, in-hospital physicians' care, rehabilitation, nursing-home services, pharmaceuticals, short-term therapy in "good prognosis" mental cases, and major appliances. Eyeglasses and dental care were not provided. The group-practice clinics provided comprehensive primary care on a prepaid basis.

18. Company doctors and fee-for-service advocates in the coal fields battled the Fund and its salaried staff for years. Non-Fund hospitals often refused to extend privileges to Fund-related physicians, and local medical societies attacked the miners' prepaid health-care medical program as socialized medicine. See Seltzer, "Health Care by the Ton," p. 8. See also Marjorie Taubenhaus and Roy Penchansky, "The Medical Care Program of the United Mine Workers Welfare and Retirement Fund," in Roy Penchansky (ed.), *Health Services Administration: Policy Cases and the Case Method* (Cambridge, Mass.: Harvard University Press, 1968); and David Katz, M.D., "Compromise of Free Practice of Medicine," 59 *Pennsylvania Medical Journal* (1956).

19. See, for example, Joseph E. Martin, Jr., "Coal Miners' Pneumoconiosis," 44 *American Journal of Public Health* (May 1954), pp. 581–591. Martin wrote that despite "authoritative opinion to the contrary. . .[coal miners suffer from a] disabling, progressive, killing disease which is related to

exposure to coal dust" (Quoted in Smith, "Digging Our Own Graves," pp. 70–71).

See also Murray B. Hunter and Milton D. Levine, "Clinical Study of Pneumoconiosis of Coal Workers in Ohio River Valley," 163 *Journal of the American Medical Association,* 1 (January 5, 1957), pp. 1–4.

20. Seltzer, *Fire in the Hole,* ch. 4.

21. Smith, "Digging Our Own Graves," pp. 145–146.

22. Jan Lieben and W. Wayne McBride, "Pneumoconiosis in Pennsylvania's Bituminous Mining Industry," 183 *Journal of the American Medical Association* 3 (19 January, 1963).

23. W. S. Lainhart et al., *Pneumoconiosis in Appalachian Bituminous Coal Miners* (Washington, D.C.: U.S. GPO, 1969).

24. Trevor Armbrister, *Act of Vengeance: The Yablonski Murders and Their Solution* (New York: Dutton, 1975), p. 49.

25. For the story of the UMWA-company partnership in the 1950s and 1960s, see Seltzer, *Fire in the Hole;* Joseph Finley, *The Corrupt Kingdom* (New York: Simon and Schuster, 1972); Brit Hume, *Death and the Mines* (New York: Grossman, 1971); and John Paul Nyden, "Miners for Democracy: Struggle in the Coal Fields" (Ph.D. dissertation, Columbia University, 1974).

26. Boyle's motives in this regard were probably not the purest. He had never before expressed any interest in dust control or lung disease. He had discouraged efforts in Pennsylvania to enact a compensation law. And the delegates were not given the opportunity to request that the UMWA seek a national compensation plan that was coupled to dust control. Armbrister writes:

> The UMW didn't want a strong black lung law because it didn't want to tackle the industry that much. But it did want to appear concerned. In actuality, the union had ignored the disease for years, and the results of its inactivity were evident everywhere. . . .[T]he trouble was that in the fall of 1968 some of the more unsophisticated delegates really believed that the union wanted to remedy this situation. When they returned from Denver, they decided to press for the sort of law that [Joseph A. (Jock)] Yablonski had helped persuade the Pennsylvania legislature to pass three years earlier. (Armbrister, *Act of Vengeance,* p. 49).

27. U.S. Senate, Committee on Labor and Public Welfare, Subcommittee on Labor, *Legislative History of the Federal Coal Mine Health and Safety Act of 1969 (Public Law 91-173) as Amended through 1974, Including Black Lung Amendments of 1972,* 94th Congr., 1st Sess. (Washington, D.C.: U.S. GPO, 1975) pt. I, p. 1123. This document will subsequently be referred to as Senate, *History.*

28. U.S. House of Representatives, Committee on Education and Labor, Subcommittee on Labor, *Coal Mine Health and Safety, Hearings,* 91st Congr., 1st Sess. (Washington, D.C.: U.S. GPO, 1969), p. 334. This document will subsequently be referred to as House, *Hearings.*

29. Congressional negligence over the years was due principally to the absence of political pressure to take on the issue of mine health and safety.

The absence of pressure was a product of the industrial partnership between the UMWA and the big unionized companies. Events in 1969 forced both the union and these companies to accept change. The big companies responded with a position that accepted some new safety and health standards. They were not unaware that these additional costs would fall most heavily on the least capitalized sector of their industry. Senator John Sherman Cooper, a spokesman for Kentucky's small coal producers, suggested the reason why Congress had done so little for so long: "Today the big coal operators and the United Mine Workers—and I'm just stating a fact and not criticizing either one of them—are together on every measure which affects their interests, such as this, to keep the big coal mines open" (Senate, *History,* pp. 376–377).

30. Senate, *History,* pp. 167–168.

31. See, for example, the testimony of Cloyd D. McDowell, president, Harlan County (Ky.) Coal Operators' Association before the House subcommittee on labor on 17 April, 1969:

> Regarding mandatory health standards for controlling dust in underground mines, we agree that some control is needed. However, there is a greater need for research and study of this problem in order to establish all the facts pertaining to it rather than setting an arbitrary limit of 4.5 milligrams of dust per cubic meter of air, which may or may not be the proper limit. . . .
>
> Coal dust per se may or may not be harmful to the health of miners but it could be other factors such as the amount of sulfur in the dust, or the silica content or some other substance. . . .
>
> We believe that the dust problem should be attacked from the standpoint of preventing dust by requiring the manufacturers of mine machinery to build dust suppressing attachments on all mine equipment rather than establishing a level of dust concentration. (House, *Hearings,* p. 498).

32. U.S. Senate, Committee on Labor and Public Welfare, Subcommittee on Labor, *Coal Mine Health Safety, Hearings, Parts 1 and 2,* 91st Congr., 1st Sess. (Washington, D.C.: U.S. GPO, 1969), pt. 2, pp. 719–720.

33. Ibid., p. 842.

34. Ibid., pp. 759–765. Dr. Gross also said that "it is extremely important to lower the dust exposure to the lowest level possible," but when asked whether he favored a 3 mg or 4.5 mg/cm^3 dust standard, he said he "was not qualified to answer that question at this time" (pp. 760, 764).

35. Note, for example, the language Dr. Gross chose to use. Chronic obstructive bronchopulmonary disease "causes disability and shortens the expectancy of life." When describing the disease he thought should be at issue he chose clear and active verbs. Cause and effect were unmistakably linked. In contrast, PMF in its advanced state is merely "associated with disability and a shortened life expectancy." Here, Dr. Gross diluted the verb, changed voice, and softened the linkage. There appears to be no functional difference between the two diseases with respect to their contributions to disability and life expectancy.

36. Senate, *Hearings, pt. 2,* p. 759.

37. Ibid., pp. 763–764.

38. Congress had good reason to be confused about the number of miners with work-related lung disease. Dr. Stewart, the Surgeon General, estimated that pneumoconiosis would be found in 100,000 active and inactive miners. This figure was based on his estimate that one of every ten of the 135,000 active miners and one of every five of the 400,000 inactive miners would show some X-ray evidence of CWP (Senate, *Hearings, pt. 2*, pp. 729–730). The UMWA's Dr. Kerr estimated that approximately 125,000 active and former coal miners had "some stage of coal workers' pneumoconiosis, commonly called 'black lung,' and about 50,000 of them are probably disabled by the disease" (House, *Hearings*, p. 309). James R. Garvey, vice president of the National Coal Association, testified that his calculations, based on the PHS prevalence studies, indicated that about "15,000 to 16,000 total [were] affected by this disease" (Senate, *Hearings, pt.* 1, p. 594). Finally, Dr. Hawey Wells stated that "at autopsy about 84 percent of the miners have some degree of pneumoconiosis" (House, *Hearings*, p. 366).

39. Senate, *Hearings, pt. 2*, pp. 857–858.

40. Ibid., p. 696.

41. Ibid., pp. 696–697.

42. Ibid., pp. 658–659.

43. House, *Hearings, pt. 1*, p. 357.

44. Senate, *Hearings, pt. 2*, p. 851.

45. House, *Hearings, pt. 1*, p. 312.

46. U.S. Bureau of Mines, "Dust Concentrations in Bituminous Coal Mines," in Senate, *Hearings, pt. 2*, pp. 1314–1328.

47. M. Jacobsen, "The Basis for the New Coal Dust Standards," 131 *The Mining Engineer*, (19 March, 1972), p. 269.

48. M. Jacobsen, S. Rae, W. H. Walton, and J. M. Rogan, "New Dust Standards for British Coal Miners," 227 *Nature* (1 August, 1970), p. 445.

49. Senate, *Hearings, pt. 2*, p. 581.

50. Ibid., p. 597.

51. House, *Hearings, pt. 1*, pp. 554–555.

52. Ibid., p. 504.

53. Senate, *Hearings, pt. 2*, p. 1356.

54. Senate, *History, pt. 1*, p. 113.

55. House, *Hearings, pt. 1*, pp. 97–98.

56. See testimony of Dr. William H. Stewart, Surgeon General, Public Health Service on 18 March, 1969 in Senate, *Hearings, pt. 2*, pp. 718ff., and testimony of Charles C. Johnson, Jr., Administrator, Consumer Protection and Environmental Health Service, Public Health Service on 26 March, 1969 in House, *Hearings, pt. 1*, pp. 273ff.

57. Senate, *Hearings, pt. 2*, p. 726.

58. Ibid., pp. 722, 734.

59. Senate, *History, pt. 1*, pp. 10–12.

60. Ibid., p. 579.

6

Regulating Asbestos: Ethics, Politics, and the Values of Science

THOMAS H. MURRAY

Science itself, the nature of scientific knowledge, the habitual ways in which scientists couch their judgments—the language of uncertainty, probability, tentativeness—have invariably become factors in the political controversies surrounding occupational health regulation. The foes of regulation often hold up a simplistic standard of "scientific certainty" and dismiss all evidence that fails to meet that standard, however powerfully it evokes the specter of an enormous human tragedy, as insufficient or irrelevant. Rather than admitting that the decision of whether or how to regulate is essentially a political or social one that can only draw on scientific evidence, the opponents of stricter occupational health regulation have tended to bemoan the intrusion of politics into what they argue should be a purely scientific matter. This conflict over the role of science in the protection of at-risk workers is forcefully demonstrated in the controversy that surrounded the federal effort to regulate asbestos.

Asbestos as a threat to human health emerged as an inescapable public issue between 1965 and 1972. The first signal event was a scientific conference held under the auspices of the New York Academy of Sciences in 1964. The second event was the first effort at formal rulemaking by the newly created Occupational Safety and Health Administration (OSHA). Both events provide us with "texts" that reveal a great deal about the relation of science and scientists to institutions, and about the usefulness and limitations of science for making public policy. They are especially revealing about values: the values of science and the values underlying decisions about how to balance risks of life and health against costs. Finally, they have much to teach us about uncertainty, including the political and moral importance of deciding where to place the burden of uncertainty.

The 1964 New York Academy of Sciences Conference on Asbestos

Although the New York Academy of Sciences (NYAS) conference was manifestly a scientific gathering to assess the health effects of asbestos, political and economic agendas lay uneasily buried just beneath the surface. Eunice Thomas Miner, executive director of the Academy, announced the social importance of the conference in her opening statement: "Hard-won data have been accumulating which indicate that neoplasms associated with asbestos exposure, especially those of the lung, are perhaps the most important industrial cancers at this time."[1] Her judgment was reinforced by J. C. Gilson, a British researcher and member of the prestigious Medical Research Council. After reminding his audience that the history of asbestos extended back over four millennia, he called asbestos "truly. . .the twentieth-century mineral. Its output has increased over a 1000-fold in 60 years."[2] He concluded that "conferences come and go. A few which happen to occur when there is a burst of new activity on the subject go down in history as a turning point. . . . It seems at least possible that this Conference will be of this type."[3]

The charge against asbestos was articulated early in the conference by Wilhelm C. Hueper, a well-known antagonist of the industry. Hueper, who would become chief of the Environmental Cancer Section of the National Cancer Institute, had more than two decades earlier warned about the manipulation of science on the part of those with strong economic interests:

> Industrial concerns are in general not particularly anxious to have the occurrence of occupational cancer among their employees or of environmental cancers among the consumers of their products made a matter of public record. Such publicity might reflect unfavorably upon their business activities, and oblige them to undertake extensive and expensive technical and sanitary changes in their production methods and in the types of products manufactured. There is, moreover, the distinct possi-

bility of becoming involved in compensation suits with extravagant financial claims by the injured parties. It is, therefore, not an uncommon practice that some pressure is exerted by the parties financially interested in such matters to keep information on the occurrence of industrial cancer well under cover.[4]

He lashed out at asbestos as a carcinogen, linked to lung cancer and mesothelioma, and at industry and physicians associated with industry: "Some commercially interested parties and their medical guardians and protectors still prefer for their own reasons and motives, to deny the existence of these dangerous and usually fatal sequelae of a respiratory contact with asbestos dust." Predictably, "no large-scale observations on the incidence, morbidity and mortality rates of asbestosis and asbestos cancers have been published from the giant American asbestos industry."[5] Continuing his denunciation, he called for "comprehensive and painstaking epidemiological procedures" as opposed to "the continued insistence of some industrial parties that reliable decisions on such aspects can be based on what is called deceptively 'sound clinical impression' [which] often merely reflects an objectionable desire to escape from an unpleasant situation into a wishful dreamland in which profits are properly protected against just compensation claims."[6] It was "regrettable," he said, "that the original plan of having a recent epidemiologic survey on these aspects of asbestos production in Canadian mines and mills to be undertaken under the aegis of the National Cancer Institute of Canada was not adhered to and that this study was carried out as an industry-dominated venture which yielded highly controversial negative results."[7]

Evidence about asbestos-related cancers was presented by researchers from around the world. William D. Buchanan, from Great Britain's Ministry of Labor, for example, reported that research on death certificates revealed that "over fifty percent of males dying with asbestosis present also have a neoplasm."[8] And he warned that "even when viewed against the steadily rising incidence of lung cancer in the population as a whole, there seems little doubt that there is a special risk of an intrathoracic tumor if asbestosis is also present in the lungs."[9] J. C. Wagner, a Welsh researcher, presented evidence linking Canadian chrysotile with mesothelioma.[10] Wagner's report represented the first evidence that chrysotile might be at least as, if not more, likely to induce mesothelioma than crocidolite—a great threat to the U.S. and Canadian asbestos industries, which wanted to cast South African crocidolite as the villain. His analysis was buttressed by reports that followed linking asbestos with mesothelioma in London, South Africa, the Piedmont region of Italy, Belfast, Dresden, and the United States.

But if exposure to asbestos posed grave risks to workers, at what level of exposure did such risks emerge? E. L. Schall of the New Jersey State Department of Health Occupational Health Program offered a critique of the then-current threshold limit value (TLV) in the United States of 5 million parts per cubic foot (5 mppcf) of asbestos dust, a standard based primarily on one seriously method-ologically flawed study published twenty-six years earlier.[11] A "point survey," it underestimated the true consequences of asbestos expo-sure, as in its analysis "the sick [were] missing and the dead [were] buried."[12] Plainly an attack on the standard reaffirmed by the Ameri-can Conference of Governmental Industrial Hygienists (ACGIH) that very year, Schall's presentation underscored a recurrent theme at the NYAS conference with regard to identifying and controlling occu-pational and environmental hazards: the problem of *allocating the burden of uncertainty* and the role of science in resolving such contro-versies.[13] But what was on the surface a methodological dispute in-volved in fact an important conflict over public philosophy, a conflict over prudence and social equity.

Scientists are taught not to make claims that overreach their evi-dence; except when generating theories, scientists assert conservatism as a principal value in science, and those who too readily extrapolate their findings to widely varying circumstances risk being accused of exaggerating, of exceeding their scientific authority. Critics making such charges may simply be defending what they view as an important scientific value. However, at the same time such critics may knowingly or unwittingly be serving the interests of those who prefer to deny the existence of a relation between a social enterprise, such as the asbestos industry, and some profound social cost, such as occupational disease. When public policy is at stake, the question of relevant scientific cer-tainty becomes more than an academic debate, and the allocation of the burden of uncertainty becomes a crucial social question.

Representatives of the asbestos industry responded to the mount-ing evidence by emphasizing scientific uncertainty. Richard Gaze, an employee of The Cape Asbestos Co., Ltd., in England, performed predictably when he argued that because concentrations of meso-theliomas usually occur in industrialized regions where many other pollutants are undoubtedly active, it was premature to blame asbestos.[14] Such reluctance to attribute responsibility for grave environmental hazards came not only from representatives of industry. G. W. H. Schepers of the U.S. Department of Health—and formerly of the industry-linked Saranac Laboratory—said:

> The facile introduction of irrelevancies and unproven suppositions, to explain an alleged prevalence of asbestos bodies in the lungs of nonindustrial workers, does more harm than good. Industry has made a splendid contribution to worker-safety through pinpointing and eradicating specific causative agents. If the contention were true that almost any urban dweller can accumulate a superabundance of asbestos particles in his lungs, through merely breathing the air of health resort cities or breathing cosmetic products, there would be no point in industry trying to reduce dust exposures within factories.[15]

Like a *leifmotif* the call for certitude was linked in these debates to a defense of industry's interests. Thus Kenneth W. Smith, medical director at Johns-Manville Corporation, asserted that "isolated studies of small selected groups may be interesting, but the true picture of the biological effects of asbestos fiber will emerge only when there is a broad study, conducted by an impartial agency, on a nation-wide scale."[16] His advice? Await evidence from the massive, long-term study, which had just now begun, and which would take many years— even decades—to complete. In the meantime, he advised conference participants to withhold judgment and (presumably) move cautiously with respect to regulation.

In a summary of the scientific findings presented at the conference, J. C. Wagner, a Welsh researcher, carefully laid out the strong case against asbestos, a case that went beyond the risks of occupational exposure. J. C. Gilson had the last word and warned against "false reassurances by medical authorities. . .[and] too great a reliance being placed on a few surveys indicating that specific jobs are dangerous, instead of insisting on environmental measurements and medical supervision wherever asbestos is used."[17] "It is abundantly clear from the evidence presented at the Conference," he said, "that in the future much greater care must be taken to eliminate unnecessary exposure to asbestos dust wherever it occurs."[18]

The proceedings of the conference, published in December 1965, quickly became the definitive source for information on asbestos and occupational disease. They also made clear the deep fissures that existed between scientists who spoke on behalf of industry and those who saw in asbestos a profound occupational and environmental threat.

The Case Builds Toward Regulation

In the years between the NYAS conference and the OSHA decision to regulate occupational exposure to asbestos, the evidence linking asbestos to cancers mounted, and word of it was widely disseminated. An article in the September 10, 1970, issue of the *New England Journal of Medicine* reported that asbestos exposure insufficient to cause asbestosis could nonetheless cause lung cancer and that mesothelioma "has been found with undue frequency in persons exposed to relatively small amounts of asbestos."[19] Mesothelioma could become a threat to the general public "as the use of this nondestructible material increases and becomes more widespread."[20]

Fifteen months later, an editorial in the same journal went further. Declaring that "asbestos workers are unintentional victims of industrial progress," the editorial called for control of asbestos emissions and protection of workers.[21] The Occupational Safety and Health Act of 1970 had set "the stage for such action."[22]

Unlike those who saw in uncertainty a basis for regulatory restraint, the editorial asserted that "more sweeping decisions on the control of asbestos must be made now, on the basis of 'reasonable probability' rather than after a delay for a precise definition of dose-response relationship."[23] Given the grave danger posed by asbestos, this conclusion would appear to have been unassailable, yet a glimpse into other quarters reveals the depth of the dispute at hand.

In 1968 Paul Brodeur, just beginning his reporting on the health effects of asbestos, interviewed Lewis J. Cralley and William S. Lainhart of the Division of Occupational Health of the U.S. Public Health Service. Both men were responsible for a large epidemiological study of asbestos exposure in workers. Cralley explained that two to four years would be needed to complete medical examinations of the 5,000 men he hoped to include in the study, who would then be reexamined at five-year intervals, funds permitting. "By following these men for the next fifteen or twenty years, we hope to establish a dose-response relationship for asbestosis. . . . Then we'll try to determine what level of exposure carries with it no discernible health hazard."[24] Asked if the study included lung cancer and mesothelioma, Cralley said he was interested only in asbestosis, that for him the "association between mesothelioma and asbestos was not yet proved."[25] This despite the many NYAS conference papers establishing the relationship of asbestos and mesothelioma in humans and animals.

William S. Lainhart stressed the need for sound scientific evidence:

> "Ideally, we'd like to take a bunch of twenty-year-olds, put them into an asbestos plant where we know the exact dust levels, and observe them for the next fifty years, or until they die. . . . Of course, we can't do that. We have to devise studies that are practical. For this reason, we estimate that it will take us from fifteen to twenty years to evaluate with any accuracy the medical effects of today's environment in the asbestos industry."[26]

This represented a very different view of how the burden of uncertainty should be allocated than other scientists were to publicly avow three years later. The position of Drs. Cralley and Lainhart was particularly curious in light of the evidence that research teams working under them had already uncovered about asbestos exposure and disease incidence in contemporary U.S. factories.

When William Johnson and Joseph Wagoner joined the newly established National Institute of Occupational Safety and Health (NIOSH), they examined the mortality data on asbestos textile workers gathered by their predecessors, including Cralley and Lainhart, which had accumulated, unanalyzed. Johnson, in dismay, declared, "Just from the most cursory look at those data, almost anyone would know that there had been a tragedy of immense proportions in many, if not all, of those factories. Why, the men working in them were dying of asbestosis and cor pulmonale—a form of heart failure that often accompanies the disease—right on the job! Men in their fifties! And some only in their *forties*!"[27]

What could account for so dramatic a failure on the part of government scientists? In attempting to answer that question, Johnson said: "I could say they were stupid, or that it was criminal negligence, or bureaucracy, or I could say they were afraid that if they did start getting concerned about this, that their right of entry [into plants] would have been cut off, but the fact is, I don't know."[28]

Regulating Asbestos: OSHA Seeks a Standard of Safety

On November 4, 1971, six months after the Occupational Health and Safety Act became effective, the Industrial Union Division of the AFL-CIO petitioned Secretary of Labor James D. Hodgson to declare an emergency temporary standard (ETS) for asbestos exposure. The Division wanted exposures limited to 2 fibers per cubic centimeter (2 f/cc), counting only fibers greater than 5 microns in length.* At this time, an informal standard of 12 f/cc was in effect.

On December 7, 1971, Secretary Hodgson put forth a "scientific compromise" and declared an ETS of 5 f/cc—2.5 times higher than requested by organized labor and 2.5 times lower than the prevailing standard. Asbestos was to be the first substance for which OSHA would go through the formal rulemaking procedure. The stakes were regarded as high by all parties in terms of life, health, and economics. Furthermore, the asbestos standard would, it was felt, establish a precedent for future OSHA standards.

The NIOSH—the successor to the Bureau of Occupational Safety and Health—was asked to evaluate the scientific evidence and prepare a Criteria Document, recommending a new standard for asbestos exposure. The report was forwarded to the Secretary of Labor on February 1, 1972. It recommended a standard of 2 f/cc, effective in two years, along with a number of other requirements involving record-keeping, monitoring, medical surveillance of workers, and labeling.

In January, Secretary Hodgson had set up an Advisory Committee on the Asbestos Standard with five members: one each from NIOSH, Raybestos-Manhattan, labor, the New York State Department of Labor, and the academic world. By majority vote, the Advisory Committee supported NIOSH's call for a 2-f/cc standard.

The problem before OSHA was to decide whether and how to control exposures to asbestos. Scientific evidence had to be evaluated; the costs, economic and otherwise, of control strategies estimated; and the two central elements—benefits in terms of health and costs in terms of lost jobs and profits—weighed against one another. Hearings were scheduled for mid-March 1972. Interested parties were asked to prepare written responses to the proposed regulations. Many came as well

---

*This is usually abbreviated as 2 f/cc. The 5-micron length limit reflects the limitations of light microscopes. Smaller particles are not reliably detectable. The ratio of smaller to larger particles varies according to the type of asbestos and the process in which it is used. There is considerable dispute about the respective health effects of fibers greater than and less than 5 microns in length.

to testify at the hearings that began on March 14. Only a few scientists testified; for the most part the hearings were dominated by representatives of business and organized labor, armed, however, with analyses that bore the mark of scientific "consultation."

There was remarkably little disagreement about one fundamental point—that the evidence available at that time could not be used to establish an uncontestably "safe" level of asbestos exposure. The NIOSH Criteria Document noted this explicitly at several points. The recommended 2-f/cc standard was "designed to protect against asbestosis. For other diseases associated with asbestos, there is insufficient information to establish a standard to prevent such diseases including asbestos-induced neoplasias by any all-inclusive limit other than one of zero."[29] Later the same report noted that "the number of studies that have collected both environmental and medical data and with a significant number of exposed workers is not sufficient to establish a meaningful standard based upon firm scientific data."[30]

George W. Wright, M.D., testified as one of a group brought to the hearings by Johns-Manville Corporation. His critique of the NIOSH Criteria Document relied upon the Institute's own acknowledgement of uncertainty: "Close examination. . .reveals in unequivocal terms that in the judgment of the authors of the Criteria Document there are no scientifically usable data on which to base a standard."[31] For Wright, insufficient data was equivalent to "no scientifically usable data." But that was not at the heart of the disagreement between the representatives of industry and those who supported labor's call for a stricter standard. The differences lay deeper: over what constituted "adequate" scientific evidence for the purpose of regulation; over how, in the face of inconclusive scientific evidence, we should allocate the burden of uncertainty; and perhaps, though this is less clear, over the weight to be assigned to the value of life and health versus economics.

George Wright was then on the staff of St. Luke's Hospital in Cleveland, Ohio. He was also chairman of the scientific advisory committee of the Institute of Occupational and Environmental Health of the Quebec Asbestos Mining Association (QAMA)—the industry-sponsored source of funds for much research on asbestos; research that typically found the risks to be minimal, at least from Canadian chrysotile (the type produced by members of QAMA). From 1939 through 1953 Wright had worked at the Saranac Laboratories. But to describe Wright, by reputation a scrupulous methodologist, as in some way "captive" to industry is to misconstrue the issues raised by his testimony, issues that were at once more subtle and less tractable. Industry executives, realizing that the demand for scientific certainty as a prerequisite for regulation would have the effect of minimizing or postponing regulation, learned to call on scientists who could be expected to speak in favor of modest and conservative science. The effect was to claim the mantle of science for those opposed to stricter control of asbestos, to tarnish proponents of stricter regulation with the stain of "politics," and to accuse the scientists among them of being less than responsible in their claims about the dangers of asbestos.

Also testifying with the group from Johns-Manville was Dr. J. C. McDonald from McGill University. McDonald's research on asbestos workers in Canada was cited in the NIOSH Criteria Document. The work, which had been supported by QAMA's Institute of Environmental and Occupational Health, was still in progress, although some data were available. NIOSH had interpreted McDonald's evidence to support its claim that a 2-f/cc standard was justified. McDonald protested that NIOSH's references to his study "are almost wholly inaccurate, out of context and seriously misleading. They were made without my knowledge or advice and I ask that they be discounted."[32]

Neither Wright nor McDonald escaped unscathed. William Nicholson of Irving Selikoff's group at Mt. Sinai Medical School questioned Wright at some length about assumptions made in the research that Wright said showed that a 5-f/cc time-weighted average exposure (TWA) "will protect workers. . .from developing asbestosis or experiencing an excess of bronchogenic cancer."[33] Others at the hearings raised additional questions about the evidence Wright embraced or dismissed. Although the questioning of McDonald at the hearing itself was not strenuous, after the hearings Nicholson submitted an extensive rebuttal of many of McDonald's claims about his own and other studies.

Selikoff submitted a statement in advance of the hearings. In it he addressed a number of concerns, among them the adequacy of the evidence for the task at hand. Speaking of the need for a numerical standard, he wrote: "We are in the unhappy position of not knowing what this number should be. Exposures have been so complex and variable and dust concentration measurements so limited, that the development of any number standard must rely on extrapolations that would hardly be countenanced in many other scientific circumstances."[34] He went on to say, however, that proposals for limits higher than 2 f/cc "are hardly even worth discussing."[35] How could he so cavalierly dismiss higher standards? For Selikoff, "the adequacy of the standard must. . .be measured against the seriousness of the hazard, since the penalties of error are heavy indeed."[36] Implicit in his statement was a judgment about how the burdens of uncertainty ought to be allocated—a judgment very different from that made by industry's proponents.

J. D. Jobe, executive vice-president for operations at Johns-Manville Corporation, announced the theme elaborated by a chorus of industry representatives: "Where there is no scientifically credible evidence demonstrating the necessity of such low standards, it would be socially irresponsible to adopt them."[37] Charles Neumann, senior vice-president of Kentile Floors, Inc. (a manufacturer of resiliant floor tile containing asbestos), argued that "unless ample medical evidence of a conclusive nature is available to show that the five fiber limit creates an undue health hazard. . .in the interest of reality and practicality. . .the five fiber limit [should] not be rejected."[38] Clifford Sheckler, chairman of the Safety and Health Committee of the National Insulation Manufacturers Association, bemoaned "the inadequacy of medical and scientific research information concerning safe exposure levels of asbestos dust" and called for a return to the old standard of 12 f/cc.[39] He also demanded "a comprehensive study of the entire asbestos industry. . .in the United States. . .to determine the effects not only of asbestos, but also of asbestos associated with other airborne contaminants and cigarette smoking."[40] Matthew M. Swetonic, executive secretary of the Asbestos Information Institute (AII) and a member of the Public Affairs Section of Johns-Manville, said, "The medical brief prepared by NIOSH in support of the 2-fiber limit, in our opinion, falls far short of establishing the necessity of such a standard. . . . The simple truth is that no one, NIOSH included, knows for sure what a safe occupational standard should be."[41] Alex Kuzmuk, a member of the Board of Governors of the Asbestos Textile Institute, was if anything less kind in his evaluation of the NIOSH report: "The information provided in this report was based on opinion and speculation rather than fact."[42] Neither did he hesitate to lay blame: "Had the USPHS Asbestos Epidemiological Study been complete as continually requested by the Asbestos Textile Institute, we might now be in a position of having factual information as to what the safe threshold limit for asbestos dust really should be."[43]

This, of course, was the same study described by Lewis Cralley; the same one that alerted William Johnson to the carnage occurring at the now infamous plant in Tyler, Texas; the same study that was years from completion; the same one from which data had lain unanalyzed for years in the files of the Public Health Service.

If industry had its view about where to place the burden of uncertainty, so did those who echoed the concerns of Selikoff. The NIOSH report itself acknowledged the problem: "It is recognized that additional data would be desirable to support an asbestos standard, but because of immediate need for worker protection, it is necessary to make a recommendation based on available studies and data."[44] In its general tone and specific judgments, NIOSH chose to err on the side of safety. William Nicholson testified that "there is no significant substantive evidence that would indicate what is a safe level of asbestos exposure that could prevent the incidence of cancer," and he concluded that it should be set as low as possible.[45] Stuart G. Luxon, Her Majesty's Superintending Chemical Inspector of Factories and director of the Industrial Hygiene Unit, Department of Employment, United Kingdom, defended the British standard set at 2 f/cc in 1969 by saying, "I think we have to keep in mind the fact that while the evidence may be scanty to arrive at a firm figure, we have a serious hazard and we must do everything within our power to reduce that hazard as far as possible."[46]

One of the ironies of the 1972 OSHA hearings was the double standard applied to evidence for the health effects of asbestos on the one hand and the economic effects of stricter regulation on the other. Although the evidence of health effects was scrutinized to the point of exhaustion, the claims about the economic effects of stricter standards, based entirely on industry's own reports of what those effects would be, went essentially unchallenged.

Clifford Sheckler, representing insulation manufacturers, offered an industry estimate that the cost of meeting even a 5-f/cc limit for a 100-person construction force (of whom twenty-five were assumed to work with asbestos) would come to $839,815—an increase in labor costs of 168 percent.[47] Albert H. Fay, president of the Asbestos Information Association of North America, said that a 2-f/cc limit would cost $200 million in new equipment and $400 million in lost sales "because of the labeling requirements and the shutdown of operations where 2 fibers is technologically unfeasible."[48] Matthew Swetonic of AII estimated that 15,000 to 30,000 jobs would be lost.[49] Sheckler understood well the interrelation of scientific uncertainty about health effects and policymaking: "Considering the supposition and assumption on which the proposed [limit] is based, it is difficult to imagine a justification for the economic stress this regulation will place upon the construction industry, Federal Government, [sic], and private enterprise."⁵⁰

For whatever reasons, supporters of a tough new standard chose not to question industry's estimates of the costs of compliance. Even a later study commissioned by Secretary of Labor Hodgson and done by the consulting firm of Arthur D. Little similarly relied on industry's own reports about what compliance would cost. That industry would benefit from exaggeratedly high estimates of cost appears, from the hearing record, to have been ignored.

What were the values at stake? Superficially, it might seem obvious that there were two sets of values—the physical well-being of workers and the economic well-being of the asbestos industry—and that these two sets of values were clearly distinct and in opposition. Sheldon Samuels of the Industrial Union Department of the AFL-CIO put it starkly: "The issue is whether human life can be traded off in the marketplace, whether workers must really face death on the job."⁵¹ George H. R. Taylor, executive secretary of the AFL-CIO Standing Committee on Safety and Occupational Health, underscored this point: "What is really before us is the specter of dead and dying workers, of workers permanently incapacitated, of unwitting victims of this deadly material exposed to it outside the plant environment."⁵² On the other side were the repetitive warnings of economic disaster offered by the industry.

J. D. Jobe of Johns-Manville gave perhaps the most nuanced analysis of the values involved. He reiterated the charge of economic harm, with interesting variations: "Achieving a standard of 5 will cost millions of dollars and cause a significant number of American jobs to be shifted to foreign workers to whom in many cases no standards apply."⁵³ Rather than preventing harm to workers, stricter regulation in the United States would merely export even greater dangers to workers in other countries. Furthermore, Jobe argued, even U.S. workers will not benefit: "Requiring a more stringent standard and requiring unnecessarily frightening labels can have catastrophic effects on the very people OSHA and the industry are trying to protect."⁵⁴ Then he cast the value conflict in a somewhat different light: "We should be concerned with two distinct goals. On the one hand, there is an obvious and recognized necessity to protect workers exposed to hazardous amounts of asbestos dust. On the other hand, our modern society requires the continued availability of a wide variety of asbestos-containing products."⁵⁵ Not only the industry would suffer; so, too, would society. Asbestos was "vital to our way of life."[56] Without it, the safety of all Americans would be placed in jeopardy. But the many benefits of asbestos could not "provide a justification for injuring those employed in the manufacture of or application of asbestos-containing products."[57] With the advantage of hindsight, we can see now that the social benefits of asbestos could be obtained by changes in processing and by product substitution. The advantages of technology-forcing, spurred by regulation, were not at that point apparent.

One of the chief questions raised in the asbestos controversy is the appropriateness of using the values underlying one social enterprise—science—to judge the work of another—OSHA. Science is concerned with the generation of knowledge and so sets very high standards for what it will accept as evidence. OSHA, charged with regulation and control of health hazards, must sift through evidence of diverse quality and cogency in order to arrive at a best estimate of the risk to human health. Having done that, institutions such as OSHA must then balance social and political values without losing sight of scientific uncertainty and come up with a reasonable administrative decision.

As long as the issue is framed narrowly in terms of knowledge of the existence of a hazard or of the precise shape of the relation between exposure and disease, then foes of stricter controls can invoke the values of science in defense of their position. But that is an epistemologically naive position. There are other kinds of knowledge that are not precisely grounded in scientific proofs but that we act on every day. We make decisions about how to raise children, for instance, and act on implicit empirical beliefs in many other situations even though the basis for the belief may be highly contestable or even intractable to scientific confirmation. Our entire system of justice rests on a combination of moral beliefs and empirical assumptions, few if any of which are scientifically confirmed or confirmable. We do not insist that judgments of guilt or innocence be withheld pending sound scientific confirmation about the facts of the crime or the state of mind of the criminal. We rightly see that as a mistaken application of standards suitable for one sort of social activity to another arena with different characteristics and demands.

Administrative decisionmaking is simply a very different social enterprise from the conduct of science and the generation of new knowledge. Administrative decisionmakers are not free to disregard the findings of science or to embrace markedly inferior evidence and to ignore superior evidence. However, their task is not to decide what has been "proved" scientifically but rather to use intelligently and in a reasonable manner whatever evidence is available in order to make an "all-things-considered" judgment. In this light the frequent calls for scientific certainty appear as naive or even as self-serving. The demand for scientific "proof," both from the NYAS conference and the OSHA hearings, functioned as a delaying tactic for opponents of regulation.

The subsequent history of asbestos regulations reveals both a growing recognition of the burdens imposed by asbestos use and a complex political process. On June 6, 1972, Secretary Hodgson and OSHA Director George Guenther announced a standard of 5 f/cc until July 1, 1976, when a 2-f/cc limit would be imposed. That rule survived court challenges. On November 4, 1983, an emergency temporary standard of 0.5 f/cc was set, but that ETS was declared invalid by a U.S. circuit court four months later. Once again, OSHA began the formal rulemaking process and proposed two possible exposure levels, 0.5 f/cc or 0.2 f/cc, on April 10, 1984. Hearings were held in the summer of 1984. OSHA announced its new standard of 0.2 f/cc on June 20, 1986. That followed by six months the January 29, 1986, published proposal of the U.S. Environmental Protection Agency to abolish all uses of asbestos over the next ten years.

The State of Occupational Medicine

Throughout the entire period of asbestos-related regulatory efforts, occupational health physicians played a strikingly limited role. An analysis of that role reveals much about the institutional restraints on professional behavior in the occupational setting.

One might have expected that physicians charged with protecting the health of employees would be among the first to notice and call attention to the dangers of asbestos. Certainly one might have expected that, when testifying at the Department of Labor's administrative hearings in March 1972, those physicians would have invoked the physicians' duty to protect the health of workers under their care by demanding a strict standard for asbestos control. In fact, the record shows that when industrial physicians did testify at the 1972 hearings, they confined their remarks to one issue—the challenge posed to their status by NIOSH's suggestion and organized labor's demand that workers be permitted to seek medical examinations from physicians of their choice at company expense. Sheldon Samuels, of the

Industrial Union Department, put it with characteristic bluntness: "We have no faith in the ability of company doctors to fulfill an unbiased patient-physician relationship."[58]

Lain Tetrick, medical director of the Midwest Steel Division of National Steel Corporation, and T. H. Davidson, medical director of Johns-Manville Corporation, testified in opposition to the recommendation for independent medical examinations. The official response of the profession, through the then-named Industrial Medicine Association, was delivered by the association's president, Norbert Roberts, a man of unquestioned integrity. Roberts acknowledged that "at some times and places deficiencies in the protection of the confidentiality of medical information have resulted in unfair action against employees. . . . We join in condemning any such practice wherever and whenever it exists."[59] But he argued that "physicians employed in industry constitute the largest reservoir of scientific knowledge and skills in existence anywhere with reference to worker health protection, a pool of professionals already figuratively deputized to work for OSHA's success."[60] Although he acknowledged the need to protect the economic interests of asbestos workers and lamented the toll of workers struck down by asbestos, Roberts nowhere called for stricter legislation. Indeed, he never mentioned the proposed limit for asbestos exposure.

The occupational medical profession, particularly those employed by or closely linked to industry, was about to face a crisis, largely as a result of the asbestos controversy. Two documents in particular seemed to engage the attention of industry physicians: Paul Brodeur's series of articles in *The New Yorker* on asbestos, appearing in 1973 and later collected in a book, and a letter to the editor by William E. Morton, a university-based physician, published in the November 1973 issue of the *Journal of Occupational Medicine*. Entitled "Are Medical Ethical Practices Sufficient in Industrial Medicine?,"[61] the letter elicited an accompanying note from the editor and triggered a flood of comments, letters, and editorials in that same journal. Morton had touched an exceedingly raw nerve.

Morton asserted that industrial physicians often were not free to publish studies of occupational illness and that censorship was exercised by business executives. Physicians typically complied "because to do otherwise would mean termination of their employment by that company and possible interference with future similar employment."[62] Morton declared that failure to warn workers about suspected hazards was a violation of medical ethics.

The editor responded to this challenge. "Dr. Morton's articulate though undocumented indictment is a serious one. Can it be substantiated? Is it justified?" Morton was right to focus "attention upon the potential tragedy of disability or death being suffered by even one worker because of the withholding of new scientific information available to physicians or other occupational health professionals in industry." Although the reluctance of management to permit "the publication of speculative and undocumented observations which might result in costly liability without real justification" is understandable, "we all join Dr. Morton in hoping that sound new knowledge will be made public consistently as soon as it is available."[63]

Just what sort of "speculative and undocumented observations" an industrial physician would want to publish and succeed in getting through the peer review system is difficult to say. There is an ingenuous view of science implicit here, as if knowledge appeared full-blown and certain rather than by the slow accretion of findings, not always clear or correct, illuminated occasionally by theory and insight. But more important, Morton had pinpointed an institutional barrier to the scientific practice of sharing information in the mutual search for knowledge. He had underscored that the firm's interests were not those of the scientist or the physician. Nor were they those of its workers. Scientific and medical professionals who accept employment under such circumstances may at some point face a choice between compromising or leaving.

Compromise may be conscious or unconscious. Professionals may come to internalize the firm's goals and soon lose awareness that a conflict even exists. Surely the process is a complex one: an initial choice because of general comfort and fit with the values of the firm and its executives is followed by socialization into the norms and world view shared by management-level colleagues. Denial and rationalization could then function to mask the tensions involved.

Whatever the process, a challenge to a profession's success in maintaining a delicate balance between professional obligation and demands for corporate loyalty can sting, especially when made publicly. And that is precisely what was done in the asbestos controversy, with the repudiation of industrial physicians in the recommendation that employees be allowed to have independent medical examinations; the unfavorable portrayal of industry physicians in Brodeur's writings; and the controversy within the pages of the *Journal of Occupational Medicine* initiated by William Morton's letter. In the October 1974 issue of this journal, William Johnson challenged the profession and the journal staff itself: "The lack of editorial activity in the *Journal of Occupational Medicine* regarding the asbestos and other problem areas in Brodeur's series could be interpreted as an act of omission designed to allow the embarrassment of the medical/industrial complex and the scandal of the U.S. Public Health Service asbestos study to 'blow over.' "[64]

Some responded to this challenge with candor, among them Clifford H. Keene, a distinguished occupational physician, president of the Kaiser Foundation Hospitals and Health Plan and a vice-president of Kaiser Industries Corporation. He understood the roots of the antagonism:

> The lack of significant positive thrust by industry and industrial medical organizations toward the enactment of recent occupational safety and health legislation undoubtedly has been contributory to these challenges. I believe that industry and industrial physicians will continue to suffer attack on the bases of motive, candor, and credibility. If these challenges do not provoke refutation or correction, industry and industrial physicians will lose all public esteem in matters related to the welfare of the worker in the industrial environment. Placed in similar jeopardy is the opinion of us held by our fellow physicians who are not involved in industrial medicine.[65]

But a decade after the debate began, there is little evidence that much has changed in occupational medicine. Although some companies and some company physicians have done excellent work in protecting workers' health, the institutional interests that push in the opposite direction remain strong, and the organization of the corporation often creates insurmountable obstacles to doing research that would prevent future tragedies.[66] Occupational medicine remains a troubled profession.[67]

Conclusion

The history of asbestos regulation gives sorry confirmation of the adage that what you see depends on where you sit. And, one might add, what you say has much to do with who owns your chair.

To a distressing degree—distressing at least to those who believe in the values of scientific objectivity and professional integrity—

industry-affiliated scientists and physicians did much to conceal, delay, and divert attention from the links between asbestos (at least the type of asbestos used by their allies within industry) and disease.

The stark silence of industrial physicians in the face of the human cost of asbestos is a reminder to us of the power of institutional incentives over and above professional norms. Undoubtedly, many physicians and scientists within the industry do act promptly to investigate and remedy occupational health hazards. But they must swim against powerful currents.

For those concerned about future threats to the health of workers, the current system of institutional controls and incentives should give scant comfort. A system for detecting and regulating occupational hazards that depends heavily on the lonesome hero or on accidental happy combinations of individual character and enlightened organizations will be a costly system indeed—costly in terms of the lives and health of American workers. Something sturdier is needed, but that might well require a general rethinking and rearrangement of the responsibility for detecting and controlling occupational health hazards in this country. However necessary, it seems unlikely at the present moment.

Notes

1. Eunice Thomas Miner, "Preface," 132 *Annals of the New York Academy of Sciences* 1 (31 December 1965): 5.

2. J. C. Gilson, "Man and Asbestos," 132 *Annals of the New York Academy of Sciences* 1 (31 December 1965): 9.

3. Ibid., p. 11.

4. W. C. Hueper, "Cancer in its Relation to Occupation and Environment," 25 *Bulletin of the American Society for the Control of Cancer* 6 (1943): 63–69.

5. W. C. Hueper, "Occupational and Nonoccupational Exposures to Asbestos," 132 *Annals of the New York Academy of Sciences* 1 (31 December 1965): 184.

6. Ibid., p. 186.

7. Ibid., p. 192.

8. W. D. Buchanan, "Asbestosis and Primary Intrathoracic Neoplasms," 132 *Annals of the New York Academy of Sciences* 1 (31 December, 1965): 517.

9. Ibid.

10. J. C. Wagner, "Epidemiology of Diffuse Mesothelial Tumors: Evidence of an Association from Studies in South Africa and the United Kingdom," 132 *Annals of the New York Academy of Sciences* 1 (31 December, 1965): 575–578.

11. W. C. Dreessen, J. M. DallaValle, T. I. Edwards, J. W. Miller, and R. R. Sayers, "A Study of Asbestosis in the Asbestos Textile Industry," *Public Health Bulletin Number 241* (Washington, D.C.: U.S. GPO 1938).

12. E. L. Schall, "Present Threshold Limit Value in the U.S.A. for Asbestos Dust: A Critique," 132 *Annals of the New York Academy of Sciences* 1 (31 December, 1965): 319.

13. I am indebted for this phrase to Professor Guido Calabresi, who employs it in a different context in his book *A Common Law for the Age of Statutes* (Cambridge, Mass.: Harvard University Press, 1982).

14. Richard Gaze, "Discussion," 132 *Annals of the New York Academy of Sciences* 1 (31 December 1965): 682.

15. G. W. H. Schepers et al., "Discussion," 132 *Annals of the New York Academy of Sciences* 1 (31 December 1965): 595–602.

16. Ibid., p. 690.

17. J. C. Gilson, "Problems and Perspectives: The Changing Hazards of Exposure to Asbestos," 132 *Annals of the New York Academy of Sciences* 1, (31 December, 1965): 698–699.

18. Ibid., p. 704.

19. Arend Bouhuys and John M. Peters, "Control of Environmental Lung Disease," 283 *New England Journal of Medicine* 11 (10 September, 1970):575.

20. Ibid.

21. B. Gee and A. Bouhuys, "Action on Asbestos," 285 *New England Journal of Medicine* 23 (2 December, 1971): 1317.

22. Ibid., p. 1318.

23. Ibid., p. 1317.

24. Paul Brodeur, *Expendable Americans* (New York: Viking Press, 1974), pp. 22–23.

25. Ibid., p. 23.

26. Ibid., p. 23.

27. Ibid., pp. 110–111.

28. Robert Sherrill, "Asbestos, the Saver of Lives, Has a Deadly Side," *The New York Times Magazine* (21 January, 1973).

29. National Institute for Occupational Safety and Health, *Criteria for a Recommended Standard: Occupational Exposure to Asbestos* (Washington, D.C.: U.S. Department of Health, Education, and Welfare, Public Health Service, 1 February, 1972); p. II-2.

30. Ibid., p. V-10.

31. George W. Wright, statement before U.S. Department of Labor Hearings on a Standard for Exposure to Asbestos Dust. The hearings, here-

after referred to as *Hearings,* were held on 14–17 March 1972. The remark cited here appears on p. 259 of the transcript.

32. J. Corbett McDonald, *Hearings,* exhibit document no. 43.

33. Wright, *Hearings,* p. 260.

34. Irving J. Selikoff, "Epidemiological Constraints in Development of a Standard for Asbestos Exposure," submitted to *Hearings,* p. 6.

35. Ibid.

36. Ibid., p. 2.

37. J. D. Jobe, *Hearings,* p. 225.

38. Charles Neumann, *Hearings,* pp. 68–69.

39. Clifford L. Sheckler, *Hearings,* p. 170-J.

40. Ibid., pp. 170-J and 170-K.

41. Matthew M. Swetonic, *Hearings,* p. 180.

42. Alex Kuzmuk, *Hearings,* p. 101.

43. Ibid.

44. NIOSH, *Criteria,* p. V-16.

45. William Nicholson, *Hearings,* p. 46.

46. Stuart G. Luxon, *Hearings,* pp. 473–474.

47. Sheckler, *Hearings,* pp. 170-I and 170-J.

48. Albert H. Fay, *Hearings,* p. 176.

49. Swetonic, *Hearings,* p. 188.

50. Sheckler, *Hearings,* p. 170-J.

51. Sheldon Samuels, *Hearings,* p. 530.

52. George H. R. Taylor, *Hearings,* exhibit document no. 52, p. 2.

53. Jobe, *Hearings,* p. 225.

54. Ibid.

55. Ibid.

56. Ibid., p. 226.

57. Ibid.

58. Samuels, transcript of statement in *Hearings,* p. 6.

59. Norbert J. Roberts, "Medical Examination of Workers Exposed to Asbestos: Confidentiality of Medical Information in Relation to Occupational Illness or Injury," 14 *Journal of Occupational Medicine,* 9 (September 1972): 707. This is the statement Roberts delivered at the March 1972 asbestos hearings.

60. Ibid.

61. William E. Morton, "Are Medical Ethical Practices Sufficient in Industrial Medicine" (Letter), 15 *Journal of Occupational Medicine* 11 (November 1973): 860–861.

62. Ibid., p. 860.

63. Irving R. Tabershaw, "Editor's Note," 15 *Journal of Occupational Medicine* 11 (November 1973): 861.

64. William M. Johnson, "Industry's Credibility," 16 *Journal of Occupational Medicine* 10 (October 1974): 645.

65. Ibid., p. 311.

66. Thomas H. Murray, "The Lethal Paradox in Occupational Health Research," *Business and Society Review* 53 (Spring 1985): 20–24.

67. Diana Chapman Walsh, "Divided Loyalties in Medicine: The Ambivalence of Occupational Medical Practice," paper presented to the Hastings Center Research Project on Divided Loyalties Dilemmas in Medicine.

Index